The Complete
THYROID
Health & Diet Guide

Understanding and Managing Thyroid Disease

INCLUDES 150 RECIPES

Dr. Nikolas R. Hedberg
DC, DABCI, DACBN, BCNP

Danielle Cook
MS, RD, CDE

Robert
ROSE

For complete cataloguing information, see page 374.

Disclaimer

This book is a general guide only and should never be a substitute for the skill, knowledge
and experience of a qualified medical professional dealing with the facts, circumstances and
symptoms of a particular case.

The nutritional, medical and health information presented in this book is based on the research,
training and professional experience of the authors, and is true and complete to the best of their
knowledge. However, this book is intended only as an informative guide for those wishing to
know more about health, nutrition and medicine; it is not intended to replace or countermand
the advice given by the reader's personal physician. Because each person and situation is unique,
the authors and the publisher urge the reader to check with a qualified health-care professional
before using any procedure where there is a question as to its appropriateness. A physician should
be consulted before beginning any exercise program. The authors and the publisher are not
responsible for any adverse effects or consequences resulting from the use of the information in
this book. It is the responsibility of the reader to consult a physician or other qualified health-care
professional regarding his or her personal care.

This book contains references to products that may not be available everywhere. The intent
of the information provided is to be helpful; however, there is no guarantee of results associated
with the information provided. Use of brand names is for educational purposes only and does
not imply endorsement.

The recipes in this book have been carefully tested by our kitchen and our tasters. To the best
of our knowledge, they are safe and nutritious for ordinary use and users. For those people with
food or other allergies, or who have special food requirements or health issues, please read the
suggested contents of each recipe carefully and determine whether or not they may create a
problem for you. All recipes are used at the risk of the consumer. We cannot be responsible for any
hazards, loss or damage that may occur as a result of any recipe use. For those with special needs,
allergies, requirements or health problems, in the event of any doubt, please contact your medical
advisor prior to the use of any recipe.

Design and Production: Kevin Cockburn/PageWave Graphics Inc.
Editors: Bob Hilderley, Senior Editor, Health; and Sue Sumeraj, Meal Plans and Recipes
Medical editor: Joanna Odrowaz
Copy editor: Sue Sumeraj
Proofreader: Sheila Wawanash
Indexer: Gillian Watts
Nutrient analysis: Magda Fahmy
Illustrations: Kveta/threeinabox.com

Cover images: © iStockphoto.com/AnjelaGr (coconuts), © iStockphoto.com/supermimicry
(seaweed), © iStockphtoo.com/digitalskillet (women walking), © iStockphoto.com/AlexPro9500
(avocados)

The publisher gratefully acknowledges the financial support of our publishing program by the
Government of Canada through the Canada Book Fund.

Published by Robert Rose Inc.
120 Eglinton Avenue East, Suite 800, Toronto, Ontario, Canada M4P 1E2
Tel: (416) 322-6552 Fax: (416) 322-6936
www.robertrose.ca

Printed and bound in Canada

1 2 3 4 5 6 7 8 9 MI 23 22 21 20 19 18 17 16 15

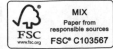

This book is dedicated to all of my patients
with thyroid problems. I have learned so much
from you, and I am honored that you trust me
to care for your health and well-being.
I am truly grateful for the opportunity
you have given me to serve you.

— *Dr. Nikolas R. Hedberg*

Contents

Foreword by Dr. R. Ernest Cohn...... 6

Acknowledgments................. 7

Introduction 8

Part 1: Thyroid Basics

CHAPTER 1
How Does the Thyroid Work? 12

Functional Anatomy 13

Thyroid Hormone Production........ 16

Thyroid Hormone Conversion 17

Thyroid Hormone Elimination....... 18

Metabolism..................... 19

Thyroid Dysfunction 22

CHAPTER 2
How Do I Know If I Have a Thyroid Disorder?............ 23

Common Symptoms of
  Thyroid Dysfunction 24

Basal Body Temperature Test........ 25

Thyroid Hormone Tests 27

Thyroid Screening................ 32

Part 2: Thyroid Dysfunction

CHAPTER 3
The Immune System and Thyroid Disorders 36

Autoimmune Thyroiditis 37

Barrier Hyperpermeability.......... 41

Vitamin D and Immunity........... 46

Nutrient Deficiencies............. 47

Treating Autoimmune Thyroiditis 49

CHAPTER 4
The Gastrointestinal System and Thyroid Disorders.......... 51

Gut–Thyroid Connections 52

GI Tract Tests 54

Food Allergies and Sensitivities 56

CHAPTER 5
The Hepatic System and Thyroid Disorders.......... 58

About the Hepatic System 59

Thyroid-Disrupting Chemicals 63

Toxic Metals 66

Body Burden.................... 68

Testing for Toxins 69

Detoxification 70

CHAPTER 6
The Adrenal Glands and Thyroid Disorders.......... 73

About the Adrenal Glands 74

Adrenal Dysfunction 76

The Blood Sugar–Adrenal–Thyroid
  Axis 78

The Hypothalamic–Pituitary–Adrenal
  Axis 80

The Adrenal–Gut Connection........ 81

Adrenal Treatment Protocol......... 81

CHAPTER 7
Hormone Imbalance and Thyroid Disorders.......... 86

Balanced Hormones............... 87

Leptin......................... 87

Testosterone 88

Progesterone 89

Estrogen 89

Pregnenolone 91

CHAPTER 8
Iodine and Thyroid Disorders 92

Iodine and Thyroid Hormones 92

Iodine Deficiency. 93

Natural Sources of Iodine 96

Halides 98

Iodine Testing 99

Part 3: Thyroid Management

CHAPTER 9
**Medications and Surgery
for Thyroid Dysfunction** 102

Prescription Medications 102

Botanical and Biologic Medicines. . . . 106

Thyroid Gland Surgery 107

Radioactive Iodine Therapy 109

CHAPTER 10
**Lifestyle Modifications
for Thyroid Dysfunction** 111

Reducing Stress. 112

Improving Sleep 113

CHAPTER 11
The Balanced Thyroid Diet 122

Thyroid Diet Principles 123

Step 1: Determine Your Body Type . . . 123

Step 2: Aim for Energy Equilibrium . . 125

Step 3: Balance Your Blood Sugar. . . . 126

Step 4: Choose Low-GI Foods 128

Step 5: Eat High-Quality Protein 132

Step 6: Optimize Your Omega Fats
Ratio 133

Step 7: Alkalize Your Body pH 135

Step 8: Improve Your Eating Habits . . 141

Part 4: Thyroid Meal Plans

4-Week Meal Plans 148

Post-Workout Meals. 152

Anytime Meals and Snacks 154

Part 5: Thyroid Recipes

Introduction to the Recipes 158

Common Ingredients for
Healing Your Body. 160

About the Nutrient Analysis 170

Breakfasts. 171

Soups 193

Salads and Dressings. 219

Dips and Sauces 239

Vegetarian Dishes 251

Fish and Seafood. 275

Meaty Mains. 295

Side Dishes 323

Snacks and Desserts 347

References. 364

Resources 372

Contributing Authors. 373

Index 375

Foreword

The concept of natural medicine dates back well over 1,000 years. In China and Greece, our ancestors used natural therapies that included diet, water and herbs to treat their patients. Even then, the most important factor in healing was the doctor–patient relationship. Health practitioners throughout the ages have looked at their patients, touched their patients and listened to their patients as part of the process of making an accurate diagnosis.

In today's medicine, the integrative physician, like Dr. Hedberg, performs diagnostic laboratory studies, such as those discussed in this book, along with the same techniques early natural medicine practitioners used. While modern medicine seems to be governed by the $7\frac{1}{2}$-minute office visit and treatment model, Dr. Hedberg teaches both clinical practitioners and patients who are ready to take charge of their own care the most appropriate testing methods to properly diagnose complicated conditions of the thyroid.

Dr. Hedberg includes actual case histories and explains the most current and thorough diagnostic testing procedures, as well as many conventional and integrative approaches to healing. He also discusses in detail the ever-growing concern of autoimmunity stemming from issues in the gut, thanks to environmental pollutants such as mercury, lead, cadmium, plastics and chemicals, and hormones that are overprescribed or accumulated through environmental exposure.

Few books include so many aspects or such a great depth of detail on the subject of thyroid dysfunction. I recommend it for both the practitioner who continues to have patients with chronic thyroid issues and the patient who has been from doctor to doctor and knows something is wrong despite being told that all the tests look normal. In my 38+ years of practice, I have never read a text with so much useful information on the thyroid.

— R. Ernest Cohn, MD, NMD, DC, FACO
Holistic Medical Clinic of the Carolinas
Holisticmedclinic.com

Acknowledgments

From Dr. Nikolas R. Hedberg

I would like to thank the following doctors, who have had the greatest influence on my understanding of thyroid disorders:

- Dr. Jeffrey Moss
- Dr. Ron Cohn
- Dr. David Brady
- Dr. Kent Holtorf
- Dr. Denis Wilson
- Dr. Michael Friedman
- Dr. Bill Kleber
- Dr. Bill Beakey

From Danielle Cook

I would like to thank the following people:

- Clarie Hollenbeck, my graduate school advisor and friend, for believing in me and pushing me to pursue nutrition and academics at a deeper level.
- Andrew Cook, for believing in me, sharing your knowledge and encouraging me to take on the world.
- Mom and Dad, for all of your love and your strong passion for education.
- All of the practitioners who have helped me on my health journey, for sharing their vast knowledge and expertise of the amazing human body.

Introduction

Until the second half of the 20th century, thyroid disease was common in North America, the effects frequently visible as a goiter on the neck or bulging, watery eyes. Iodized salt has reduced the incidence of thyroid disorders, but 12% of North Americans still develop some form of thyroid disease.

There are almost fifty types of thyroid disorders. Incidence is five to eight times higher in women than in men, and one in every eight women will develop a thyroid disorder. However, not everyone with thyroid disease recognizes the problem, despite how difficult it is to function when your thyroid is out of balance. Many suffer in silence — needlessly, in most cases.

> Not everyone with thyroid disease recognizes the problem, despite how difficult it is to function when your thyroid is out of balance.

The most widely recommended treatment for thyroid disease today is the synthetic drug levothyroxine (Synthroid). Levothyroxine also happens to be the most commonly prescribed medication in North America. Despite the widespread use of medications, outcomes remain poor for many individuals.

This book is meant for you if

- you have been told that conventional treatments should cure your thyroid problems, but you are still enduring thyroid dysfunction
- standard blood tests, such as thyroid-stimulating hormone (TSH) assays, look normal, but you still have symptoms
- your doctor has referred you for psychological counseling, the theory being that if your TSH test is normal, your symptoms *must* be in your head
- you need to constantly adjust your thyroid medication, as you just can't seem to find the right dose
- you are doing fine on your prescription medication but want some nutritional advice to optimize your health

If you are reading this book, you or a family member, or someone you are close to, probably has a thyroid disorder.

Perhaps you are looking for alternatives to the conventional standards of care that have failed you or them. Many people with thyroid disorders are seeking alternatives and supplements to their current treatment. You could be feeling extremely frustrated, wanting someone to take a serious look at your case and figure out your health issues. We all want answers — and to feel better again.

We wrote this book to help you understand why your thyroid glands may be out of balance and what you can do to normalize them.

In this book, we

- briefly describe the anatomy and function of the thyroid
- explain how thyroid disease is diagnosed
- analyze causes of thyroid dysfunction by body system
- review standard treatments
- discuss diet as a therapy that complements standard care
- provide thyroid-healthy recipes and nutritional strategies to maximize your metabolism

If you are lucky enough to do well on conventional medical treatment, this book can still provide you with nutritional strategies to help your thyroid work even better. You may even find that your doctor can lower your dose of thyroid hormone replacement.

We hope this book inspires you to get well and stay well!

> Many people with thyroid disorders are seeking alternatives and supplements to their current treatment.

Caution

Continue to take any medication you have been prescribed. Discuss any changes to your treatment plan, including dietary changes and supplements, with your doctor, to ensure that nothing interferes with your medication. Do not make any changes until after discussing them with your doctor. Make sure you are examined and treated by a licensed medical professional, so that nothing serious, such as thyroid cancer, is overlooked.

PART 1

Thyroid Basics

CHAPTER 1

How Does the Thyroid Work?

CASE STUDY

A New Diagnosis

When Elisabeth first came to our clinic, she had just been diagnosed with hypothyroidism and Hashimoto's thyroiditis. Her doctor had put her on levothyroxine to treat her hypothyroidism, but she was told there was nothing to be done about the thyroiditis. The medication really wasn't working, so she began searching for answers on the Internet. She was extremely confused about the "pro-iodine" group versus the "anti-iodine" group. Should she go gluten-free? What about infections and leaky gut syndrome? Did she also need T3 (triiodothyronine, a thyroid hormone)?

We explained to Elisabeth that a lot of the information on the Internet is suspect and requires knowledge of how to interpret the data, that the answers to her questions were all strictly individualized and that there are no single best answers for everyone. She learned that, in many cases, thyroid imbalances can be corrected with a few simple treatments once the underlying causes of disease are identified. We then did a series of laboratory tests to find out exactly what was contributing to her thyroid disease, so that there would be no further guesswork or frustration.

Elisabeth needed only to make a few simple dietary changes and add some supplements to replenish the deficiencies that showed up in her lab tests. Her medication immediately started to work more effectively. Her doctor was extremely pleased with the results and, as a result, became interested in functional medicine approaches to health and disease.

Elisabeth is now doing fine.

Functional Anatomy

The thyroid, a small, butterfly-shaped gland that weighs approximately 1 ounce (30 g), wraps around your throat at about the level of the Adam's apple. Despite its small size, the thyroid has a powerful impact on your well-being. The main role of thyroid hormone is to control energy production inside the cell. The hormones that the thyroid secretes function as primary metabolic agents, prompting our bodies to maintain our basal metabolic rate and temperature, and convert food into energy when we need it for any activity.

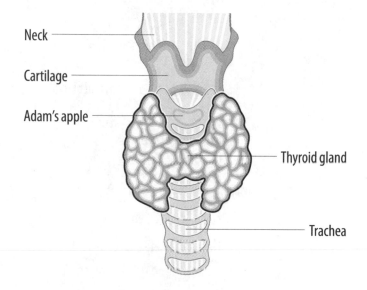

Neck

Cartilage

Adam's apple

Thyroid gland

Trachea

The Endocrine System

The thyroid gland is part of the endocrine system, a complex signaling system that sends messages via the circulatory system to tissue and cells in your body. The endocrine system maintains homeostasis, or a state of balance, so that all your organs and systems work at their best.

The Hypothalamic–Pituitary–Thyroid Axis

The thyroid gland cooperates with the hypothalamus and pituitary in a feedback axis, or loop, to maintain a state of metabolic balance in your body. The hypothalamus, which is located in the brain, tells the endocrine glands when to start and when to stop secreting hormones. If the hypothalamus detects low levels of thyroid hormones in the bloodstream, it releases thyrotropin-releasing hormone (TRH). TRH stimulates the pituitary, a pea-sized gland just under the hypothalamus, to produce thyroid-stimulating hormone (TSH). TSH, in turn, stimulates the thyroid to produce thyroxine (T4) and triiodothyronine (T3) until their levels in the blood return to normal.

When the hypothalamus detects higher levels of these thyroid hormones in the bloodstream, it stops releasing TRH, which signals the pituitary to stop releasing TSH.

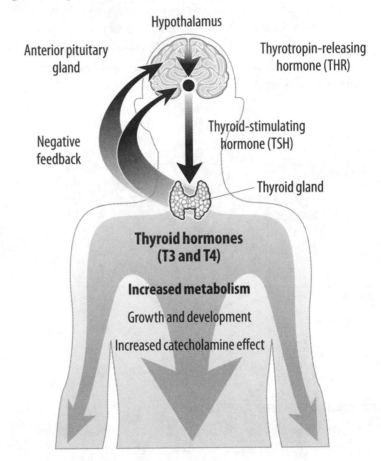

Other Endocrine Glands
The endocrine system includes a number of glands that are connected through the circulatory system. Many are affected by or affect the thyroid:

- the pineal gland, which secretes melatonin, a hormone that governs sleep
- the thymus gland, where immune cells are formed, mature and multiply
- the adrenal glands, which secrete
  - adrenaline, the hormone that prepares your body for "flight or fight" by increasing your heart beat, helping you to breathe more deeply and diverting blood to your limb muscles

- cortisol, which plays a role in how the immune system functions, as well as in the stress response, including blood pressure control and metabolism of carbohydrates
- the islets of Langerhans, which secrete insulin, a hormone that promotes sugar uptake by cells and the deposit of fats
- the gonads, which secrete androgens in males and estrogens in females, hormones that are involved in sexual development

In addition to these specialized endocrine glands, many organs have roles to do with hormone metabolism. For example, the liver detoxifies the body of used hormones.

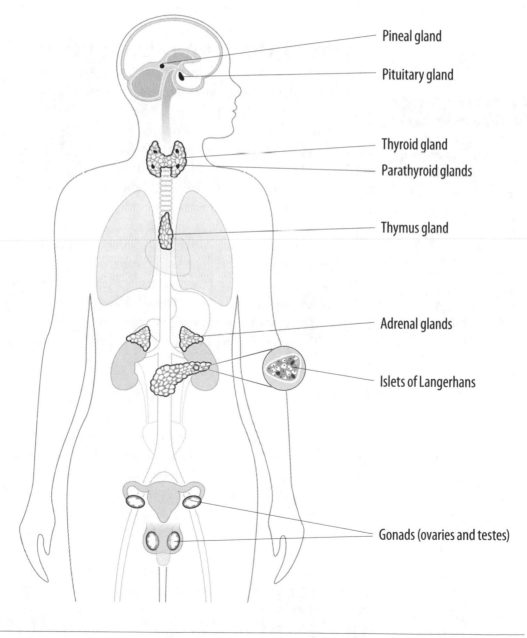

Pineal gland

Pituitary gland

Thyroid gland

Parathyroid glands

Thymus gland

Adrenal glands

Islets of Langerhans

Gonads (ovaries and testes)

Q. What are hormones?

A. Hormones are proteins that carry messages through the bloodstream from the endocrine glands to cells within tissues in your body. Hormones act as catalysts for chemical changes in the cells, to balance out chemical levels and help achieve homeostasis, a state of stability in your body that is necessary for growth and development, and for life itself.

Hormones circulate freely in the bloodstream, waiting to be recognized by the specific target cells that are their intended destination. The target cell has a receptor that can be activated only by a specific type of hormone.

If hormone production and transportation are impeded, we become prone to acute health disorders and chronic disease conditions.

Thyroid Hormone Production

T3 (triiodothyronine) and T4 (thyroxine) are the main hormones produced by the thyroid gland. The numbers "3" and "4" indicate the number of iodine atoms in the molecule. About 95% of thyroid hormones is T4, but T3 is about five times more active than T4.

T3 is synthesized when one iodine atom is split off a T4 molecule by a deiodinase enzyme. This process, which takes place mainly in the liver, is the key to understanding how the thyroid works (see "Thyroid Hormone Conversion," page 17).

Both T4 and T3 are transported through the bloodstream bound to one of the carrier proteins: thyroxine-binding globulin (TBG), transthyretin or albumin. Despite its low concentration, TBG carries most of the T4 in the blood because it has the highest affinity for this hormone and for T3. Once T4 and T3 reach their target cells, they become unbound and work their metabolic magic.

Iodine

Both T4 and T3 molecules contain iodine. Your body cannot synthesize (create) iodine, so you must get it from your food or from supplements. Too little iodine can result in hypothyroidism, while too much can cause hyperthyroidism.

According to the Institute of Medicine, the recommended dietary allowance (RDA) for iodine is 150 micrograms per day for adult men and women. Almost three times that amount (400 micrograms) can be found in a teaspoon (5 mL) of iodized salt. The RDA for pregnant women is higher, at 220 micrograms per day, and even higher for breastfeeding mothers, at 290 micrograms per day.

DID YOU KNOW?

INCREASED OR DECREASED TBG

The reasons for increased TBG could be genetic; pregnancy or neonatal state; hepatitis; porphyria; the use of selective estrogen receptor modulators (e.g., tamoxifen); the use of perphenazine, mitotane or 5-fluorouracil; or the use of heroin or methadone. Decreased TBG may also be genetic or may be due to the use of anabolic steroids, glucocorticoids, nicotinic acid or L-asparaginase, or to a severe illness such as liver failure or nephrosis.

Thyroid Hormone Conversion

Although 95% of thyroid hormone is T4, T3 is responsible for most of the hormonal action on cells. About 60% of T4 is converted into T3, 20% is converted into an inactive form of thyroid hormone known as reverse T3 (rT3), and the remaining 20% is converted into triiodothyronine sulfate (T3S) and triiodothyroacetic acid (T3AC). Many factors, including radiation, chemotherapy, growth hormone deficiency and cigarette smoking, can inhibit this vital conversion process, but the most common causes of reduced hormone conversion are nutrient deficiencies, hormone imbalance and depleted glutathione.

Nutrient Deficiencies

As you age, you lose your ability to convert thyroid hormone, possibly due to decreased vitamin and mineral absorption. Your gastrointestinal (GI) tract becomes less able to absorb nutrients, so supplementation becomes necessary. Deficiencies in selenium, antioxidants, iron, magnesium, zinc, vitamin A, vitamin B_6 or vitamin B_{12} can lead to poor conversion of T4 into T3.

Hormone Imbalance

Excess estrogen from xenoestrogens in the environment, birth control pills and hormone replacement therapy can lead to poor conversion of T4 to T3. Estrogen increases the amount of thyroxine-binding proteins that bind to thyroid hormones, thereby decreasing the number of free hormones circulating in the bloodstream. The seemingly low levels of thyroid hormones stimulate the hypothalamus to start the feedback loop process that produces more thyroid hormones.

Cortisol, a hormone produced by the adrenal glands, is a major factor in converting thyroid hormone. Both too much and too little cortisol can inhibit the activation of thyroid hormones. Excess cortisol suppresses detoxification and clearance of rT3 and hence TSH production by the anterior pituitary, resulting in low thyroid function. Exhausted adrenals that do not produce enough cortisol cause symptoms of low thyroid hormones.

Insulin, a hormone released by the pancreas to handle the amount of sugar in the blood after consumption of carbohydrates, can also inhibit hormone conversion.

Reverse T3

About 20% of T4 is converted by the liver into rT3, an inactive form of thyroid hormone. Although rT3 itself is inactive, it binds to T3 receptors, thus blocking T3 action, and prevents the conversion of T4 into T3, slowing down metabolism and inhibiting T4 and T3 from entering your cells.

Too much or too little cortisol, which is produced by the adrenal glands, increases circulating levels of rT3. Elevated insulin levels due to a diet high in refined carbohydrates also increase rT3 production, as do toxic metals, including mercury, cadmium and lead.

Immune system activation, high adrenaline, excess free radicals, aging, fasting, stress, prolonged illness and diabetes all drive the inactivation of T3 to rT3.

Depleted Glutathione

Glutathione is the most abundant antioxidant in the body. It is involved in detoxification and is also important for healthy conversion from T4 to T3. Glutathione can be depleted by large amounts of toxins and/or drugs passing through the liver, as well as by starvation or fasting. Glutathione levels also drop when you have a chronic viral infection, potentially leading to autoimmune thyroiditis.

Thyroid Hormone Elimination

Your body eliminates expended T3 through two chemical processes that take place in the liver:

- *Glucuronidation* occurs when toxins are bound to glucuronic acid produced by the liver. Your body needs vitamin B complex, glycine and magnesium for this process.
- *Sulfation* involves binding toxins to sulfur-containing amino acids, such as methionine, glycine and N-acetylcysteine, so that the toxins can be excreted. The enzyme used in this step is dependent on molybdenum.

An inability to metabolize and detoxify T3 can make thyroid hormone replacement therapy difficult if you have symptoms of excess T3. You may need a careful evaluation of your ability to detoxify. Certain medications, including phenobarbital, rifampin, carbamazepine, rifabutin and phenytoin, can increase the elimination of T4 and T3 by up to 20%. Drugs that lower T3 levels include any type of corticosteroid and beta blockers, such as metoprolol, prescribed for high blood pressure.

✳ RESEARCH SPOTLIGHT

Low T3 and Heart Disease

Chronically low levels of T3 have been shown to be directly connected with coronary artery disease (CAD). Researchers have investigated whether low levels of T3 in euthyroid (normal TSH) patients are associated with the presence of and prognosis for CAD. Researchers assessed data from 1,047 euthyroid patients who had undergone coronary angiography for suspected CAD. The authors concluded that, even in patients with no history of myocardial infarction or chronic heart failure, low free T3 levels were associated with either single-vessel or multivessel CAD, and low T3 syndrome was associated with an adverse prognosis for CAD.

Metabolism

"Metabolism" is a term used to describe all of the chemical and physical reactions involved in maintaining the living state of cells and organisms. Our cells contain mitochondria, which produce energy from carbohydrates, proteins and fats. Thyroid hormones control the function of the mitochondria, determining how much energy needs to be produced to keep us alive and how much is needed to initiate and sustain activity.

Your body needs a specific amount of each nutrient to stay healthy. You can synthesize some nutrients, but others, including the chemical elements that make up thyroid hormones, must be ingested through food or supplements.

Q What does "synthesis" mean?

A Synthesis is a process your body performs to create compound substances, such as nutrients and hormones, by combining simpler substances through chemical reactions. The body is able to synthesize many of the substances it needs for optimal health, but others must be obtained through diet or supplements. When the body cannot synthesize a particular nutrient, that nutrient is known as an "essential" nutrient because we must get enough of it from external sources. Examples are essential amino acids and essential fatty acids.

The nutrients derived from food are commonly classified as either macronutrients or micronutrients. Macronutrients are needed in large quantities for normal growth and development. They include carbohydrates, proteins and fats. Micronutrients include chemical elements (minerals) and vitamins.

Carbohydrates

Carbohydrates (or "carbs") make up about half of all the foods we eat as part of a standard North American diet. Carbohydrates are digested in the mouth and gastrointestinal tract, and are metabolized into energy. They include:

- raw sugars, such as glucose and fructose
- refined starches, such as rice, wheat, potatoes and pasta

Proteins

Proteins are composed of amino acids. Amino acids are metabolized by our bodies to make more proteins, including:

- enzymes, which are involved in all aspects of metabolism
- hormones, messenger molecules that help your body maintain homeostasis
- carrier molecules, such as TBG, which carries T4 and T3 in the bloodstream
- structures, such as muscles, ligaments, tendons, hair and nails

Of the twenty amino acids, your body is unable to synthesize eight. As a result, you must get these "essential" amino acids from food.

Fats

Fats are concentrated sources of energy. The same weight of fat produces twice as much energy as either carbohydrate or protein. Storing fat (in the abdomen or under the skin) is an efficient way to store excess energy. Your body also uses fats to synthesize hormones and other substances needed for its activities.

Fats are complex molecules composed of fatty acids and glycerol. Your body can synthesize many fats, but you must get essential fatty acids through your diet. Essential fatty acids include omega-6 fatty acids, such as linoleic and arachidonic acids, and omega-3 fatty acids, such as linolenic acid.

Chemical Elements (Minerals)

The chemical elements, or minerals, we absorb from food are important for regulating blood pressure, for building bones and teeth, for transporting oxygen to all of your cells and for enabling the function of nerves, muscles and hormones. The body contains more than fifty elements, twenty-five of which are essential because the body cannot synthesize them. A deficiency in one of these essential elements causes specific symptoms. For example, a deficiency in calcium can cause rickets and, in later life, osteoporosis.

Of the chemical elements, your body needs iodine, magnesium, iron, selenium, zinc and copper to synthesize thyroid hormones.

> The body contains more than fifty elements, twenty-five of which are essential because the body cannot synthesize them.

Vitamins

Vitamins are essential organic compounds, many of which your body cannot synthesize and must get from food or supplements. Generally, we get enough vitamins from a well-balanced diet. However, older people may suffer from a vitamin D deficiency, and vegans may get too little vitamin B_{12}.

Your body needs vitamins A, B complex, C, D and E to synthesize and secrete thyroid hormones, to regulate their production and to transport them.

Q What is autoimmune thyroiditis?

A The immune system defends your body against pathogens (bacteria, viruses, parasites and fungi). If you are immunodeficient, your immune system is too weak to fight pathogens and you are more prone to infections. About one-quarter of people with an immunodeficiency disorder also have an autoimmune disorder, in which the immune system attacks normal tissues as if they were foreign organisms. Common autoimmune disorders include Hashimoto's thyroiditis, rheumatoid arthritis, type 1 diabetes mellitus and systemic lupus erythematosus (lupus).

In the case of autoimmune thyroiditis, the body's immune system attacks thyroid cells, causing chronic inflammation and gradual destruction of the thyroid gland. Many people with autoimmune thyroiditis take synthetic thyroid hormone but still have symptoms of hypothyroidism — fatigue, irritability and nervousness. However, health-care professionals rarely address the role of autoimmunity in thyroid dysfunction. This does you a great disservice because the attack on the body can be greatly reduced with treatment that spares the thyroid gland.

Thyroid Dysfunction

There are many types of thyroid dysfunction. Most can be classified as hypothyroidism (too little thyroid hormone produced) or hyperthyroidism (too much thyroid hormone produced). Other types of thyroid dysfunction can be classified as thyroiditis and thyroid cancers. The causes appear to be primarily nutrient deficiencies or excesses, suppressed detoxification, lack of balance with other hormones, and autoimmune reactions.

Some Types of Thyroid Disorders

Hypothyroidism	Hyperthyroidism	Thyroiditis	Thyroid Cancer
• Infantile hypothyroidism • Subclinical hypothyroidism • Hereditary hypothyroidism • Primary hypothyroidism • Secondary hypothyroidism • Tertiary hypothyroidism • Postpartum hypothyroidism • Acquired hypothyroidism • Hypothyroid goiter • Medication-related hypothyroidism	• Graves' disease • Thyroid nodules • Subclinical hyperthyroidism • Thyroid storm • Postpartum hyperthyroidism • Thyroid eye disease • Hyperparathyroidism • Hyperthyroid osteoporosis	• Hashimoto's thyroiditis • Subacute granulomatous thyroiditis • Postpartum thyroiditis • Myxedema coma • Pretibial myxedema	• Papillary cancer • Medullary carcinoma • Familial medullary cancer • Anaplastic cancer • Follicular adenocarcinoma • Multiple endocrine neoplasia

▷ DOC TALK

Understanding how the thyroid gland functions and how thyroid hormones are produced is challenging. When you next meet with your doctor, ask questions on any topics you feel unsure about. Taking control of your own health is essential in thyroid care.

You can run several tests, such as the basal body temperature test, on yourself if you suspect you have a thyroid disorder. If these at-home tests reveal concerns, your doctor can conduct other hormone tests. Some are more reliable than others.

CHAPTER 2

How Do I Know If I Have a Thyroid Disorder?

CASE STUDY

Reverse T3 Test

Maria was referred to our clinic complaining of weight gain, chronic depression, hair loss and constipation. She felt cold all the time. Her doctors kept telling her that all of her thyroid lab tests looked normal, but she knew something was wrong.

Maria's doctors had run a thyroid-stimulating hormone (TSH) test, and even when she requested more extensive testing, such as free T4 and free T3, the values appeared normal. Finally, her doctors tried her on levothyroxine, but her symptoms only got worse, at which point the doctors said, "I told you so."

After carefully reviewing Maria's lab tests, we agreed with her doctors that her thyroid levels looked good. However, a reverse T3 (rT3) test revealed extremely high levels of this metabolite. RT3 is an inactive form of T3 that is also made from T4. It binds to T3 receptors, causing symptoms of hypothyroidism despite normal-looking lab test results. Administering T4 would further increase rT3 levels. She bypassed this problem by starting on T3 replacement therapy, as T3 cannot be converted into rT3. After a few months, her rT3 levels were reduced to normal, her thyroid had "reset" and was functioning at its best, and her symptoms had improved significantly. Maria was able to discontinue taking T3, and her thyroid has remained stable since.

Common Symptoms of Thyroid Dysfunction

Hypothyroidism and hyperthyroidism each have specific symptoms, but the disorders also share common indications with each other and with other health conditions, making diagnosis difficult. If you recognize one or more of these symptoms, talk with your doctor about them and ask about laboratory tests.

Disorder	Symptoms	Associated Conditions
Hypothyroidism: too little thyroid hormone produced by the thyroid gland	Symptoms of hypothyroidism relate to a decrease in energy production. • Unrefreshing sleep; fatigue • Depression; anxiety • Weight gain or inability to lose weight; water retention • Dry and itchy skin; dry, brittle hair and nails • Hair loss; lateral third of eyebrow thinning • Voice deepens or sounds hoarse • Headaches; muscle aches and cramps • Cold intolerance; cold hands and feet • Low sex drive (libido) • Depressed immune system; chronic infections; slow wound healing • Constipation; digestive problems due to low stomach acid	Hypothyroidism is also involved in a number of conditions often overlooked by clinicians: • Carpal tunnel syndrome • Chronic fatigue syndrome • Depression • Fibrocystic breasts • Fibromyalgia • Heart disease • High blood pressure • High homocysteine • Infertility • Insulin resistance (diabetes, obesity) • Polycystic ovarian syndrome (PCOS) • Premenstrual syndrome (PMS) • Sleep apnea
Hyperthyroidism: too much thyroid hormone produced by the thyroid gland	Excess thyroid hormone results in symptoms of excessive metabolism: • Rapid heart rate • Sweating at rest • Headaches • Weight loss • Increased appetite • Anxiety	Hyperthyroidism is caused mainly by the autoimmune condition known as Graves' disease.

Basal Body Temperature Test

Testing your basal body temperature — your body's resting temperature — is a convenient way to evaluate your metabolic status and assess how well your thyroid functions. It is generally measured immediately after awakening, before any physical activity and 12 hours after having eaten; that is, when you are in a post-absorptive state. If your temperature is below the norm, your thyroid hormones may be out of balance.

Measure your temperature using a glass/mercury thermometer either in the armpit (axillary temperature) or under your tongue (oral temperature). A normal axillary temperature is between 97.8°F and 98.2°F (36.6°C and 36.8°C); a normal oral temperature is between 98.2°F and 98.6°F (36.8°C and 37.0°C). Basal body temperature should reflect a "sleeping state" of bed rest for at least 3 hours.

Keep a 5-day basal temperature diary (see page 26), along with any notable symptoms. If scheduling allows, women should record their axillary temperature during the first 3 to 5 days of their menstrual cycle. Otherwise, use any consecutive 5 days.

> If your temperature is below the norm, your thyroid hormones may be out of balance.

1. Shake down a glass/mercury thermometer to below 96.0°F (35.6°C) the night before the test. (If you don't have a glass/mercury thermometer, you can use an ear or digital thermometer.) Leave the thermometer near your bed so you can reach it easily without getting out of bed.
2. Place a clock or watch nearby to time your temperature test.
3. When you wake up, stay as still as possible. Place the thermometer in your armpit (or mouth/ear) and hold it against your skin for 10 minutes. Press your arm against your body to hold the thermometer firmly in place. Avoid rolling over onto that side, so you don't break the thermometer.
4. After 10 minutes, check the temperature reading. Log the temperature to the nearest tenth of a degree, for example, 97.8°F (36.6°C).
5. Show the completed diary to your doctor at the next visit.

5-Day Basal Temperature Diary

Normal Axillary Temperature: 97.8°F to 98.2°F (36.6°C and 36.8°C)
Normal Oral Temperature: 98.2°F to 98.6°F (36.8°C and 37.0°C)

Day 1 Temperature: _____
Notable Symptoms: _____

Day 2 Temperature: _____
Notable Symptoms: _____

Day 3 Temperature: _____
Notable Symptoms: _____

Day 4 Temperature: _____
Notable Symptoms: _____

Day 5 Temperature: _____
Notable Symptoms: _____

Common Symptoms

Your answers to the following questions may indicate whether you have a thyroid disorder.

Do you use extra blankets at night to stay warm?
YES / NO
Feeling consistently cold at night is a common symptom of a thyroid disorder.

Do you have a chronic sore throat, cold or other infection?
YES / NO
Chronic colds and infections can indicate a thyroid problem.

Do you have a chronic sinus problem and/or post-nasal drip?
YES / NO
Sinus problems can signal a thyroid disorder.

SOURCE: COURTESY OF DR. ROBBAN SICA.

Thyroid Hormone Tests

The blood tests listed in the table below can provide more information about your thyroid. Make sure to follow the instructions about food and permitted medications before the tests. Prescribed thyroid hormones, for example, will alter test results. Free T4 levels will increase up to 20% after you take L-thyroxine, peaking after 3.5 hours and remaining high for 9 hours. Total T4 levels will increase 1 hour after you take this medication and peak at 2.5 hours.

T3 and T4 levels may also increase if you are seriously ill or otherwise under stress, even if your thyroid is working effectively. For that reason, thyroid testing should be avoided when you are ill or are recovering from an illness if you want the most accurate picture.

Thyroglobulin and calcitonin tests are mainly used in the diagnosis of more serious thyroid diseases, such as cancer.

> Thyroid testing should be avoided when you are ill or are recovering from an illness if you want the most accurate picture.

TSH (thyroid-stimulating hormone)	TSH is produced by the pituitary to stimulate the thyroid into secreting hormones. TSH above 2.5 µIU/mL may indicate decreased thyroid function. Conventional medicine uses a broad range of about 0.5 to 4.5 µIU/mL to diagnose hypothyroidism.
Total T4 (thyroxine)	Measures the amount of bound and free T4. This test is not considered very accurate and has been largely replaced by free T4 testing.
Free thyroxine index	Calculated by multiplying total T4 by the percent of T3 uptake. The result is the amount of unbound, or free, T4.
Free T4	Measures the amount of unbound T4.
T3 uptake	Measures the amount of available binding sites for free T3 on the thyroxine-binding proteins: TBG, transthyretin and albumin. This test has largely been replaced by free T3 and free T4 testing.
Total T3 (triiodothyronine)	Measures the total amount of T3, including free T3 and T3 bound to transport proteins.
Free T3	Measures the total amount of circulating T3 (bound and free), i.e., the amount of active thyroid hormones.
Reverse T3 (rT3)	Measures the amount of T3 that has been inactivated. The rT3 test is no longer widely used, in favor of methods that measure free T4 and T3 directly.
Thyroid antibodies	An increase in thyroid peroxidase antibodies, TSH receptor antibodies, thyroid-stimulating immunoglobulin (TSI) or antithyroglobulin antibodies indicates autoimmune thyroiditis, such as Hashimoto's thyroiditis or Graves' disease.

Understanding Hormone Test Results

TSH is made in the pituitary, so any disease or dysfunction in that gland will affect TSH levels and, as a result, thyroid function. In primary hypothyroidism, where the issue lies within the thyroid gland, TSH levels are elevated but the thyroid gland is not functioning at its best. In central hypothyroidism, where the issue originates in the pituitary gland, TSH levels are normal or low and the thyroid gland does not get enough stimulation.

TSH	T4	T3	Interpretation
High	Normal	Normal	Mild hypothyroidism
High	Low	Low or normal	Hypothyroidism
Low	Normal	Normal	Mild hyperthyroidism
Low	High or normal	High or normal	Hyperthyroidism
Low	Low or normal	Low or normal	Non-thyroidal illness, pituitary hypothyroidism

The Inadequacy of TSH Tests

Conventional medicine relies mainly on TSH blood tests to measure thyroid function. If thyroid hormone levels drop, TSH production increases to stimulate the thyroid to make more hormones. If circulating thyroid hormone levels increase, the pituitary responds by decreasing TSH production. If TSH levels are elevated, most doctors will prescribe synthetic T4, which usually reduces TSH into the normal range.

However, TSH testing alone cannot assess thyroid function for several reasons:

- TSH testing does not consider the conversion of T4 into its active form, T3, which occurs primarily in the liver, as well as the kidneys and lungs.
- TSH testing does not take into account that thyroid hormone receptors can become resistant to thyroid hormones as a result of chemical exposure. With resistance, levels of thyroid hormones stay normal but symptoms of hypothyroidism develop.
- TSH testing does not account for the impact of cortisol produced by the adrenal gland when you are under stress. Cortisol can inhibit TSH production, further throwing off the accuracy of the test.

- TSH testing does not take into account peripheral thyroid hormone conversion or receptor binding, that is, the action in target tissues and not at the level of the thyroid gland. If your body cannot effectively convert T4 into T3, taking T4 supplements may not stimulate your metabolism.
- TSH testing does not account for the adrenal glands being out of balance. If they are, thyroid function will probably also be out of balance. In addition, if thyroid hormone receptors are desensitized, TSH testing may be deceptive.
- TSH levels can vary up to 50% over a 24-hour period, so the time of the blood draw may not accurately reflect thyroid function. TSH values tend to be lowest in the afternoon and highest before bed. The early morning is considered the best time to measure TSH.
- TSH testing does not account for elevated levels of rheumatoid factor. Usually present in rheumatoid arthritis, rheumatoid factor may cause a falsely elevated TSH level reading.
- TSH levels tend to increase with age, especially for people over 80. TSH values above 3.0 µIU/mL and ranging from 2.5 to 4.5 µIU/mL may be a normal part of aging that does not require treatment.

> TSH values tend to be lowest in the afternoon and highest before bed. The early morning is considered the best time to measure TSH.

✳ RESEARCH SPOTLIGHT

TSH Test Controversy

The upper limit of TSH values is considered to be 4.5 µIU/mL, based on a reference population study. This is further supported by the Hartford Thyroid Disease Study. However, the National Academy of Clinical Biochemistry indicates that 95% of individuals without evidence of thyroid disease have TSH concentrations below 2.5 µIU/mL. It has been suggested that the upper limit of the TSH test be changed to 2.5 µIU/mL. Should we be basing our testing guidelines on large masses of the population and on a hormone that is not even made by the thyroid gland? There are too many factors to "throw all of our eggs in one basket."

TSH and T3 Levels

The TSH picture becomes even more complex when we look at differences between T3 levels in the pituitary and in the rest of the body. TSH is normally a reflection of T3 levels in the pituitary. However, T3 levels can be different in the rest of your body's cells and tissues, for a number of reasons, including aging, calorie restriction/fad dieting, chronic fatigue syndrome,

T3 levels often appear normal in hypothyroidism due to overstimulation of the thyroid tissue by elevated TSH and increased response to deiodinase, the enzyme that converts T4 to T3. Conventional medicine does not recognize the issue of decreased peripheral conversion of T4 into T3, except in "severe illness." Thus, T3 is rarely used in conventional medicine despite its rapid and positive effects on so many people.

ACHILLES TENDON TEST

One of the original ways of assessing thyroid function was by measuring the speed of the Achilles tendon reflex. A slow Achilles tendon reflex can be a sign of hypothyroidism. A study in the *Journal of Clinical Endocrinology and Metabolism* actually found this test to be more accurate than TSH testing.

depression, fibromyalgia, inflammation, insulin resistance (diabetes, obesity), premenstrual syndrome (PMS) and stress.

In response to any of these conditions, your body increases the amount of T3 in the pituitary, which lowers TSH levels, but T3 levels in the rest of your body's tissues and cells actually decrease. Your blood tests will appear normal even though the most active form of thyroid hormone, T3, is low in the rest of your body. This is another reason why people have symptoms of hypothyroidism even though their blood tests look normal.

Medications

TSH levels can also be suppressed by various medications:

- bexarotene, used to treat cutaneous T-cell lymphoma (a type of skin cancer)
- dopamine and dopaminergic agonists, used to treat Parkinson's disease
- glucocorticoids
- interleukin 6
- metformin, used to treat type 2 diabetes
- opiates, such as heroin
- somatostatin analogs, used to regulate cell growth
- thyroid hormone analogs

TSH levels can be increased by:

- amphetamines
- dopamine receptor blockers, used to treat schizophrenia, bipolar disorder, nausea and vomiting
- interleukin 2, used to treat cancers
- ritonavir, used to treat HIV infection
- St. John's wort, used for depression and associated conditions (anxiety, tiredness, loss of appetite and trouble sleeping)

Thyroid Hormone Levels During Pregnancy

When you are pregnant, blood protein levels change substantially. TSH levels may drop to below 0.1 µIU/mL during the first trimester because human chorionic gonadotropin, a hormone secreted by the placenta, stimulates the thyroid. TSH levels usually return to normal in the second trimester. Thyroid hormone requirements usually increase during pregnancy and return to base levels after you give birth.

Measuring total T4 is recommended over measuring free T4 during pregnancy because free T4 levels may show lower than normal, especially in the third trimester. Total T4 levels will increase during the first trimester.

If possible, get thoroughly evaluated before conceiving. Untreated hypothyroidism can lead to preterm delivery, miscarriage, preeclampsia, high blood pressure, stillbirth, low birth weight or impaired psychomotor and intellectual development of the fetus. Treatment with thyroxine ensures that these issues don't occur.

T4 Levels

Although T4 levels usually decrease during chronic illnesses, they can also increase or even stay the same. If T4 levels don't change, it could be because T4 is not being converted into T3 or because higher levels of rT3 are increasing thyroid hormone resistance.

This shows that, like TSH, T4 is an unreliable marker because T3 levels can decrease when T4 levels are high, normal or low.

✳ RESEARCH SPOTLIGHT

Tumor Necrosis Factor Alpha

A study in the *Journal of Clinical Endocrinology and Metabolism* showed that injecting people with tumor necrosis factor alpha, which increases inflammation, also lowers TSH and T3 levels and increases rT3 levels. Simply by increasing inflammation, T3 levels drop and rT3 levels increase. But the drop in TSH levels would normally indicate that thyroid hormone is not needed.

Euthyroid Sick Syndrome

Euthyroid sick syndrome occurs as a result of a non-thyroidal illness that creates inflammation and suppresses the anterior pituitary and TSH production, lowering T3 and increasing rT3. Non-thyroidal illness can include gastrointestinal, pulmonary, cardiovascular and renal diseases; inflammatory conditions; myocardial infarction; starvation; sepsis and burns; trauma and surgery; and bone marrow transplantation.

Unfortunately, some of these conditions, such as chronic gastrointestinal issues due to infection, dysbiosis (imbalance in the ratios of healthy and unhealthy bacteria), leaky gut and food sensitivities/intolerances (for example, to gluten or dairy) are often overlooked.

Thyroid Screening

Currently there is no consensus about population screening for hypothyroidism, but people with the following conditions merit further investigation for screening:

- abnormal thyroid physical examination
- autoimmune disease
- history of neck radiation exposure
- history of thyroid surgery or imbalance
- pernicious anemia (vitamin B$_{12}$ deficiency)
- psychiatric disorders

Other people who merit screening may include:

- those taking amiodarone, used to treat cardiac arrhythmias
- those taking lithium, used to treat some psychiatric conditions
- those with a first-degree relative with autoimmune thyroiditis

Q What is the best way to diagnose a thyroid condition?

A Let's set out this procedure in stages for easy reference:

Stage 1: Screening

A standard thyroid profile that includes TSH, T4, free thyroxine index and T3 uptake is usually offered as a single test by most commercial labs. In addition, you should be tested for:

- a lipid panel that includes cholesterol, triglycerides, high-density lipoprotein (HDL), or "good" cholesterol, and low-density lipoprotein (LDL), or "bad" cholesterol, which can also give you a good idea of the state of your thyroid
- levels of sex hormone–binding globulin (SHBG), which tend to be low in hypothyroidism
- thyroid peroxidase and antithyroglobulin antibodies, which will indicate whether you have Hashimoto's thyroiditis
- total T3, free T4, free T3 and rT3

If you have symptoms of hyperthyroidism, request the test for thyroid hormone receptor antibodies or thyroid-stimulating immunoglobulin (TSI).

Stage 2: Follow-up Monitoring

Once a thyroid condition is diagnosed, follow-up tests should monitor TSH, free T4 and free T3 levels and any other levels that were abnormal to begin with, such as reverse T3.

People who have any of the following diagnoses are justified in having a thorough thyroid evaluation:

- adrenal fatigue or insufficiency (Addison's disease)
- alopecia (hair loss)
- anemia
- cardiac dysrhythmia, prolonged QT interval on an electrocardiogram (EKG) or congestive heart failure
- constipation
- dementia
- dysmenorrhea (menstrual cramps)
- fatigue/malaise and myopathy
- high blood pressure
- high cholesterol
- mixed hyperlipidemia
- type 1 diabetes mellitus
- vitiligo and changes in skin texture
- weight gain

▷ DOC TALK

All licensed health-care practitioners, including chiropractic physicians, medical doctors, osteopathic physicians and naturopathic physicians, as well as physician assistants and nurse practitioners, can examine you and do the necessary diagnostic testing. Finding a health-care practitioner who will run all the tests recommended in this chapter may be difficult, however. If your TSH is normal but you still have thyroid symptoms and your doctor does not take into account how you feel, get a second opinion from a doctor who knows about integrative or functional medicine approaches to thyroid disorders.

Consider seeing an endocrinologist if you have thyroid symptoms and:

- you are pregnant or are planning to conceive
- you have a history of cardiac disease
- your thyroid hormone levels fluctuate, despite following your recommended treatment, or your thyroid hormone test results are otherwise unusual
- you have goiter, thyroid nodules or other structural changes to the thyroid gland
- you have medication-induced hypothyroidism or hypothyroidism stemming from other unusual causes

PART 2

Thyroid Dysfunction

CHAPTER 3

The Immune System and Thyroid Disorders

CASE STUDY

Infection Connection

Brandy was suffering from many common symptoms of hypothyroidism, including fatigue, cold hands and feet, anxiety, sleep problems, loss of drive and zest for life, poor digestion and dry skin. She had also lost a significant amount of hair. Brandy had seen many doctors, who adjusted her thyroid medication frequently because the dose she was prescribed never stabilized her body. Based on lab tests and symptoms, she appeared to swing from hypothyroidism to hyperthyroidism. She had tried a gluten-free diet and was taking a large number of supplements, chiefly vitamin D and fish oil. Nothing helped.

   Like most people with thyroid problems, Brandy had never been tested for autoimmune thyroiditis. After diagnosing Brandy with Hashimoto's thyroiditis, we immediately tested her for the three most common infections associated with this autoimmune disease: Epstein-Barr virus, *Helicobacter pylori* and *Yersinia enterocolitica*. Her Epstein-Barr virus titers (antibody concentrations) and *Yersinia* antibodies were elevated. Her *H. Pylori* breath test was negative.

   We started Brandy on a herbal combination product designed for intestinal parasites and infections: selenomethionine, monolaurin and reishi mushroom extract for the Epstein-Barr virus and an herbal combination for the *Yersinia enterocolitica*. We also added the yeast *Saccharomyces boulardii* to help fight off *Yersinia*. She reported improvement of all her symptoms after the first 3 weeks, and her hair stopped falling out. The *Yersinia* infection was successfully treated after about 8 weeks, and her Epstein-Barr virus titers came down to normal after about 3 months.

Brandy was a perfect example of the "infection connection" to autoimmune disease. Treating the infections brings the immune system back into balance so it has no reason to attack its own tissues. Another consideration was Epstein-Barr virus, which can reactivate in those who are genetically susceptible to autoimmune diseases due to an inability to control this virus. Brandy was also a good example of the many individuals we see who have tried gluten-free diets for months and even years, often with no benefit, because they were never thoroughly checked for infections.

Brandy continues to do extremely well as long as she controls her stress levels and follows the specific nutrition recommendations we gave her.

Autoimmune Thyroiditis

Autoimmune thyroiditis is not a single disease process but a symptom of an immune system that has broken down as a result of one or more possible causes. Autoimmune thyroiditis is a common response when your immune system fights off pathogens and allergens too enthusiastically. Many people do not receive a thorough evaluation of their thyroid gland and are put on thyroid medication without being adequately tested for autoimmune thyroiditis.

Hashimoto's Thyroiditis

The number one cause of hypothyroidism worldwide is Hashimoto's thyroiditis. Hashimoto's thyroiditis is also the most common undiagnosed autoimmune disease in the world. More women than men are diagnosed with this condition.

DID YOU KNOW?

COEXISTING DISEASES

Hashimoto's thyroiditis tends to coexist with other autoimmune diseases, such as type 1 diabetes, rheumatoid arthritis or lupus. Most doctors focus on these other autoimmune diseases, ignoring the possibility that the thyroid is also being attacked.

Molecular Mimicry

Your immune system works by recognizing amino acid sequences on foreign "invaders." But in some cases, the surface protein of the pathogen looks just like your own tissues and your immune system attacks your tissues as well as the pathogen. This process is known as molecular mimicry, and it is a likely cause of Hashimoto's thyroiditis.

Amino acids are the building blocks of protein. They make up body tissues, foreign invaders and dietary proteins, such as gluten from wheat and casein from milk. Molecular mimicry occurs when your immune system attacks a dietary or infection-related protein and then identifies and attacks the same protein in body tissues, such as thyroid cells. According to research published in the journal *Endocrine Reviews*, "Molecular mimicry has long been implicated as a mechanism by which microbes can induce autoimmunity."

Hashimoto's thyroiditis is not routinely evaluated, which leaves some people in limbo for months and even years before they finally receive an accurate diagnosis.

People with Hashimoto's thyroiditis usually do not respond to thyroid medication. Their doctors continually adjust their medication based on thyroid-stimulating hormone (TSH) test results. However, TSH can fluctuate significantly in an autoimmune disease state as the thyroid gland becomes inflamed.

Graves' Disease

Graves' disease is another form of autoimmune thyroiditis and is the number one cause of hyperthyroidism. If you have Graves' disease, your thyroid produces too much hormone, initially increasing metabolism. With time, your thyroid hormone receptors become saturated and your body shows signs of hypothyroidism. Symptoms include anxiety, insomnia, bulging eyes, weight loss, swelling in the thyroid gland and either increased or decreased energy depending on the stage of the disease.

Graves' disease is eight times more common among women than among men. It usually occurs between the ages of 20 and 40.

Graves' disease is treated with medications that shut down thyroid function, including methimazole, propylthiouracil and radioactive iodine. Regrettably, instead of trying to find the cause of the autoimmunity, many traditional doctors destroy the thyroid gland with radioactive iodine or surgically remove it. Once this is done, you must remain on thyroid hormone indefinitely.

✳ RESEARCH SPOTLIGHT

L-carnitine

L-carnitine shuttles fat into the cells' mitochondria (energy-producing "furnaces") to convert into energy. L-carnitine is an antagonist of thyroid hormone action in target tissues when there is too much thyroid hormone. L-carnitine inhibits entry of both T3 and T4 into cell nuclei. This is relevant because thyroid hormone action is mainly mediated by specific receptors in the cell nuclei.

A recent report in the *Annals of the New York Academy of Sciences* found that 2- and 4-gram doses of carnitine were equally effective in reversing symptoms of hyperthyroidism. The symptoms that benefited the most were asthenia (weakness), nervousness and palpitations. Amelioration occurred 1 or 2 weeks after commencement of carnitine.

Thyroid Infections

Most patients with autoimmune thyroiditis have a chronic infection that is driving their autoimmunity. In a nutshell, autoimmune thyroiditis is a common response when your immune system fights off pathogens and allergens too enthusiastically.

The most common infections associated with Hashimoto's thyroiditis are the Epstein-Barr virus, *Yersinia enterocolitica* and *Helicobacter pylori*. Others include:

- *Borrelia burgdorferi* and other Lyme disease spirochetes, bacteria transmitted via tick bites that cause Lyme disease
- *Rickettsia* bacteria, transmitted by biting insects
- hepatitis C virus, which causes liver disease that affects thyroid function
- parvovirus B19, which causes fifth disease
- influenza B virus, which causes the flu
- rubella virus, which causes German measles

Epstein-Barr Virus

People with autoimmune thyroiditis have been shown to have significantly larger amounts of Epstein-Barr virus inside the thyroid gland. As long as the virus is active in the thyroid gland, they will have autoimmunity and resultant inflammation.

Although the drug rituximab destroys the cells that are infected with Epstein-Barr virus, alternative and less drastic approaches to deactivating this virus include using the following minerals, vitamins, amino acids and medications. Consult your doctor before using any of these approaches.

- curcumin
- *Larrea tridentata*
- monolaurin
- N-acetylcysteine
- quercetin
- reishi mushroom extract
- selenomethionine and glutathione
- vitamin C
- zinc

Yersinia enterocolitica

Yersinia enterocolitica, an infectious agent found in contaminated food and water, can trigger autoimmune thyroiditis. The protein that makes up the outer shell of *Yersinia* can lead to cross-reactivity, or molecular mimicry, of thyroid tissue, resulting in an immune attack on the thyroid gland.

> **DID YOU KNOW?**
>
> **CD8+ T-CELL DEFICIENCY**
> One of the common conditions in people with autoimmune disease is known as a CD8+ T-cell (or cytotoxic T-cell) deficiency. These cells control the Epstein-Barr virus, but if you have a genetic deficiency, the virus can remain active. Excess estrogen levels can exacerbate Epstein-Barr virus reactivation by affecting CD8+ T-cells.

As long as the *Yersinia* infection is in your intestine, your body will produce antibodies that attack this bacteria and the thyroid. Eradication of the infection through antibiotics or herbal medicines eliminates or significantly reduces the autoimmune attack on the thyroid gland.

Helicobacter pylori

Helicobacter pylori is found in the gastrointestinal (GI) tract of about two-thirds of the population. It causes ulcers in susceptible people. The presence of *H. pylori* is best determined through a breath test. Stool analysis and blood testing for *H. pylori* are also available, but these are not as sensitive as the breath test.

H. pylori has been shown to be more common in patients with Graves' disease. Treatment of this infection can reduce autoimmunity. *H. pylori* is treated with antibiotics or a variety of natural agents, such as mastic gum, zinc carnosine, deglycyrrhizinated licorice root, berberine, quercetin and probiotics and *Saccharomyces boulardii*.

> *Helicobacter pylori* causes ulcers in susceptible people.

Q What is dysbiosis?

A "Dysbiosis" means an imbalance in the ratio of healthy and unhealthy bacteria in the body, most commonly in the GI tract. In a healthy intestine, "good" bacteria have many functions in the digestion and absorption of food, the manufacture of vitamins and the control of harmful microorganisms, and no single strain dominates. If you are sick, one strain can become dominant, a situation that may become chronic. Dysbiosis is often caused by antibiotics, which can kill both "bad" and "good" bacteria. You can support the healthy bacteria by taking supplements of prebiotics (such as fructooligosaccharides) that bacteria in the GI tract feed on.

Candida albicans

Candida albicans and other yeasts can contribute to the development and perpetuation of autoimmune thyroiditis. Yeasts that grow in the intestine impair absorption of the nutrients required for optimal immune function and further acidify the digestive environment. In some cases, if overgrowth is very bad, the yeast regurgitates into the stomach, causing chronic heartburn and impaired digestion. Constipation can further worsen the problem of overgrowth, as yeasts feed on sugars produced as a result of food fermenting in its transit through the intestine. Decreasing transit time is a first order of priority when eradicating yeast overgrowth.

A stool analysis provides data on what type of yeast is present and what natural compounds can be used to kill it. Undergoing this test is essential, as some yeasts are resistant to a number of natural medicines. A stool analysis also indicates whether you have any dysbiotic (abnormal) flora or intestinal parasites. Dysbiotic flora can also contribute to autoimmunity and intestinal dysfunction. Parasites can further stress the immune system and lead to deficiencies in those minerals that are important for healthy thyroid function, such as iron and the vitamin B complex. Both dysbiotic flora and intestinal parasites must be treated.

People with yeast overgrowth also have impaired intestinal barrier function, so toxins can freely leak into the bloodstream, further taxing the immune system. In some cases, the yeast must be killed slowly while the immune system is supported. Multiple probiotic strains of at least 50 billion viable organisms are ingested each day during this process. However, if your immune system is still weak, the diet is poor and supplements are not taken, the yeast can quickly regrow.

Barrier Hyperpermeability

Autoimmune thyroiditis is a sign that your blood–thyroid barrier has been breached, that substances that should not enter the thyroid gland are doing so and that white blood cells have entered the thyroid gland and are attacking it. This increased permeability indicates that your body can no longer keep up with repairing the damage caused by your immune system.

Thyroid hyperpermeability can sometimes be traced to an intestine that is also hyperpermeable, allowing unwanted substances and toxins into the blood, further exhausting your body's ability to repair itself. As your gut becomes more permeable, or "leaky," so do the rest of your tissues and organs. When the intestinal barrier is broken, autoimmune thyroiditis may result.

Four barrier systems protect your body from pathogens and allergens that potentially trigger the onset of autoimmune diseases:

- gut barrier
- lung barrier
- skin barrier
- blood–brain barrier

Gut Barrier

The gut has a mucosal barrier that prevents pathogens and allergens from entering your body from the intestinal lumen. This barrier makes up 70% of your body's immune system. However, dietary proteins, digestive enzymes, allergens (such as gluten) and environmental toxins can all break down the intestinal barrier, as can health conditions such as cirrhosis of the liver, hepatitis, irritable bowel syndrome (IBS), inflammatory bowel disease (IBD), ulcers, colon cancer, low stomach acid and diverticulosis.

When the gut barrier breaks down, the result is a localized or systemic inflammatory cascade in the immune system. This condition is known as gut hyperpermeability, or leaky gut. Leaky gut is involved in the pathogenesis of autoimmune thyroiditis, as well as skin conditions (psoriasis, eczema and dermatitis), allergies, asthma, malabsorption and inflammatory bowel disease.

Leaky gut can be diagnosed by an assessment of the symptoms and severity of food sensitivities that show up on immunoglobulin G (IgG) food sensitivity testing.

Food Allergies and Sensitivities

Nutrients from our food pass into the bloodstream through tight gap junctions in the intestinal barrier. When the intestinal barrier breaks down, these tight junctions expand, allowing larger particles to pass through easily. These larger particles include undigested food particles, pathogens and antigens.

This constant "invasion" overloads the immune system, over time leading to immune system dysfunction. As the intestinal barrier breaks down, food sensitivities begin to proliferate and the overwhelmed immune system starts to function abnormally.

To determine your food allergies and sensitivities and help your body recover:

1. **Run a blood panel** that measures a large number of different foods and the level of reaction your body has to each. This method quickly pinpoints what foods you should avoid while your intestinal barrier is healing. It is also an excellent measure of the integrity of the intestinal barrier and immune function: the more food sensitivities you have, and the stronger the severity, the more permeable the gut barrier. Each food is graded on a scale of mild, moderate or strong response. As the foods are eliminated and the

barrier heals, the immune system no longer reacts to these foods as before. However, to prevent a relapse, some foods may need to be avoided indefinitely or placed on a rotation, even when the barrier is healed.

2. **Follow an elimination diet** by avoiding the most common food allergens, which include dairy, gluten, soy, tomato, peanuts, corn and eggs, for 3 to 6 months. The purpose of this diet is to remove immune stresses on the intestine so it can heal.

Celiac Disease

People with celiac disease are allergic to gluten, a protein found in wheat and many other grains. This devastating autoimmune condition breaks down the intestinal barrier, causing immune dysfunction, malabsorption of nutrients and many problems outside the GI tract. In fact, up to 70% of the effects of gluten occur outside the intestine. One of the serious effects, multiple organ dysfunction syndrome, results in simultaneous dysfunction of many organs, such as the thyroid, liver, adrenal glands, pancreas, sex organs, heart, brain, bones and kidneys.

People with celiac disease are about 10 times more likely to have autoimmune thyroiditis. Approximately one-quarter of people with celiac disease have autoimmune thyroiditis.

> **DID YOU KNOW?**
>
> **CONSTIPATION**
> Diets high in simple sugars, low in fiber and high in meat content can cause constipation, which increases the amount of time that the gut barrier is exposed to toxins.

Gluten Intolerance (Non-Celiac Gluten Sensitivity)

Celiac disease and gluten intolerance are not the same thing. People who have celiac disease must avoid gluten for life, but gluten intolerance can be reversed. Gluten intolerance does not necessarily have an autoimmune component, so its effects are not as devastating as in celiac disease. It can still damage the intestine and other organs, but usually not as severely.

Conventional medicine does not recognize gluten intolerance as a medical condition, although celiac disease is recognized.

Many people live their entire lives with gluten intolerance without being aware of it. They may suffer from mild to moderate health problems, such as osteoporosis, nutritional deficiencies, hypothyroidism, digestive problems and even autoimmune thyroiditis. Their degree of gluten intolerance depends on their genetic makeup, the environment, their overall nutrition and, of course, how much gluten they consume.

Gluten intolerance does have a potential link to autoimmune thyroiditis. If you are gluten-intolerant, your body produces antibodies to gluten that also cross-react and attack the thyroid gland. This is called molecular mimicry.

It is a mistake to assume that if you don't have any digestive problems, you don't have gluten intolerance. Remember, 70% of gluten's negative effects occur outside the intestine, affecting other tissues, including the thyroid gland.

Medications

Certain medications can contribute to the breakdown of the gut barrier.

- **Antacids** block hydrochloric acid production in the stomach. Although this suppression is an effective treatment for heartburn, or gastroesophageal reflux disease (GERD), it compromises protein digestion. As a result, large undigested proteins pass from the stomach into the small intestine. If your intestinal mucosa is leaky, these protein particles can be absorbed into the bloodstream, taxing the immune system. Chronic inadequate stomach acid production can also lead to depressed intestinal immune function, bacterial overgrowth in the small intestine, nutrient deficiencies (such as calcium and magnesium deficiencies), protein malnutrition and greater susceptibility to GI infections and dysbiosis.
- **Antibiotics** disrupt normal flora not only in the GI tract, but also in the skin, vagina and mouth, potentially leading to yeast infections in these areas. The yeast that overgrows in the intestine can result in bloating, gas, chronic fatigue, depression and gut inflammation.
- **Nonsteroidal anti-inflammatory drugs (NSAIDs)**, such as Aspirin or ibuprofen, are anti-inflammatory medications mainly used for pain and inflammation. NSAIDs may inhibit the COX-1 enzyme, which is important for intestinal barrier health. They cause bleeding and inflammation in the GI tract, resulting in significant damage to the mucosal barrier.

Q What is the difference between an antibiotic, a probiotic and a prebiotic?

A Antibiotics are drugs that kill bacteria. A nonspecific antibiotic can eliminate not only the "bad" but also the "good," or "friendly," bacteria, causing an imbalance that results in yeast overgrowth, which adversely affects the intestinal barrier.

Probiotics are beneficial bacteria that should live in healthy colonies within the gut, to "crowd out" bad bacteria and maintain immune system health and digestion. An imbalance caused by antibiotic use can be corrected by replenishing probiotics with supplements of *Lactobacillus* and *Bifidobacteria*.

Prebiotics are substances that bacteria in the intestine can feed on, such as fructooligosaccharides (FOS). If you have an overgrowth of "bad" bacteria, prebiotics should not be used, because they will further feed the bad bacteria.

Lung Barrier

Your lungs are constantly exposed to a variety of toxins, including air pollution, second-hand smoke, emissions from new automobiles (that new car smell is not a good thing!), carpeting, dry-cleaned clothes, paint, solvents, furniture, wrinkle-free clothes, new plastics and many building materials. These toxins place excessive stress on the lung barrier and break it down, and the toxins leak into the bloodstream as a result.

Skin Barrier

The main enemy of the skin barrier is too much washing. Many of the commercial products available today are loaded with chemicals that break down the skin barrier. Soaps, body washes, shampoos, conditioners, lotions, aftershaves, cosmetics and other personal hygiene products can be extremely toxic, and a broken skin barrier allows them to be absorbed into the bloodstream.

Blood–Brain Barrier

The blood–brain barrier is extremely selective in what it allows to pass in and out of the brain. However, once this barrier begins to break down after the gut barrier starts to leak, substances that wouldn't normally enter the brain end up doing so, causing an immune response and inflammation in the very delicate cerebral tissues. Your immune cells begin to attack the invaders, but they don't always limit the attack and can harm normal brain tissue as well.

Toxins

Toxins get into the bloodstream by passing through the gut barrier, lung barrier and skin barrier. If the blood–brain barrier is leaky, toxins can enter the brain and cause immune cell dysfunction in cerebral tissues.

Toxins can alter tissue proteins, making them look foreign to the immune system cells. Mercury, for example, binds to proteins and enzymes, altering their structure, which confuses the immune system. Continuous exposure to a toxin can lead to immune system dysfunction that culminates in autoimmune disease.

We are all exposed to environmental toxins every day, but our overall health and genetic makeup determine how we handle and detoxify them. Some people can live a long healthy life despite constant exposure, while others will suffer from severe debilitating sickness with even the smallest exposure.

Treating the barrier systems of the body with natural medicine is an integral part of overcoming the negative effects of autoimmune disease.

Vitamin D and Immunity

Vitamin D is not actually a vitamin but rather a type of hormone known as a secosteroid. Your body synthesizes vitamin D_3 from the sunlight (ultraviolet B rays) that hits your skin. Vitamin D_3 is also found in fish and egg yolks, while D_2 is found in enriched dairy products and plants.

Vitamins D_3 and D_2 are similar in many ways, except that D_3 is metabolized much more efficiently than D_2. Vitamin D_3 is converted in the liver into 25-hydroxycholecalciferol (also known as calcidiol or calcifediol), while vitamin D_2 is converted into 1,25-hydroxycholecalciferol (also known as calcitriol). 25-hydroxycholecalciferol is a vitamin D receptor antagonist, and 1,25-hydroxycholecalciferol is an agonist. The kidneys also play a part in vitamin D metabolism, converting 25-hydroxycholecalciferol into 1,25-hydroxycholecalciferol, the active part of vitamin D.

Vitamin D is best known for its role in regulating calcium absorption and utilization. However, it is also involved in regulating hormone secretion, cellular proliferation and differentiation, and immune system function. Vitamin D receptors are found in cells of the immune, neuromuscular, cardiovascular and endocrine systems. When vitamin D levels drop, parathyroid hormone levels increase, which increases calcium absorption. Calcium can even be pulled from bone in an attempt to maintain a balance of this mineral.

1,25-hydroxycholecalciferol inhibits adaptive immunity (the immunity that develops over your lifetime) and activates the innate immune system (the immunity already encoded at birth). This may explain the role of 1,25-hydroxycholecalciferol in fighting off acute infections. But a problem can arise if you have one of the following infections with links to autoimmune thyroid disease:

- Epstein-Barr virus
- *Borrelia burgdorferi* (which causes Lyme disease)
- hepatitis C
- cytomegalovirus

Such an infection can deactivate the vitamin D receptor, with the result that 1,25-hydroxycholecalciferol is unable to bind to its receptor. If 1,25-hydroxycholecalciferol can't bind to the vitamin D receptor, it binds to the T3 receptor. When 1,25-hydroxycholecalciferol levels rise, thyroid hormone resistance can develop because the thyroid hormone receptor is bound by 1,25-hydroxycholecalciferol instead of T3.

It takes a highly skilled doctor to identify any existing chronic stealth infections so that vitamin D supplementation can be avoided or used appropriately. Vitamin D supplementation is currently extremely popular, to the point that virtually everyone is advised to take it. However, anyone with a chronic stealth infection or autoimmune disease should use caution when considering vitamin D supplementation. If you have no infections, it may be safe to supplement with vitamin D to regulate the immune system.

Nutrient Deficiencies

A variety of nutrient deficiencies can affect autoimmune thyroiditis.

Vitamin B₁₂

You need a substance called intrinsic factor, secreted by the intestinal mucosa, to absorb vitamin B_{12}, but your body sometimes produces antibodies to intrinsic factor, resulting in a B_{12} deficiency. People with Hashimoto's thyroiditis are deficient in vitamin B_{12}, which results in a condition known as pernicious anemia. Gluten intolerance and B_{12} deficiency often go hand in hand.

Your doctor will order a test for intrinsic factor antibodies if you are unresponsive to vitamin B_{12} supplementation.

Iodine

Although iodine is essential for the health of the thyroid gland, too much iodine leads to an increase in the thyroid peroxidase antibody in people with autoimmune thyroiditis, which in turn leads to an increased attack on the thyroid gland.

Until more definitive research is available, we do not recommend iodine supplementation in most cases of autoimmune thyroiditis, as it may worsen the condition.

> **DID YOU KNOW?**
>
> **B₁₂ SUPPLEMENTS**
> Sublingual B_{12} bypasses the gut and is an excellent way to raise B_{12} levels, although injections are the most efficacious route of administration.

Q What is an antibody?

A An antibody is a protein produced by plasma cells that the immune system uses to identify and destroy foreign objects, such as bacteria and viruses. People with symptoms of thyroid dysfunction should be tested for two antibodies: thyroid peroxidase and antithyroglobulin.

Thyroid peroxidase is the enzyme required for thyroid hormone synthesis. Increased levels of thyroid peroxidase antibodies indicate that your immune system is attacking this enzyme. Similarly, increased levels of antithyroglobulin antibodies mean that your immune system is attacking antithyroglobulin in the thyroid gland. Levels of these two antibodies are elevated in 85% to 90% of people with chronic autoimmune thyroiditis.

Antibodies involved in Graves' disease include thyroid-stimulating immunoglobulin (TSI) antibody and TSH receptor antibody. Anti-nuclear antibody (ANA) can also be elevated in Graves' disease.

DID YOU KNOW?

CRETINISM

When your body is low in iodine and selenium, a condition known as myxedematous cretinism can occur. "Cretin" became a medical term in the 18th century and saw widespread medical use in the 19th and early 20th centuries, actually being a "tick box" category on Victorian-era census forms in the United Kingdom. The term came to be used popularly as a derogatory term for a person who behaves stupidly. Because of the pejorative connotation, today's health-care workers no longer use terms like "cretin," "lunatic," "idiot" or "retarded."

Selenium

Your body needs selenium to produce thyroid hormone. Selenium is a cofactor for deiodinase, the enzyme that converts T4 to the more active T3 and degrades rT3. Selenium reduces inflammation in the thyroid gland during Hashimoto's thyroiditis and Graves' disease. Because of its antiviral properties, selenium can be an excellent supplement for those with Epstein-Barr virus reactivation. Moreover, selenium binds to mercury, rendering the heavy metal completely inert so that your body can easily excrete it.

Selenium has been shown to reduce thyroid antibodies and improve the well-being of those with autoimmune thyroiditis. It also slows the progress of Graves' ophthalmopathy, which is the classic bulging of the eyes.

Selenium is best taken as selenomethionine, at 200 micrograms per day. Avoid higher doses, and avoid selenium selenite or selenate, as these have been linked to toxicity and the development of diabetes and prostate cancer.

Caution

Brazil nuts contain high amounts of selenium. To avoid selenium toxicity, do not consume more than two or three per day.

Treating Autoimmune Thyroiditis

If you have autoimmune thyroiditis:

1. Get checked for the following infections:
   - Epstein-Barr virus
   - *Helicobacter pylori*
   - *Yersinia enterocolitica*
2. Request a stool analysis for:
   - *Candida albicans* and other yeasts
   - fungi
   - parasites
3. Get your estrogen levels checked, as elevated estrogen levels can exacerbate an Epstein-Barr virus reactivation.
4. Get tested for IgG (immunoglobulin G) food sensitivities and eliminate these foods from your diet to reduce stress on your immune system and help heal a leaky gut.
5. Go gluten-free.
6. Have your antibody levels tested.
7. Use caution with vitamin D supplements until any chronic stealth infection is no longer active. If you have no infections, 1,000 IU per day of vitamin D may be beneficial if taken under your doctor's supervision.
8. Avoid iodine supplementation unless recommended and supervised by a doctor.
9. Take selenomethionine (200 micrograms per day) with food. This is a safe and effective dose to reduce thyroid antibodies and improve your symptoms.

▷ DOC TALK

Autoimmune thyroiditis responds to lifestyle changes. Changing your habits is not always easy, but you will see much more rapid improvements in your health if you make the following adjustments to your lifestyle:

1. Consider alternatives to NSAIDs, as these drugs contribute to the breakdown of the gut barrier.
2. Treat constipation by increasing fiber intake, drinking half your body weight (in pounds) in ounces of water each day and taking probiotics and magnesium supplements. If these measures do not resolve the constipation, other underlying causes need to be evaluated.
3. Sleep 7 to 8 hours each night, as most healing takes place during sleep.
4. Eliminate or severely restrict coffee, tea and soft drinks, as they can disrupt sleep. In addition, sugar can create immune system imbalances.
5. Take the following supplements to help heal the gut barrier:
   - aloe vera
   - deglycyrrhizinated licorice root (DGL)
   - L-glutamine
   - marshmallow root
   - methylsulfonylmethane (MSM)
   - N-acetyl glucosamine
   - okra
   - quercetin
   - slippery elm bark
   - zinc or zinc carnosine

CHAPTER 4

The Gastrointestinal System and Thyroid Disorders

CASE STUDY

Gut Health

Chantal's gut problems included bloating, gas, cramping, heartburn and diarrhea six to seven times a day. She also felt fatigued, slept a lot, felt depressed, found it difficult to lose weight and felt cold all the time. The condition of her skin made her look like she was aging rapidly.

Chantal's previous thyroid tests had showed hypothyroidism, but she had decided to try to treat her condition herself with some natural thyroid supplements. Unfortunately, these hadn't helped at all.

We ran a functional stool analysis to look for bacterial, fungal and parasitic infections and discovered one of each, as well as significant dysbiosis. Chantal's thyroid antibody tests showed Hashimoto's thyroiditis, and her infection connection tests showed active *Helicobacter pylori*. We tested her for food sensitivities, which can be very stressful to the gut and immune system, and found sensitivities to dairy, eggs, yeast, gluten and soy.

We started Chantal on a natural antimicrobial protocol to get rid of the infections. She also started taking supplements and eliminated the foods she was sensitive to. Her symptoms began improving almost immediately and, after about 4 weeks on the treatment plan, her gut felt almost 100% better.

We discussed some long-term nutrition strategies to help keep her gut healthy and emphasized that it was important to avoid eating the same foods all the time so that she wouldn't develop new sensitivities. Chantal continues to do well.

Gut–Thyroid Connections

Apart from its obvious functions — digestion, nutrient absorption, elimination — the gastrointestinal (GI) tract is involved in many aspects of overall health, including detoxification, hormone metabolism and energy production. Surprisingly, 99% of brain neurotransmitters are formed in the intestine. A healthy GI system is very important in achieving optimal thyroid health, and many people find that thyroid function is normalized after imbalances in the GI tract are treated.

T4 Conversion

Thyroxine (T4) is inactive until it is converted into triiodothyronine (T3). Although most of this conversion takes place in the liver, approximately 20% of thyroid hormone is converted into T3 in the GI tract by the enzyme sulfatase. This conversion of inactive T4 into active T3 depends on healthy colonies of beneficial bacteria in the GI tract.

Infections

All intestinal infections can have a negative effect on thyroid hormone metabolism, because one-fifth of hormone activation takes place in the GI tract. Infections also contribute to autoimmune thyroiditis by constantly stressing the immune system.

Many diseases can be traced to a breakdown in the GI tract, where 70% of the immune system resides.

Hydrochloric Acid

Optimal thyroid function is also extremely important for the production of hydrochloric acid in the stomach. Hydrochloric acid breaks down protein and any supplements or medications and prepares food to pass into the small intestine. Low hydrochloric acid levels may cause insufficient absorption of thyroid medication.

In addition to hypothyroidism, low levels of hydrochloric acid can lead to:

- gastroesophageal reflux disease (GERD), or heartburn
- gas, bloating, belching and constipation
- deficiencies in vitamin B_{12}, minerals (calcium, magnesium, zinc and iron) and protein
- increased food sensitivities
- GI infections (fungal, parasitic and bacterial)

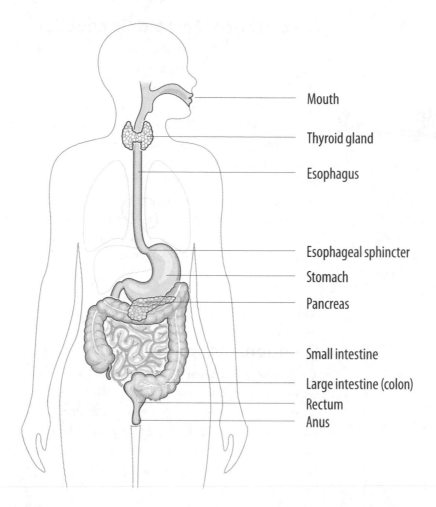

Mouth

Thyroid gland

Esophagus

Esophageal sphincter

Stomach

Pancreas

Small intestine

Large intestine (colon)

Rectum

Anus

- poor gallbladder function
- intestinal dysbiosis
- a weakened immune system

Gut-Associated Lymphoid Tissue

Your digestive tract is lined with lymph tissue known as gut-associated lymphoid tissue (GALT). GALT is responsible for localized immunity to bacteria, yeast, viruses and parasites. Food sensitivities, undigested proteins, leaky gut and pathogens can cause a major stress response in GALT, which in turn increases cortisol production by the adrenal glands. Cortisol causes a shift in thyroid hormone metabolism, inhibiting conversion of T4 to T3 and increasing levels of reverse T3 (rT3), the inactive form of T3.

Chronic elevations of cortisol as a result of stress suppress the immune system in the GI tract, which can lead to dysbiosis, parasites, excess yeast and leaky gut, creating a vicious cycle that further disrupts thyroid function.

GI–Estrogen–Thyroid Connection

The GI–estrogen–thyroid relationship is essential to having your thyroid working at its best. The GI tract contains an enzyme called beta-glucuronidase that can reactivate estrogen that has been metabolized in the liver. This metabolized form of estrogen would normally be excreted in the feces, but if beta-glucuronidase levels are too high, estrogen can be reabsorbed into the bloodstream. Beta-glucuronidase levels depend on optimal nutrition and healthy gut bacteria ratios.

Estrogen can suppress thyroid hormone function by increasing the amount of thyroid hormone–binding proteins in the blood. In autoimmune thyroiditis, excess estrogen can exacerbate Epstein-Barr virus reactivation.

GI Tract Tests

Functional Stool Analysis

The best way to determine whether you have digestive tract issues is to complete a functional stool analysis, which your doctor must order. Many conventional doctors are unfamiliar with these types of tests and may not consider them valid diagnostic tools. Find a doctor who will order a test that looks for all types of infections, including bacteria, parasites and fungi, and for dysbiosis.

Functional stool analysis tests are vital for identifying the underlying causes of many people's health problems. Another advantage of these tests is their sensitivity. If the lab identifies a bacteria or yeast, it will test a number of medications and herbal medicines to determine which one eradicates the infection, so you know exactly what to use to address the infection. For example, oil of oregano may test well for *Candida* infection, but garlic may not.

Testing labs generally require three samples, taken at different times and on different days, because parasites can be difficult to identify on a single sample.

Transit Time Test

A quick way to determine whether you have a GI problem is to complete a transit time test, such as the activated charcoal test. Food should pass through your intestines within 18 to 24 hours. If it takes more than 24 hours or less than 18 hours, there is something wrong with your digestive tract.

1. Swallow four capsules of an inert product called activated charcoal with a meal. Note the day and time that you take the capsules.
2. Examine your stools until you excrete a black or dark gray one. Note the day and the time.
3. Work out the difference, to the nearest hour, between the time you swallowed the charcoal capsules and the time you saw the black stool. If passing the stool took more than 24 hours or less than 18 hours, see your doctor.

The 4R Protocol

In the early 1990s, Dr. Jeffrey Bland devised a model known as the 4R protocol to address infections and imbalanced digestive system function. The 4R protocol involves the following:

- **Remove** foods to which you are sensitive. Simple blood testing can pinpoint food sensitivities, such as to gluten, dairy, eggs, soy or peanuts. Alcohol, caffeine and sugar should also be avoided, because they put further stress on the immune system in the gut.
- **Repair** the intestinal barrier by taking supplements, including:
  - aloe vera
  - deglycyrrhizinated licorice root (DGL)
  - L-glutamine
  - marshmallow root
  - methylsulfonylmethane (MSM)
  - N-acetyl glucosamine
  - okra
  - quercetin
  - slippery elm bark
  - zinc or zinc carnosine
- **Replace** hydrochloric acid and pancreatic enzymes to offer digestive support. Betaine hydrochloride is the recommended digestive aid. Herbs known as Swedish bitters can also stimulate digestion. In addition, support hydrochloric acid production by making sure zinc and B complex vitamin levels are not depleted.
- **Reinoculate** by taking probiotics that contain "friendly" bacteria, such as *Lactobacillus* and *Bifidobacterium*, to reinoculate the right bacterial colonies. *Saccharomyces boulardii* is a beneficial yeast that helps restore the immune system in the GI tract and helps fight infections.

Food Allergies and Sensitivities

Food allergies and sensitivities can lead to inflammation, and inflammation can lead to hypothyroidism. Each time you eat a food to which you are sensitive, there is an inflammatory response in your digestive system and in the rest of your body. Reactions to the food you cannot tolerate may occur within 45 minutes of consuming the food, or may take days to show up. You could eat eggs for breakfast on Monday morning, then have an energy crash on Wednesday afternoon and not know why.

Food allergies and sensitivities also lead to leaky gut syndrome, which can be a trigger for autoimmune thyroiditis.

To heal your digestive tract, it is important to know which foods you are sensitive to. You can find this out through simple blood tests that determine which of approximately 100 foods you should avoid. Suspect foods can also be tested using the skin-scratch method, in which a visual cue, such as a wheal, appears on the skin after it is scratched with a needle contaminated with a small amount of the suspected allergen. These tests can also show how "leaky" your gut is based on how many strong reactions you have.

Conventional medicine only recognizes as allergens those foods, airborne substances, mites, pet dander and so forth that induce an immunoglobulin E (IgE) antibody response. IgE is only a tiny part of the immune system, but the emphasis on it is partly due to the fact that an IgE response can kill you. IgE responses, known as anaphylactic reactions or anaphylaxis, can occur immediately or up to 2 hours after exposure. Peanuts and bee stings are two common and potentially deadly allergens.

The Paleo Diet

Until recently, we ate only what was available to us locally and seasonally. When we consume specific foods seasonally, our immune systems are given a break from them for months at a time. Seasonal consumption prevents food sensitivities.

Modern agricultural technology now allows us to eat pretty much any food we want 365 days a year. Despite this access to a wider variety of foods, the average North American eats the same ten to fourteen foods all year long. This is not good for either the digestive system or the immune system.

Eggs, wheat and other grains, dairy, corn, peanuts, soy, cereals, oranges, legumes and nuts are not only the most commonly eaten foods but also the most problematic. One reason why the paleo diet has become so popular is because it excludes many of these foods, thus reducing stress on the immune system and digestion.

Food sensitivities affect a much larger part of the immune system, specifically IgG, IgA and even IgM antibodies. These antibodies make up about 99% of the immune system and can give us valuable information on how your body reacts to the foods you eat. Like IgE responses, IgG responses can cause anaphylaxis.

Food sensitivities can also be described as "intolerances," meaning that the immune system responds abnormally to the food because of overexposure or compromised digestive tract function. Eating the same food over and over can result in sensitivity to that food. This is why we recommend eating foods that are in season and trying to eat a variety of different foods.

> Eating the same food over and over can result in sensitivity to that food. This is why we recommend eating foods that are in season and trying to eat a variety of different foods.

Immunoglobulin A

IgA is the "glue" that lines your mucous membranes, including your sinuses, lungs and GI tract. Food sensitivities can affect IgA levels, impairing the immune system function of your GI tract. IgA serves as the first line of defense against unwanted infection, and also prevents undigested food particles from entering your bloodstream. As the gut barrier wears down, more and more undigested food particles leak through the intestinal mucosa into the bloodstream, which significantly stresses the immune system, resulting in inflammation and more food allergies and sensitivities.

▷ DOC TALK

Take the following steps to prevent and treat GI dysfunction that may be affecting your thyroid:

1. Test the health of your GI with an activated charcoal test.
2. Request a functional stool analysis to identify whether you have dysbiosis or any bacterial, parasitic or fungal infections.
3. Follow the 4R protocol if you have dysbiosis or any infections.
4. Request IgG food sensitivity testing to learn what foods may trigger your GI symptoms and stress your immune system.

CHAPTER 5

The Hepatic System and Thyroid Disorders

CASE STUDY

Iron Stores

Mumtaz had many of the symptoms of hypothyroidism: fatigue, dry and brittle nails and hair, depression, low zest for life, constipation and dry skin. She had read a lot about various cleanses and detoxes to help her thyroid, and had tried a bunch of them, but they seemed to just make her more sick.

Mumtaz was a vegetarian, and as we reviewed her diet history, we discovered that her protein intake was extremely low. Blood tests showed that her ferritin levels, a marker of how much iron your body has stored, were also very low. Her TSH levels were high, while her free T3 levels were on the low end of normal.

We explained to Mumtaz that, while there is nothing wrong with being a vegetarian, she needs to combine proteins to maximize their benefits. We recommended a hemp- and pea-based protein powder to help her get extra protein. We told her that, for detoxification to be effective, you need to consume plenty of protein and amino acids, and that the programs she had tried were deficient in protein. After explaining that the thyroid needs healthy levels of iron to make the right amount of hormones, we started her on an iron supplement (chelated, for better absorption) to get her ferritin levels back to normal.

Once Mumtaz was getting enough protein and her iron stores were back to normal, her thyroid symptoms significantly improved. She is now able to maintain her health. We check her ferritin levels twice a year, as well as some other markers, such as vitamin B_{12}, to make sure they don't fall below normal.

Mumtaz now understands that her body is perfectly capable of ridding itself of toxins as long as it gets all the building blocks it needs from food.

About the Hepatic System

The hepatic system includes the liver and related biliary functions (bile ducts, the gallbladder and structures involved in the production and transportation of bile).

The liver is the organ of detoxification, but it is also involved in blood sugar homeostasis, immune system function, amino acid metabolism and cholesterol production. Everything you absorb through your intestines is first transported to the liver before circulating through your bloodstream.

The bile the liver produces is released from the gallbladder onto digested food in the small intestine when you eat. Bile acts like a detergent, breaking down fat for optimal absorption.

The Hepatic System and Thyroid Hormone

Most thyroid hormone is converted into its active form in the liver when an iodine atom is split off a T4 molecule to make T3. If the liver is not functioning at its best, signs and symptoms of hypothyroidism may arise.

DID YOU KNOW?

LIVER FACTORS
A number of factors, including blood sugar levels, insulin resistance, adrenal gland health, immune system function, gut health and thyroid function, affect liver function. Your doctor should be evaluating these systems to ensure that they are working well. Any issues with your liver should begin to resolve once these systems are working well.

LIVER DETOXIFICATION PATHWAYS AND SUPPORTIVE NUTRIENTS

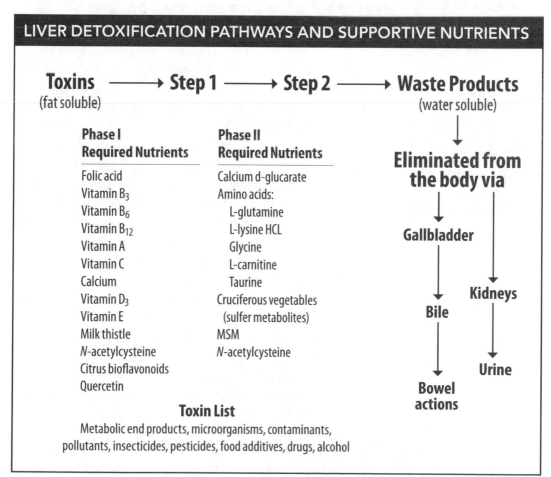

Toxins (fat soluble) ⟶ **Step 1** ⟶ **Step 2** ⟶ **Waste Products** (water soluble)

Phase I Required Nutrients

Folic acid
Vitamin B3
Vitamin B6
Vitamin B12
Vitamin A
Vitamin C
Calcium
Vitamin D3
Vitamin E
Milk thistle
N-acetylcysteine
Citrus bioflavonoids
Quercetin

Phase II Required Nutrients

Calcium d-glucarate
Amino acids:
    L-glutamine
    L-lysine HCL
    Glycine
    L-carnitine
    Taurine
Cruciferous vegetables
    (sulfer metabolites)
MSM
N-acetylcysteine

Eliminated from the body via

Gallbladder

Bile → Bowel actions

Kidneys

Urine

Toxin List
Metabolic end products, microorganisms, contaminants, pollutants, insecticides, pesticides, food additives, drugs, alcohol

At the other end of the chain, the liver eliminates expended T3 through a two-step detoxification process. It also metabolizes other hormones and toxins and excretes these by-products in the feces, through the gastrointestinal (GI) tract, as well as in urine and sweat.

The liver is also important for balancing sex and adrenal hormones in its role of metabolizing hormones and detoxifying thyroid-disrupting chemicals.

If the liver is not detoxifying optimally, you will have virtually no success in treating any disease, including thyroid and other hormone imbalances. Unfortunately, many patients are given hormones without a thorough analysis of their liver's ability to metabolize them. Unmetabolized or partially metabolized hormones circulating in the bloodstream can do more harm than good, as they can cause abnormal hormone responses. Partially metabolized hormones can bind to hormone receptor sites, blocking hormone receptors and preventing normal hormones from binding.

> If the liver is not detoxifying optimally, you will have virtually no success in treating any disease, including thyroid and other hormone imbalances.

Detoxification and Elimination

The liver plays several roles in detoxification:

1. It filters the blood to remove large toxins, including metabolic end products, microorganisms, environmental toxins and contaminants (pollutants and pesticides, among others), drugs and alcohol.
2. It synthesizes and secretes bile, which acts like a detergent, carrying fat-soluble substances, including hormones, environmental toxins, drugs, pesticides and allergy-causing complexes, into the gut. The bile and its contents are absorbed by fiber in the gut and excreted in feces. (If you consume too little fiber, the eliminated compounds might not be adequately bound and may be reabsorbed. Bacteria in the intestine can further alter these toxins to more damaging forms.)
3. It breaks down toxins and unwanted metabolites, usually in two distinct phases:
   - In Phase I, the cytochrome P450 group of enzymes directly neutralizes chemicals or converts them into water-soluble waste products that you can easily excrete, or modifies them to form activated intermediates that are neutralized by one or more of the Phase II enzyme systems.
   - Phase II involves six pathways through which various liver enzymes attach chemicals to the toxic compounds produced in Phase I to neutralize them.

Both phases of detoxification need to be functioning optimally to counteract the effects of toxins, but especially Phase II, which can be very delicate in people whose genetic anomalies make them sensitive to everyday toxins, such as perfumes.

Phase II Pathways

The following pathways must be supported for proper detoxification. This can be important for thyroid patients who have thyroid imbalances due to excess testosterone, estrogen, toxic metals or thyroid-disrupting chemicals.

Phase II Pathway	Necessary Nutrient Support
Glucuronidation	B vitamins, glycine and magnesium
Acetylation	Vitamin B_1 (thiamine), vitamin B_5 (pantothenic acid) and vitamin C
Sulfation	Molybdenum
Methylation	Betaine, choline, folate, magnesium, methionine, S-adenosylmethionine, trimethylglycine, vitamin B_6, vitamin B_{12}, vitamin C and vitamin E
Glycine conjugation	Glycine and protein
Glutathione conjugation	Cysteine, glutamic acid and glycine (the three peptides that make glutathione); selenium, vitamin B_6 and zinc

Glutathione

Although each detoxification pathway is essential, the "king of detoxification" is glutathione. Glutathione is the most abundant and powerful antioxidant in your body. It is used to neutralize free radicals produced in Phase I detoxification and is the key to detoxifying mercury, lead and other toxic metals. Your body can synthesize glutathione, and you can also get it from fresh fruits and vegetables, fish and meat. Although dietary glutathione appears to be efficiently absorbed into the blood, the same may not be true for glutathione supplements.

As long as you are eating the optimal amount of protein, your body will likely make enough glutathione. But glutathione can be depleted by large amounts of toxins and/or drugs passing through the liver, as well as by starvation or fasting. Glutathione levels will also drop when you have a chronic viral infection. Such a decrease in glutathione levels will contribute to any autoimmune thyroiditis caused by the infection.

Some people have a genetic defect in their ability to make glutathione. Genetic testing, through blood or saliva, can identify whether you have such a genetic issue. If you do, your doctor will guide you toward the steps you'll need to take to support your body's production of glutathione.

DID YOU KNOW?

RESTORING GLUTATHIONE
If your glutathione is depleted, you can restore it by consuming a good-quality whey protein supplement that is high in the amino acid leucine, as well as N-acetylcysteine and selenomethionine. Glutathione can also be taken orally in a reduced or acetylated form.

Liver Stress

An imbalanced GI tract, whether it's a result of dysbiosis, inflammation, leaky gut, infections or food allergies, puts a major strain on the liver's ability to metabolize hormones and thyroid-disrupting chemicals. This can lead to a toxic liver, impairing its ability to activate thyroid hormone.

Nutrition, toxin exposure and your genetic makeup are all key factors in effective liver detoxification. Detoxification can be impeded by inflammation, insulin resistance and leaky gut syndrome, all of which can also affect the thyroid. In addition, many studies have shown that impaired liver detoxification can lead to fatigue and autoimmune disease — both major factors in thyroid health.

Inflammation

Inflammation can put undue stress on the liver, impairing its function. L-carnitine, L-methionine, choline and inositol all help to metabolize fat and can reverse fatty liver disease. Phosphatidylcholine (from lecithin) can protect against alcoholic cirrhosis.

Insulin Resistance

Insulin resistance — when insulin becomes less effective at lowering blood sugar levels — puts major stress on the liver, because fatty acids produced from the excess sugar are deposited in the liver. Over time, this leads to fatty liver disease, when the liver becomes an insulin-resistant organ. At this point, major steps, such as eliminating sugar, alcohol and processed carbohydrates from your diet, must be taken to repair it.

Leaky Gut Syndrome

A leaky gut puts undue stress on the liver as a constant flow of toxins passes through the gut barrier into the bloodstream and then enters the liver, which must subsequently detoxify them. An imbalanced GI tract also increases the chances of thyroid-disrupting chemicals recirculating and impairing thyroid function. This exacerbates the vicious cycle involving the enzyme beta-glucuronidase, which undoes the liver's work, reactivating estrogen that has been metabolized in the liver. Instead of the inactive, metabolized form of estrogen being excreted in the feces, excess beta-glucuronidase can cause reactivated estrogen to be reabsorbed into the bloodstream.

Thyroid-Disrupting Chemicals

Approximately 100,000 synthetic chemicals are in commercial use today, and roughly 4,000 to 6,000 new ones are produced each year. Eighty percent have never been tested in relation to human safety or their effects on unborn children.

Some synthetic chemicals can disrupt normal production of thyroid hormones, causing circulating levels to decrease. Others can block hormone receptors, preventing hormones from binding, or can mimic the actual hormones. These thyroid-disrupting chemicals — including polychlorinated biphenyls (PCBs), polybrominated diphenyl ethers (PBDEs), phthalates and bisphenol A (BPA) — are used extensively in common household objects, such as plastics, paints, synthetic textiles and home electronics.

Evidence that certain toxic chemicals can disrupt hormone synthesis — including sex hormones, such as testosterone and estrogen — has increased over the past decade. We now know that certain synthetic chemicals can significantly affect thyroid hormone production and metabolism, carrier proteins and cellular uptake mechanisms. Some even resemble T4 and T3, and bind to receptor sites, inducing symptoms of hypothyroidism even when blood levels are normal.

If your thyroid is producing adequate amounts of hormones but the thyroid receptors are blocked by chemical binding, the cells in your body cannot respond to the thyroid hormones. As a result, your doctor may tell you that your thyroid hormone levels are fine when you aren't feeling fine at all.

Polychlorinated Biphenyls

Polychlorinated biphenyls (PCBs) can accumulate in fatty tissue in your body. A number of studies have found that adults, adolescents, children and even newborn babies living in areas of high PCB exposure have reduced levels of circulating thyroid hormones, including T4, free T4, total T3 and thyroxine-binding globulin, and increased levels of TSH. Adults were found to have significantly larger thyroids compared with people who were not exposed.

Abundant in the environment despite being banned in the 1970s, approximately 200 different PCBs are still found in high concentrations in human tissues, particularly the fetal brain, liver and plasma, because mothers who are exposed to PCBs

DID YOU KNOW?

BILE PRODUCTION

Bile production and flow must be optimal for effective detoxification. Taurine, vitamin C, betaine (beets), lecithin (phosphatidylcholine), methionine, inositol and L-carnitine have been shown to support bile production and flow.

DID YOU KNOW?

TERATOGENS

Many thyroid-disrupting chemicals are teratogens, which means they can harm a fetus. Some may have delayed effects that show up later as impaired cognitive function and behavioral problems. Since thyroid hormones directly influence the effects of genes, thyroid-disrupting chemicals may alter gene expression (the detectable effect of a gene).

transfer the chemicals to their fetuses. In addition, breastfed 6-week-old infants were found to have higher levels of PCBs than bottle-fed infants, indicating that PCBs are also transferred from mothers to their infants in breast milk.

A child whose developing brain was exposed to high levels of PCBs is extremely vulnerable to both impaired brain development and impaired thyroid function. Early exposure results in neuropsychological deficits, such as lower IQ, attention deficit disorder, impaired coordination and reduced ability to remember what has been seen. These negative effects are the result of PCBs (whose structure resembles that of T4) binding to thyroid hormone receptors.

Polybrominated Diphenyl Ethers

Polybrominated diphenyl ethers (PBDEs) — flame retardants added to furniture, carpeting and other household items — have been shown to reduce circulating thyroid hormone levels in rodents. In addition, PBDEs upregulate (increase the response of) liver enzymes used in detoxification processes and cause changes in thyroid tissue, indicating hypothyroidism.

Phthalates

Phthalates are found in plastics, such as plastic water bottles, food storage containers and plastic food wraps, and in cosmetics and personal products, including nail polish remover, hair spray, perfume and eye shadow. The glow sticks that are popular among children are loaded with phthalates.

Rodent studies have shown that exposure to phthalates results in changes in thyroid gland tissue, with resultant hyperactivity. Some studies show that phthalates increase circulating hormone levels; others have shown that they decrease them.

Bisphenol A and Other Phenols

About 5 to 6 billion pounds of bisphenol A (BPA) are produced every year. They are used in food containers and bottles, including baby bottles, and dinnerware, the lining of food cans and even some dental sealants. Phenols have also been used in antifungals, wood preservatives and biocides, compact discs, powder paints and adhesives. BPA can also be chemically altered to make flame retardants by adding bromine or chlorine, which are also known thyroid disrupters.

DID YOU KNOW?

LITHIUM
Studies have shown that lithium, used in the treatment of various bipolar disorders, inhibits the uptake of iodine by the thyroid and the secretion of thyroid hormone. Because of these effects, as many as half of the people taking lithium may have hypothyroidism and even goiter. Unfortunately, lithium is concentrated in the thyroid gland and, even when discontinued, the hypothyroidism and goiter do not always return to normal.

BPA behaves like a weak estrogen and has been shown to bind to thyroid receptors, inhibiting the binding of T3. This could lead to someone having all the symptoms of hypothyroidism despite normal levels of circulating thyroid hormone.

Dioxins and Dioxin-Like Chemicals

Dioxins are used in the production of herbicides and industrial burning processes. 2,3,7,8-tetrachlorodibenzo-p-dioxins (TCDDs), the most toxic of the dioxins, was shown to transfer from female rats to their offspring across the placenta and through breast milk. A single dose of TCDDs resulted in decreased T4 and free T4 levels and increased TSH levels, as well as in enlargement of the thyroid glands.

Effects in animals include a toxic liver and altered immune and thyroid function. In human studies, TCDD exposure resulted in increased levels of TSH and T4. Developmental effects are a particular concern.

Parabens

Parabens are widely used as a preservative in cosmetics and as antimicrobial agents in foods and prescription drugs. Parabens have estrogen-like effects that can inhibit thyroid function and cause symptoms of excess estrogen. Methylparaben has been shown to inhibit iodine.

Pesticides and Fungicides

Of the pesticides and fungicides that affect the thyroid, dichlorodiphenyltrichloroethane (DDT) and hexachlorobenzene (HCB) have been the most extensively studied.

DDT exposure has been shown to decrease T4 and increase the weight of the thyroid in birds. The amount of DDT in the blubber of seals was inversely proportional to total T3 and free T3 levels.

Many studies have shown that HCB exposure decreases T4 and T3 levels. Prenatal exposure reduces T4 and free T4 levels and increases the response of enzymes that metabolize thyroid hormone in the fetal brain. Our thyroid glands enlarge when we are exposed to HCB, which causes a reduction of T4. Animal studies have shown a link between exposure and cancer of the liver and thyroid.

Q How do thyroid-disrupting chemicals inhibit thyroid function?

A Each chemical affects thyroid function in its own way:

- Perchlorates, such as HCB, impede the uptake of iodine by the thyroid cells, inhibiting hormone production.
- Phthalates may stimulate the uptake of iodine into the thyroid, resulting in too much hormone production.
- Phenols inhibit the enzyme deiodinase, which is required to make thyroid hormone.
- DDT and PCBs block TSH receptors.
- PCBs, phthalates, phenols and HCB have been shown to bind to thyroxine-binding globulin (TBG), which transports thyroid hormones in the bloodstream.
- Phthalates and chlordanes impede cellular uptake of thyroid hormones.
- PCBs, phenols, BPA and HCB inhibit thyroid hormone receptors and gene expression (the detectable effects of a gene) in the cell.
- PCBs, dioxins, phenols, HCB and BPA affect the metabolism of thyroid hormones and the rate of excretion of the by-products.

Toxic Metals

DID YOU KNOW?

DENTAL AMALGAMS

Amalgams in teeth do not have their own blood supply, so all mercury exposure comes directly from emitted mercury vapors that you inhale or absorb through the mucous membranes of the mouth.

We all have toxic metals in our systems. Every day we are exposed to lead and mercury in car exhaust, in industrial emissions and through the burning of coal, oil and gas. Although many more dangerous metals exist, lead and mercury are the most heavily researched because we have such frequent exposure to them.

Toxic metals attach to deiodinase, the enzyme that converts T4 into the more active T3, inhibiting its activity. In addition, they can block thyroid hormone receptors, preventing hormones from binding. Toxic metals can also enter the mitochondria and inhibit energy production. They tend to accumulate in body tissues, specifically the thyroid, brain, heart, liver, pancreas and bone. Some metals have a higher affinity for specific tissues; of all the toxic metals, mercury has the highest affinity for the thyroid.

Heavy Metal	Thyroid Action	Sources
Aluminum	• Inhibits T4 production (in rats)	• Aluminum and coke production (while many products contain aluminum, they are not necessarily sources)
Arsenic	• Affects mitochondrial enzymes and therefore energy production	• Asphalt, car batteries, electronics, fungicides, glass, herbicides, insecticides, pesticides, pigments, rodent poisons, seafood and shellfish, semiconductors, smog, well water, wood preservative • Chicken feed may have arsenic in it, so source your food carefully
Cadmium	• Accumulates in the thyroid, as well as in the liver, kidneys and pancreas • Causes oxidative stress and damage to mitochondria and decreases blood levels of T3 and T4 (in rats)	• Asphalt, batteries, cigarette smoke, drinking water, fertilizer, fungicides, industrial exposure, liver and kidney meat, metal plating, paints, photoconductors, photography, pigments, plastics, printing, rubber, semiconductors, shellfish, textiles
Lead	• Inhibits the conversion of T4 to T3 • Is associated with elevated levels of blood TSH in mine workers	• Mining, smelting, manufacturing and recycling activities • Leaded paint and loaded gasoline • Ammunition, batteries, brass, bronze, ceramic glazes, some conventional medicines, some cosmetics, crystal, electrical devices, jewelry, pesticides, pigments, pipes, plastics, solder, stained and TV glass, toys
Mercury	• Disrupts the hypothalamic–pituitary–thyroid axis by accumulating in all three glands, as well as in the liver and kidneys (although mercury tends to accumulate mainly in the liver and kidneys, it also has a high affinity for the endocrine system) • Can either increase or decrease TSH, T4, T3 and rT3 levels • Leads to an increase in the size of the thyroid gland • Increases rates of thyroid cancer • Inhibits thyroid peroxidase enzyme, required for thyroid hormone production • Inhibits the uptake of iodine into the thyroid gland • Increases the rate that iodine is excreted through the kidneys • Binds to deiodinase, inhibiting the conversion of T4 to T3	• The burning of fossil fuel (coal) for power and the by-products of heating and waste incineration • Mining for mercury, gold, etc. • Tuna, marlin and swordfish (large predatory fish contain the highest levels of methylmercury; the smaller and younger the fish, the less mercury) • Agricultural chemicals, antibacterial products, antiseptic creams, asphalt, batteries, dental amalgams (these account for the largest percentage of non-occupational mercury exposure), electrical equipment, electroplating, explosives, felt, fireworks, fungicides, hemorrhoid preparations, hospital wastes, interior paint, paper industry, pesticides, photography, pigments, skin-lightening creams, taxidermy, textiles, thermometers, waste incineration

Methylmercury

Mercury tends to be the most problematic toxic metal for the thyroid gland. Three main types of mercury affect people and animals: methylmercury, mercury chloride and elemental mercury. You are most likely to be exposed to methylmercury. In a report published in *Critical Reviews in Toxicology* entitled "The Endocrine Effects of Mercury in Humans and Wildlife," the authors concluded that mercury influences the thyroid–adrenal and reproductive systems by accumulating in the endocrine system; by being specifically toxic to endocrine tissue cells; by changing hormone concentrations; by interacting with sex hormones; and by changing the response of cells to the enzymes involved in making steroids.

Body Burden

We are exposed to a large number of environmental chemicals every day. Some may disrupt thyroid function. We need to reduce the burden of toxic chemicals in our bodies by avoiding our exposure to them and by supporting the detoxification action of the liver.

"Body burden" refers to the total amount of environmental chemicals in your body at a particular time. It does not take into account which chemicals are passing through quickly (such as arsenic, which is largely excreted 72 hours after ingestion) and which are stored in fatty tissues for a long time (such as DDT, which can stay in your body for 50 years). Body burden is merely a snapshot of the current situation.

Q What can you do to reduce exposure to thyroid-disrupting chemicals?

A Start in the bathroom by avoiding any cleaning product containing the chemical triclosan, including antibacterial soap, hand sanitizer, toothpaste, cosmetics, body wash, mouth wash and deodorants. Triclosan may not affect TSH levels directly but can affect other thyroid hormone levels and even thyroid hormone receptors.

Keep a close eye on all household and cosmetic products that may come into contact with the skin. Check all the cosmetic products you use in the Environmental Working Group's online cosmetics database: www.ewg.org/skindeep.

Testing for Toxins

Although doctors can test for toxic metals and chemicals in a variety of ways, none of them are accurate for body burden.

Blood Testing

Blood testing is the gold standard in conventional medicine, but it works well only for recent or ongoing exposure (for example, children who have recently eaten lead paint). It works best for some (but not all) toxic metals and in certain compounds (for example, mercury from methylmercury). The tests are not reliable for chronic contamination, however. Once you are exposed to a toxic metal, it clears from the blood within 72 hours, on average, and is excreted or deposited in your tissues. If blood levels are high, you can assume that exposure to the metal was recent.

Hair Analysis

Despite the claims of some medical practitioners and clinics, hair analysis is not an accurate way to test for toxic metal body burden. A test result that shows low metal excretion in hair shows what is being excreted in the hair, and not how much metal is in the body. Hair tests can indicate a high degree of environmental exposure or a genetic disposition, which can be helpful in managing some thyroid conditions. Confirm the results of hair analysis with a blood test.

Stool Testing

Stool analysis is a good way to measure what is being excreted through the liver and gallbladder, but it does not reflect body burden. Stool tests are sometimes recommended for the very young because stools are easy to collect.

Urine Challenge

The urine challenge is the most widely used and accepted test for toxic metals. It involves ingesting or injecting a chelator, such as dimercaptosuccinic acid (DMSA), 2,3-dimercapto-1-propanesulfonic acid (DMPS), d-penicillamine (D-pen) or ethylenediaminetetraacetic acid (EDTA), and collecting the urine for anywhere from 2 to 24 hours. The chelator pulls metals out of the bloodstream, but it cannot enter the cell or cross the blood–brain barrier. That means the test results really only show what may be in the upper GI tract, liver, blood and kidneys. So again, the urine challenge is not an accurate test for body burden.

> **DID YOU KNOW?**
>
> **PORPHYRIN TESTING**
>
> Porphyrin does not test for levels of metals, but it does test for how certain metals may be disrupting your biochemistry at the cellular level. This type of testing was considered very promising, but it does not yield useful clinical information, and we recommend avoiding it.

Detoxification

Eliminating toxic metals is an art, and no clinical gold standard exists at this point. There are two basic theories on how to get rid of toxic metals:

1. Support your body's detoxification systems through diet, supplementation and other therapies, such as infrared saunas, colonics and salt and soda baths.
2. Use chemical-based chelators with a high affinity for metals, such as DMSA, DMPS, D-pen and EDTA, which bind to the metals and are excreted with them.

Chelation

Certain minerals bind to metals and make them inert so that they can be safely excreted in the feces or urine. Chelators include:

- dimercaptosuccinic acid (DMSA), which the U.S. Food and Drug Administration has approved for the treatment of lead poisoning in children
- 2,3-dimercapto-1-propanesulfonic acid (DMPS), which is non-toxic, can be given orally and has been shown to reduce blood lead levels in children
- d-penicillamine (D-pen), which binds to copper
- ethylenediaminetetraacetic acid (EDTA), which is infused directly into the bloodstream to treat lead poisoning and, as a result, works very quickly
- dithiocarb (DTC), which is used to treat nickel carbonyl poisoning; it may be administered orally for mild toxicity and transfused into the blood for acute or severe poisoning
- zinc and selenium, which have been shown to decrease cadmium and lead toxicity in the thyroid gland; selenium also binds to and completely deactivates mercury

If you undergo chelation, be prepared for some side effects. For example, if you have leaky gut syndrome, many of the toxins that are being dumped via chelation into the intestine from the liver/gallbladder complex may reabsorb into the bloodstream and may leave you feeling ill. In addition, you need healthy bacterial colonies in the GI tract to adequately eliminate toxins.

Make sure you consult a medical practitioner who understands chelation thoroughly. Chelation is not a home remedy.

DID YOU KNOW?

DETOX SUPPLEMENTS

Exposure to mercury rapidly depletes your stores of selenium. If you have been exposed to mercury, supplement with 200 micrograms of selenomethionine a day. Vitamin C has been shown to increase the excretion of mercury and lead in the urine.

Cleansing Programs

Clinically supervised detoxification and popular bowel cleansing routines must not be confused. No "miracle" cleanse can detoxify your body more effectively than sound nutrition that supports Phase I and II detoxification in the liver.

However, many people seem to prosper when they follow a bowel cleansing regimen. They feel better not because of any products or supplements, but because the program eliminates all of the things that are making them sick and promotes foods that make them feel better: fruits, vegetables and other healthy foods. Most programs:

- call for the elimination of sugar and processed carbohydrates
- encourage eating lean protein, such as wild-caught fish or a high-quality protein shake, with each meal
- eliminate foods that often cause sensitivities, such as gluten, dairy, soy, peanuts and corn
- eliminate caffeine and alcohol from the diet
- recommend high-quality "detox" powder that has extra protein and anti-inflammatories
- encourage people to exercise regularly
- encourage people to meditate or engage in other relaxation practices

So why don't we recommend following a bowel cleansing program? The issue is that some people feel worse, or get extremely ill, because some cleansing programs:

- do not provide enough protein and amino acids, especially glutathione, to support Phase I and II liver detoxification
- do not supply enough calories to fuel healthy metabolism
- do not test patients for genetic defects in glutathione production

If you follow the dietary guidelines in this book, you will be on your way to healthy detoxification.

> No "miracle" cleanse can detoxify your body more effectively than sound nutrition that supports Phase I and II detoxification in the liver.

▷ DOC TALK

Take the following steps to prevent and treat hepatic dysfunction:

1. Eliminate or reduce your intake of caffeine, alcohol, sugar and other obvious offenders, to decrease the stress you put on the liver.
2. Eat organic foods as often as possible to avoid exposure to synthetic pesticides and herbicides.
3. Make sure you eat sufficient protein to enable your body to make enough glutathione to safely and effectively neutralize and rid your body of mercury and other heavy metals and toxic chemicals.
4. Get tested for genetic anomalies, such as glutathione enzyme defects, if you are not responding to care. These are usually not checked until doctors hit a sticking point.
5. Take infrared saunas to help reduce toxic body burden.
6. Consume plenty of sulfur-rich foods, including garlic and onions, and eat vegetables from the Brassica family, such as broccoli and Brussels sprouts, which help to eliminate toxic metals.
7. Eat plenty of fruits and vegetables so that you get enough vitamin C. Alternatively, supplement with buffered vitamin C.
8. Use plastics as little as possible. Carry water in glass or stainless steel bottles.
9. Avoid products, carpeting and furniture that are treated with flame retardants.
10. Learn about cosmetic products and the harmful chemicals they contain (visit www.ewg.org/skindeep, the Environmental Working Group's excellent cosmetics database).
11. Avoid antibacterial products.

CHAPTER 6

The Adrenal Glands and Thyroid Disorders

Adrenal Fatigue

Liam had never been able to stabilize his thyroid hormone levels. In addition to having many of the classic symptoms of hypothyroidism, Liam also craved salt, had difficulty recovering from exercise, urinated frequently at night, was a slow starter in the morning and felt like he was "aging really fast."

Liam tested negative for Hashimoto's thyroiditis, but his adrenal hormone profile indicated classic adrenal fatigue. His cortisol levels were low, as were his metabolized cortisol and cortisone levels. In addition, his DHEA levels and those of its metabolites were extremely low.

We explained that cortisol is necessary for healthy thyroid function, and that his thyroid levels would continue to fluctuate as long as he had adrenal fatigue. We emphasized that some people need their adrenal glands supported before or during thyroid treatment; otherwise, the glands further exhaust themselves as thyroid hormones begin to stimulate the metabolism.

We started Liam on adrenal adaptogens, pregnenolone and DHEA, which immediately resulted in his symptoms improving, and we recommended that he stay on adrenal adaptogens to help his body adapt to stress in the future.

We helped him eliminate caffeine, sugar and foods to which he was sensitive, and emphasized that he needed to eat more protein. We explained that he must do his best to avoid physical and emotional stressors. Light exercise, meditation and plenty of self-care played a large role in his recovery.

Liam was a perfect example of someone with imbalances in another organ that impacted his thyroid function.

About the Adrenal Glands

The adrenal glands are each about the size of a walnut and lie on top of the kidneys. The adrenal cortex (the outer portion of the gland), makes up 80% of the gland and produces many hormones, including cortisol (the stress hormone) and dehydroepiandrosterone (DHEA), which is extremely important for immune system function and anabolic function, and is a sex hormone precursor. The adrenal medulla (the inner tissue) produces adrenaline and noradrenaline, also known as norepinephrine and epinephrine. While the adrenal cortex is under the control of hormones produced in the brain, the adrenal medulla is governed by the autonomic (involuntary) nervous system.

THE ADRENAL GLANDS

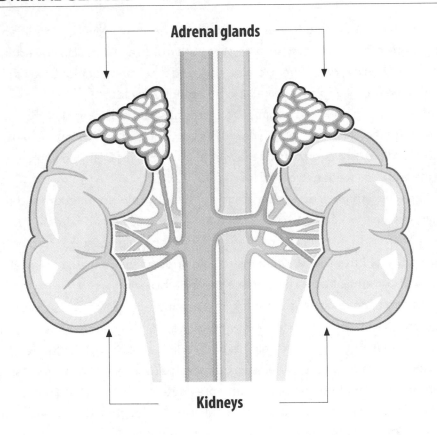

Adrenal glands

Kidneys

Adrenal Hormones
Adrenaline

Adrenaline, which is secreted by the adrenal medulla, stimulates increases in blood sugar if your body is under stress. Adrenaline also increases the circulation of fat in the blood so that more is available for energy production. This built-in survival mechanism is not ideal if you are desk-bound or otherwise sedentary. Large amounts of circulating fat and sugar are meant to be used when you are running from a saber-toothed tiger or other danger. If you are not active, the excess sugar is converted into fat and is stored mainly around your midsection, hips and thighs. Chronic stress, coupled with inactivity, can lead to continually high blood sugar levels and, hence, insulin resistance.

Aldosterone

Aldosterone, a hormone produced by the adrenal cortex, supports sodium absorption and potassium excretion as part of blood pressure regulation. Low-sodium diets and high water intake put a major stress on your adrenal glands as they work to retain the maximum amount of salt when your blood becomes more dilute from the extra water. In turn, low aldosterone levels can lead to excessive thirst, salt cravings and low blood pressure.

Cortisol

Cortisol, produced by the adrenal cortex, is a glucocorticoid hormone that slows down digestion, suppresses immune function and raises blood sugar. This response is a survival mechanism to deal with stress. The problem arises when stress becomes chronic. Cortisol will induce the liver to produce glucose (sugar) and will even strip muscle tissue, the gut lining and your skin of protein to maintain blood sugar levels. Cortisol can suppress TSH secretion, inhibit the conversion of T4 into T3 and disrupt thyroid hormone receptors. In addition, excess cortisol over long periods of time can increase the risk of diabetes, thanks to the prolonged blood sugar elevation.

DHEA

DHEA, which is also produced by the adrenal cortex, is a precursor (a substance from which other things are made) of estrogen, progesterone and testosterone. In men, it converts mainly into estrogen; in women, it converts mainly into testosterone. It is extremely important for immune system function and anabolic processes. DHEA levels begin to decline after you turn 35. Low DHEA levels are also found in people with multiple sclerosis, cancer, fibromyalgia, lupus, rheumatoid arthritis, Crohn's disease, ulcerative colitis and, of course, thyroid disorders.

Pregnenolone

Pregnenolone, which is synthesized mainly in the adrenal glands, is known as the "mother of all hormones because it converts into cortisol, DHEA, testosterone, estrogen and progesterone. Some studies suggest that pregnenolone may be a powerful antioxidant, and may boost mood and improve memory and brain function. People with low thyroid function also have low pregnenolone levels.

Adrenal Glands and Menopause

Healthy adrenal glands are vital for women who are peri- and postmenopausal. The adrenal glands are responsible for producing most sex hormones in menopause once the ovaries stop functioning. If the adrenal glands are fatigued and unprepared for menopause, menopausal symptoms such as hot flashes, weight gain, sleep problems, bone loss, mood swings, depression, anxiety, loss of sex drive and vaginal dryness will be more pronounced. Healthy adrenals ensure an easy transition into menopause and beyond.

Adrenal Dysfunction

Causes of adrenal stress include:

- acidic pH
- alcohol consumption
- anemia
- caffeine consumption
- emotional traumas
- food sensitivities, leaky gut
- infections of all types
- isolation/lack of companionship
- lack of sleep/staying up too late
- stressful or "toxic" relationships
- too much exercise
- too much sugar and processed carbohydrates, and insufficient protein intake
- work stress

Adrenal Fatigue

People who need caffeine and/or sugar to get going in the morning likely have adrenal fatigue, also known as adrenal insufficiency: their adrenal glands can't make enough cortisol to raise their blood sugar. They also "crash" many times throughout the day, especially in the afternoon, when they need a pick-me-up, such as a cup of coffee, or crave something sweet. This further disrupts their blood sugar and hormone levels, leading to weight gain, insomnia, fatigue and an underactive thyroid gland.

Although adrenal-fatigued people can usually fall asleep without a problem, they may have trouble staying asleep. They do not produce enough cortisol to stabilize their blood sugar, so their adrenals release adrenaline to raise blood sugar, which stimulates them into waking up.

The opposite happens when the adrenals are in overdrive, producing too much cortisol. Excess cortisol has an excitatory effect on the nervous system, so people with adrenal hyperfunctioning usually have trouble falling asleep and, when they do, are "light sleepers" easily shocked awake by even the quietest noises. Increased cortisol secretion eventually leads to adrenal fatigue.

Symptoms of Adrenal Dysfunction

If you have adrenal gland dysfunction, you may notice the following symptoms:

- allergies
- chronic infections
- dark pigmentation on the skin
- depression, anxiety, irritability
- digestive system issues
- fatigue
- flabby muscles, difficulty building muscle
- insomnia
- joint and muscle pain
- low sex drive
- osteoporosis
- poor appetite
- salt and/or sugar cravings
- weakness, dizziness when standing up or straightening quickly
- weight gain around the midsection and/or unexplained loss of muscle mass throughout the body

Adrenal Hormone Testing

A urinary spot hormone profile, or urinary cortisol test, measures cortisol at four different times of day, as well as the total load of cortisol produced by the adrenal gland. This test tells you about the hormones in the urine, and all of their metabolites, so you can learn how your body is breaking down cortisol and DHEA, which can provide further valuable information. For example, if cortisol levels look normal but metabolized cortisol levels are low, this could indicate hypothyroidism.

The Blood Sugar–Adrenal–Thyroid Axis

Blood sugar, the adrenal glands and the thyroid gland are a closely connected triad. The adrenal glands are stressed when blood sugar is out of balance, and vice versa. When both blood sugar and adrenal function are out of balance, the thyroid also suffers.

The main function of thyroid hormone is to regulate metabolism. That, however, is easier said than done, as both insulin resistance and the adrenal hormone cortisol can get in the way.

Blood Sugar Imbalance and Insulin Resistance

Blood sugar imbalances are key factors in thyroid and adrenal health, and insulin plays an enormous role in blood sugar balance, binding to cell receptors to allow blood sugar to enter the cells. Insulin resistance prevents blood sugar from being transported into your cells, decreasing the "fuel" available for energy production. When insulin binds to cell receptors, the receptors no longer respond. The pancreas then releases more insulin, putting added strain on it and further feeding the vicious cycle.

Insulin resistance is caused by chronically elevated levels of cortisol due to adrenal stress. It is at the core of many health issues in our society, especially diabetes, and is a growing concern as North Americans continue to consume large amounts of sugar, high-fructose corn syrup and processed carbohydrates. Insulin resistance leads to inflammation and many other imbalances in the body. It increases the strain on the thyroid, which makes more hormones to balance out the loss in energy, and can eventually lead to hypothyroidism. Other systems will also be stressed when the excess sugar is converted into fatty acids and stored in the liver and in the fat around the abdomen, hips and thighs.

If you have insulin resistance, talk to your doctor about a protocol for managing it.

Diabetes and Thyroid Hormone

Research published in the medical journal *Diabetologia* found that people with untreated diabetes had low levels of T4 and T3 but high levels of rT3. Once treated, their levels of thyroid hormone returned to normal. This indicates a direct connection between how well your body uses blood sugar and T3 levels. The more insulin-resistant you are, the lower your T3 levels.

Symptoms of Insulin Resistance

The following symptoms may indicate insulin resistance:

- abdominal obesity and inability to lose weight
- aches and pains
- brain fog
- fatigue after meals
- general fatigue
- high total blood cholesterol and low-density lipoprotein (LDL) cholesterol, high glucose and triglycerides, and low levels of high-density lipoprotein (HDL) cholesterol
- high blood pressure
- sugar cravings and constant hunger

Thyroid Inhibition by Cortisol

Cortisol inhibits the thyroid in a number of ways:

- About 95% of the hormone produced by the thyroid is the inactive thyroxine (T4). T4 is activated to triiodothyronine (T3) by the enzyme 5'-deiodinase, mainly in the liver. However, cortisol directly inhibits 5'-deiodinase, which can lead to low T3 levels.
- Higher cortisol levels cause thyroid hormone receptors to become less sensitive. Even if T3 levels are adequate, molecules of the hormone may not be able to bind normally to receptor sites.
- Cortisol increases the production of reverse T3 (rT3), which binds to and blocks T3 receptors.

DID YOU KNOW?

HYPOGLYCEMIA

If you have hypoglycemia, your cortisol levels are too low to raise blood sugar into the normal range. Adrenal fatigue and hypoglycemia are, therefore, often seen together. People with hypoglycemia develop symptoms of low blood sugar and need to eat to normalize blood sugar levels. They may feel shaky, irritable, light-headed or fatigued, or they may crave sugar. Once they rejuvenate their adrenal glands, their symptoms usually improve.

- Cortisol can lower the levels of thyroxine-binding globulin (TBG), which transports T3 and T4 in the bloodstream.
- High levels of cortisol increase the excretion of iodide (an iodine compound the body uses) from the kidneys. Iodine is vital to thyroid health.
- Elevated cortisol levels inhibit the production of thyroid-stimulating hormone (TSH) by disrupting hypothalamic–pituitary feedback.

Impaired Liver Detoxification

High cortisol levels also inhibit liver detoxification, which can lead to abnormal thyroid function. Signs of impaired liver detoxification include nausea, constipation, bloating, lack of response to treatment, acne (throughout the month or just during the menstrual cycle) and medication sensitivity, as well as poor elasticity and greater permeability of blood vessels (the latter can be confirmed by pressing the skin and noting a pale patch that lingers).

To optimize metabolism of toxins, excess hormones and thyroid-disrupting chemicals, it is often necessary to support liver detoxification pathways while treating the adrenal glands and thyroid.

The Hypothalamic–Pituitary–Adrenal Axis

The adrenal cortex communicates with the pituitary gland and hypothalamus in the brain via a hypothalamic–pituitary–adrenal (HPA) axis that works like the feedback loop of the hypothalamic–pituitary–thyroid (HPT) axis (see page 13).

If the hypothalamus detects low levels of cortisol in the bloodstream, it secretes two hormones: vasopressin and corticotropin-releasing hormone (CRH). These hormones stimulate the anterior (front) lobe of the pituitary to produce adrenocorticotropic hormone (ACTH). ACTH, in turn, stimulates the adrenal cortex to produce cortisol. Once the hypothalamus detects that blood levels of cortisol have been restored, it stops secreting vasopressin and CRH.

Your doctor may order an ACTH stimulation test to determine how well your adrenal glands are working. The test compares the amount of cortisol in your blood before and after you are injected with cosyntropin, a synthetic version of ACTH, to determine how well your adrenals respond to stimulation from the pituitary gland.

The Adrenal–Gut Connection

The adrenal–gut connection is also powerful:

- Elevated levels of blood cortisol slowly break down gut-associated lymphoid tissue (GALT), which is part of the mucosal lining of the gastrointestinal (GI) tract. Allergens and foods you are sensitive to, undigested proteins and bacterial, fungal and parasitic infections can cause a major stress response in the GALT that, in a vicious cycle, further increases cortisol production, which inhibits activation of T4 to T3.
- Chronic elevation of cortisol as a result of stress suppresses the immune system in the GI tract. This leads to dysbiosis, parasites, excess yeast and leaky gut, which in turn lead to further increases in cortisol levels. In leaky gut, gaps open in the intestinal barrier, allowing undigested proteins and toxins to enter the bloodstream uninhibited. Leaky gut puts a major stress on your immune system and can lead to immune dysfunction, adrenal stress, chronic fatigue and thyroid hormone imbalance.
- High cortisol levels increase inflammation in the GI tract, preventing the cells that line it from regenerating. This heightens the risk of ulcers as a result of *Helicobacter pylori* infection, which leads to increased infections from parasites, mold, fungi, viruses and bacteria, which further stresses the adrenal glands in a vicious cycle.

> Leaky gut puts a major stress on your immune system and can lead to immune dysfunction, adrenal stress, chronic fatigue and thyroid hormone imbalance.

Adrenal Treatment Protocol

When your adrenal glands have reached a state of fatigue, they no longer produce sufficient cortisol or DHEA. This leaves you more susceptible to chronic diseases, because you are unable to compensate for your daily stresses. It is essential to treat the adrenal glands before or at the same time as treating the thyroid. Increasing thyroid hormone production while the adrenals are fatigued can overwhelm the adrenal glands and lead to further exhaustion.

In some cases, once the adrenal glands are healthy and the other factors associated with thyroid imbalance are optimized, thyroid function returns to normal.

Adaptogens

Adaptogens are compounds that strengthen your body systems and help them to normalize if they are in a state of fatigue, high stress or both. They have many health benefits and have long been used to improve energy and stamina, brain function, immune system health, mood, sleep and sex drive.

Adaptogens for the HPA Axis

- **Ashwagandha:** Ashwagandha (*Withania somnifera*) is similar to Korean ginseng in its ability to normalize adrenal stress syndromes and the many adverse effects stress has on health.
- **Korean ginseng:** Korean ginseng (*Panax ginseng*) optimizes the functioning of the HPA axis and enhances physical performance, stamina and energy production. It shifts metabolism into a fat-burning state (as opposed to a sugar-burning state) by increasing the oxygen available for muscles. Studies have also seen decreases in fasting blood glucose and postprandial sugar, suggesting a possible hypoglycemic effect; however, the results were uncertain.
- **Magnolia and phellodendron:** Magnolia (*Magnolia officinalis*) is native to the rainforests of China. The bark has been used for a variety of medicinal purposes, including the regulation of stress and anxiety. Phellodendron (*Phellodendron amurense*) grows in northeastern China and Japan. Together, extracts from magnolia and phellodendron restore cortisol and DHEA production. They bind to stress hormone receptors, promoting relaxation and feelings of well-being.
- **Pantethine:** You need pantethine to produce adrenal hormones. However, it does not overstimulate cortisol production during times of stress; instead, it has the opposite effect.
- **Perilla oil and medium-chain triglycerides:** Perilla oil is rich in anti-inflammatory omega-3 fatty acids, which stimulate repair. Medium-chain triglycerides reduce cell acids and help to produce energy in the cells' mitochondria. These essential oils have natural stress-reducing effects. Medium-chain triglycerides are easy to assimilate and metabolize, which is extremely important for those with delicate stomachs and impaired absorption.
- **Rhodiola:** Popular in traditional Eastern and northern European medicines, rhodiola (*Rhodiola rosea*) has been shown to enhance immunity and brain function. It prevents the adrenaline roller coaster rides caused by high stress. In addition, rhodiola has antidepressant properties and protects against cancer.

- **Eleuthero:** Eleuthero (*Eleutherococcus senticosus*) supports the HPA axis under times of stress and enhances physical capacity and athletic performance as well as brain function.

Supplements to Balance Blood Sugar

Blood sugar imbalance greatly influences the ability of your thyroid to function at its best. There are many supplements vital for balancing blood sugar when you have insulin resistance. The following list includes the ones we use clinically.

Botanical Medicines

- **Berberine:** Berberine has been compared to metformin, and its action has been found to be equally effective in people with diabetes. Berberine is derived from goldenseal (*Hydrastis canadensis*) and Chinese goldthread (*Coptis chinensis*). It is also an excellent antimicrobial for the GI tract and works well against yeasts, parasites and bacterial infections.
- **French lilac:** French lilac (*Galega officinalis*) has been used since the Middle Ages to treat diabetes. It lowers blood sugar by decreasing insulin resistance. Prescription medications used to control blood sugar, such as metformin, are derived from the active ingredients in French lilac.

Minerals

- **Chromium:** Chromium stabilizes blood sugar and insulin levels after meals. It also ensures optimal delivery of blood sugar into your cells. Deficiencies in this nutrient can lead to insulin resistance, high cholesterol and abnormalities in sugar's ability to bind to red blood cells.
- **Magnesium:** Magnesium is involved in approximately 350 reactions in your body, and deficiencies in our society are rampant. Magnesium deficiency leads to insulin resistance and abnormal sugar metabolism. Magnesium appears to enhance insulin secretion by the pancreas.
- **Vanadium:** Vanadium improves transportation of sugar into your cells because of its insulin-like effects on cell receptors.
- **Zinc:** The role of zinc in blood sugar management may include optimizing insulin metabolism, protecting the insulin-producing beta cells of the pancreas and improving insulin sensitivity, which ensures optimal uptake of sugar into your cells.

Other Nutrients

- **Alpha lipoic acid:** A strong antioxidant, alpha lipoic acid (ALA) increases energy production by your cells, optimizes sugar metabolism and lowers lactic acid levels.
- **Biotin:** Biotin is important in supporting the liver's utilization of sugar. It enhances the effects of insulin and lowers blood sugar levels after a meal.
- **L-carnitine:** L-carnitine is a dipeptide compound that shuttles fatty acids into the cells' mitochondria to convert into energy. Similarly, L-carnitine lowers blood sugar by transporting sugar into cells.
- **Vitamin E:** Vitamin E improves insulin sensitivity, lowers blood fats, is a powerful antioxidant and lowers low-density lipoprotein (LDL) cholesterol.

Time-released pregnenolone restores exhausted adrenal glands. Patients tend to notice an instant increase in energy, improved memory and a greater feeling of well-being once they start taking it.

Caution

Vitamin E should not be taken in its alpha tocopherol form. Mixed tocopherols, including gamma and delta tocopherol, are the preferred form of delivery.

Hormone Supplements

Pregnenolone

Time-released pregnenolone restores exhausted adrenal glands. Patients tend to notice an instant increase in energy, improved memory and a greater feeling of well-being once they start taking it.

DHEA

Research suggests that DHEA may resensitize insulin receptors, boost the immune system, prevent bone loss, enhance memory, build muscle and lower cholesterol. When under stress, your body makes cortisol at the expense of DHEA. Topical magnesium gel or oil can increase DHEA levels naturally.

Caution

Pregnenolone and DHEA are powerful hormones and should never be taken without having your existing levels tested, and then only under the supervision of your doctor.

▷ DOC TALK

Take the following steps to prevent and treat adrenal thyroid dysfunction:

1. Go to bed at the same time every night, preferably no later than 10:30 p.m., to help balance your adrenal glands. Aim for a minimum of 7 hours of sleep every night.
2. Wean yourself off caffeinated drinks if you use them for false energy.
3. Take ¼ to ½ teaspoon (1 to 2 mL) of unrefined sea salt (such as Celtic salt) in a large glass of water every morning to support your adrenal glands if they are fatigued.
4. Follow the dietary guidelines in chapter 11 to begin to balance your blood sugar.
5. As long as your blood sugar levels are out of balance, restoring adrenal function will be extremely difficult. Follow these guidelines to ensure stable blood sugar levels:
   - Snack on proteins and fats, such as nuts, eggs and seeds, not on carbohydrates.
   - Consume protein at every meal.
   - Consume vegetables at every meal.
   - Avoid sugar, processed carbohydrates and fruit juice.

CHAPTER 7

Hormone Imbalance and Thyroid Disorders

CASE STUDY

Excess Estrogen

Ilsa was frustrated because her doctor kept telling her that her thyroid levels looked fine, that there was nothing wrong with her and that all she had to do was diet and exercise. But she was having a hard time losing weight, no matter how much she dieted, and she was still suffering from fatigue, depression, dry skin, bloating and insomnia.

We reviewed Ilsa's lab tests, and found that her T3 uptake was on the low side, which can indicate too much estrogen. She also reported a history of uterine fibroids, which can be caused by too much estrogen, secondary to hypothyroidism. We ordered tests of her sex hormones, which did show high estrogen levels. We explained that too much estrogen in the body can inhibit thyroid function, and that healthy thyroid levels are required to metabolize estrogen well. So she was stuck in a vicious cycle.

With a focus on ridding her body of the excess estrogen, we started Ilsa on doses of diindolylmethane (DIM), which is found in cruciferous vegetables and helps the body metabolize estrogen. She did not have Hashimoto's thyroiditis, so it was relatively safe to start her on an iodine supplement that contained iodine and iodide, again to help the body metabolize estrogen. We recommended that she increase her fiber intake, as fiber binds to estrogens in the GI tract in the excretion process. We also suggested that she eat more cruciferous vegetables to maximize estrogen metabolism and excretion. In addition, she started taking calcium d-glucarate, which helps the body rid itself of too much estrogen.

When we revaluated Ilsa 6 weeks later, her T3 uptake had increased into a healthier range and her estrogen levels were back to normal. She was starting to lose weight and looked a lot less "puffy," and her clothes were fitting more loosely. In addition, her symptoms of hypothyroidism had improved without resorting to thyroid medication.

We told her she could keep her estrogen levels in check through diet and by continuing to take the DIM supplement. We also explained that the more body fat a woman has, the higher her estrogen levels. Now that she could burn fat efficiently, she was able to implement long-term weight-loss strategies.

Ilsa is a great example of how sex hormones can disrupt thyroid function.

Balanced Hormones

A number of hormones, including leptin, testosterone, progesterone, estrogen and pregnenolone, need to be balanced for the thyroid to work at its best. Unfortunately, many doctors tend to view the thyroid gland in isolation. Yet these hormones can provide us with indirect clues about thyroid function and about what happens to thyroid hormones in the rest of your body.

Thyroid hormones can also affect the levels of these other hormones. For example, estrogen can significantly increase in cases of hypothyroidism, resulting in uterine fibroids, endometriosis, mood disorders, weight gain and other problems. In a vicious cycle, excess estrogen further suppresses thyroid function.

Leptin

Leptin regulates body composition and metabolism by signaling to the hypothalamus that you have plenty of fat storage to use for energy. The hypothalamus normally regulates appetite, satiety and metabolism, but your body views leptin resistance as starvation and holds on to as much fat as possible for survival. Leptin resistance is closely linked to insulin resistance, which also results in weight gain, a sluggish metabolism, appetite issues such as craving sweets and difficulty losing weight. The more weight you gain, the more insulin-resistant you become and the more likely you are to develop leptin resistance as well.

DID YOU KNOW?

HORMONE TESTING

Leptin, testosterone, progesterone, estrogen and pregnenolone do not need to be tested in everyone who may have a thyroid problem. However, if standard treatment doesn't seem to be effective, these hormones may be the missing link. Always have your hormone levels tested before taking any hormones.

Leptin resistance may be associated with increased levels of reverse T3 (rT3) and decreased response to deiodinase, the enzyme used to convert thyroxine (T4) to the more active triiodothyronine (T3). This results in low intracellular T3 levels and suppressed thyroid-stimulating hormone (TSH). Leptin levels above 10 nanograms per milliliter (ng/mL) are a sign that intracellular T3 levels are low, which explains why you cannot lose weight. Reversing leptin resistance by correcting insulin resistance solves the problem.

Testosterone

Testosterone is made in the testes and adrenal glands of males and in the ovaries and adrenal glands of females. It is essential for metabolism, and low testosterone causes reduced thyroid function. When thyroid function optimizes, testosterone levels also return to normal.

For men, testosterone replacement can help many conditions, including hypothyroidism and autoimmune diseases, but simply giving patients testosterone without addressing the reason for their low testosterone is ineffective in the long run. Testosterone replacement suppresses the pituitary hormone that signals the testes to make testosterone. Once the patient comes off testosterone, natural production may be suppressed for a time, resulting in dependence on continued hormone replacement.

Men can increase their testosterone levels by weight training and reducing their body fat. As men gain fat mass, an enzyme called aromatase is upregulated (response to it increases), which increases the conversion of testosterone into estrogen.

If lab results show low levels of the testosterone precursor dehydroepiandrosterone (DHEA), women can usually increase their testosterone levels by taking a small amount of DHEA supplement. Weight training 2 to 4 days a week, with a focus on building lean muscle mass, also increases testosterone levels.

Elevated testosterone levels can decrease T4 levels and increase the amount of T3 entering your cells, which can give an initial boost of energy and well-being. (In contrast, excess estrogen from hormone replacement therapy or birth control pills can cause high T4 levels and low T3 uptake.) Be careful, however, of oversaturating T3 receptors and creating thyroid hormone receptor resistance. We often see increased T3 uptake in women with PCOS who have high testosterone levels or those taking a testosterone supplement.

Progesterone

In women, progesterone is produced primarily during the second half of the menstrual cycle. The hormone is made mainly in the ovaries, which are signaled to increase production by luteinizing hormone, secreted by the pituitary. Some progesterone is also made in the adrenal glands. In men, progesterone is made in the adrenal glands and in the testes.

Progesterone has a calming effect on the nervous system and, in women, increases levels of free T4. While progesterone enhances thyroid hormone production, low levels of thyroid hormones can result in too little progesterone being produced.

A combination of estrogen and progesterone can be extremely helpful for women who suffer from the standard symptoms of menopause: hot flashes, mood swings, bone loss, sleep problems, low sex drive and vaginal dryness. Progesterone is best applied as a cream to the vaginal labia or taken as oral sublingual drops. Creams applied anywhere other than the vaginal labia are very poorly absorbed. Like all other hormones, progesterone should be used only for a short time, especially by women who are menstruating, and only in minimal doses. Over-the-counter progesterone cream often does more harm than good.

> ## Caution
>
> Synthetic progesterone, commonly known as Provera or Depo-Provera, is not the progesterone that your body makes but a chemically modified form. It has been shown to increase the risk of breast cancer.

Estrogen

Estrogen, a group of hormones made in the ovaries of menstruating women and mainly in the adrenal glands of menopausal women, includes three types: estrone (E1), at 10% to 20%; estradiol (E2), at 10% to 20%; and estriol (E3), at 60% to 80%. The proportion of these hormones varies depending on whether women are menstruating, pregnant or menopausal.

Synthetic estrogens, on the other hand, are given in very high doses of estrone or estradiol, with little or no estriol, which throws off the natural balance. In fact, the Women's Health Initiative study was terminated early in part because of the many

HORMONE REPLACEMENT THERAPY

A current theory is that hormone levels should be the same when you are 60 as when you were 20. As a result, many women who are experiencing menopause-related symptoms such as hot flashes, mood swings, weight gain, low sex drive and osteoporosis consider hormone replacement therapy. Although bioidentical hormones may be safer and more effective than conventional synthetic hormone replacements, it is unwise to dump hormones into your body without a thorough look at the rest of your biochemistry. Gut health, liver function, adrenal health, thyroid health and many other factors are important in hormone metabolism, but are often overlooked.

side effects of too much estrogen, especially an increased risk of breast cancer.

Estrogen is important for healthy bones, enhances serotonin levels and sex drive, and may protect against heart disease. However, excess estrogen can lead to hypothyroidism, because estrogen inhibits conversion of T4 into T3 and binds to the proteins that transport thyroid hormones. Women who take synthetic estrogen, such as Premarin, Prempro or the birth control pill, often become hypothyroid as a result of the excess estrogen.

Excess Estrogen

The more body fat you have, the more likely your estrogen levels are high, regardless of whether you are male or female. Elevated estrogen levels can also be due to hypothyroidism, diet, estrogen exposure or impaired hormone detoxification systems. Stress causes the conversion of inactive estrogen to active estrogen, leading to water retention, breast cysts, moodiness, weight gain and other side effects.

Many women with menstrual problems have too much estrogen because of low thyroid function. Excess estrogen may result in heavy bleeding, longer bleeding and many of the symptoms associated with premenstrual syndrome (PMS), including cramping, bloating, irritability, breast tenderness and menstrual acne. Excess estrogen secondary to low thyroid function may also cause uterine fibroids and endometriosis. Many women have unnecessary hysterectomies as a result of the effects of undiagnosed, subclinical hypothyroidism.

During the second half of a woman's cycle, progesterone levels should be higher than estrogen levels, but if these levels fluctuate, women may get PMS. Some practitioners recommend taking progesterone during the second half of the menstrual cycle to correct the estrogen dominance, but a better approach is to lower excess estrogen in the body. Fat tissue can produce estrogen, so the best approach is to reduce body fat through a healthy diet and exercise. If your thyroid is working properly, weight loss will be much easier to achieve.

Eating cruciferous vegetables also helps you eliminate excess estrogen, as does increasing your fiber intake, eliminating dairy products and meat from the diet, liver detoxification and stress reduction. Diindolylmethane (DIM), which occurs naturally in cruciferous vegetables, is the preferred method of supplementation to eliminate excess estrogen, but calcium d-glucarate can also work well.

Pregnenolone

Pregnenolone, the "mother of all hormones," is the precursor of all the sex hormones, including testosterone, estrogen, progesterone and DHEA, as well as cortisol. Pregnenolone is made from cholesterol, mainly in the adrenal glands. It is found in high concentrations in the brain and may be important for memory and brain function. Research has shown that those with low thyroid function also have low pregnenolone levels.

We prescribe time-released pregnenolone to restore the adrenal glands when they are exhausted. Most of this pregnenolone converts into cortisol, which is good if the adrenal glands are not producing enough cortisol, as you need some (but not too much) cortisol to convert inactive T4 into active T3. Patients tend to notice an instant increase in energy, improved memory and a greater feeling of well-being once they start taking pregnenolone. However, as with all other hormones, never take pregnenolone without knowing exactly what your levels are.

> Patients tend to notice an instant increase in energy, improved memory and a greater feeling of well-being once they start taking pregnenolone.

▷ DOC TALK

If your hormones are unbalanced and are interfering with your thyroid function, or low thyroid function is interfering with your hormone levels, take the following steps:

1. Exercise caution with sex hormones if you haven't had your levels tested first. Sex and adrenal hormones are best tested through a urinary spot hormone profile, which provides the levels of both the hormones themselves and all of their metabolites. Metabolite levels can be just as important as hormone levels.
2. Although hormone replacement therapy may seem like a fast and easy solution, first try reducing your body fat into a healthy range: about 12% to 18% for men and 22% to 28% for women.
3. Address insulin resistance to correct leptin resistance and high levels of SHBG.
4. Eat plenty of cruciferous vegetables and take DIM and calcium d-glucarate to help eliminate excess estrogen.
5. As much as possible, eat organic foods to avoid exposure to estrogens in pesticides. Avoid widely used synthetic xenoestrogens, such as PCBs, BPA and phthalates.

Iodine and Thyroid Disorders

Iodine Deficiency

Tomiko showed signs of iodine deficiency — fatigue, feeling cold all the time, lack of motivation, dry skin, brittle nails and hair, constipation and depression. Her blood tests showed normal levels of thyroid-stimulating hormone (TSH), but her T4 levels were quite low. She tested negative for Hashimoto's thyroiditis, and no other systems in her body appeared to be out of balance. However, her health history revealed fibrocystic breast disease and a uterine fibroid. She was also a regular user of a hot tub that was treated with bromide, a potent anti-iodine chemical.

Basing our decision on Tomiko's history of fibrocystic breast disease and fibroids, both of which can be connected to abnormal estrogen metabolism, we started her on an iodine supplement that contained iodine and iodide. After 6 weeks, her T4 levels were normal and her symptoms had abated.

Iodine deficiency is rare in North America, but Tomiko had definitely become deficient. We told her to stop using the hot tub and to continue taking the iodine supplement for another 6 weeks. Later follow-ups showed that her thyroid levels stayed healthy as long as she avoided the hot tub and ate iodine-rich foods, such as seaweed salad, in moderation.

Iodine and Thyroid Hormones

Both triiodothyronine (T3) and thyroxine (T4) contain iodine, with the numbers "3" and "4" indicating the number of iodine atoms in the molecule. T3 is synthesized when one iodine atom is split off a T4 molecule by the enzyme deiodinase. This process mostly takes place in the liver.

Your body cannot synthesize iodine, so you must get it from food or from supplements. Too little iodine can result in hypothyroidism; too much can cause hyperthyroidism. About 20 to 30 milligrams of iodine is usually circulating in your body at any given time, and three-quarters is stored in the thyroid.

You need adequate amounts of vitamin C and magnesium for iodine to enter the thyroid gland. You also need iron, selenium, zinc, copper, magnesium and vitamins A, B_2, B_3, B_6 and C to synthesize thyroid hormones. Drugs that can affect thyroid uptake of iodine include lithium, dexamethasone, sex steroids, RU486, amiodarone, bromide, ketoconazole, retinoic acid, hydrocortisone and adenosine.

Caution

Although iodine supplementation is often effective for treating thyroid dysfunction, in some cases it can be dangerous, and even life-threatening. Iodine supplements can create symptoms of hyperthyroidism when the patient has a hot nodule on the thyroid gland (see page 96). Some individuals will also experience acne, lung congestion, sinus headache, fatigue, rash and a bad taste in the mouth when supplementing with iodine. Iodine should always be taken under the supervision of a physician. Overdoses of more than 1 gram of iodine can cause burning in the mouth and throat, abdominal pain, nausea, vomiting, diarrhea, weak pulse and coma.

Iodine Deficiency

Iodine deficiency is the most common cause of hypothyroidism. Approximately one-third of the world's population lives in areas where iodine is lacking in the soil and water. In North America, the amount of iodine in the water supply and in locally grown food decreases from the Atlantic coast to the Great Lakes.

Iodine deficiency leads to thyroid tissue enlarging into goiter in an attempt to synthesize thyroid hormones. At one time, people who lived in the "goiter belt" in North America were more likely to have goiter than those living in other areas. Since the 1950s, iodine has been added to table salt to correct this deficiency. Although iodized table salt has indeed decreased the incidence of goiter in North America, some populations are still deficient in iodine. In addition, thanks to recent recommendations to reduce salt intake, many people's iodine intake has also been reduced.

The symptoms of iodine deficiency are closely related to those of hypothyroidism. They include weight gain, fatigue, insomnia, tenderness around the breast bone, cold hands and feet, dry eyes and cracking heels. Iodine deficiency can also cause your thyroid gland to develop thyroid nodules (see page 95).

Conversely, high levels of iodine can cause thyroid papillary cancer and iodermia, a severe skin disorder.

(see page 95)

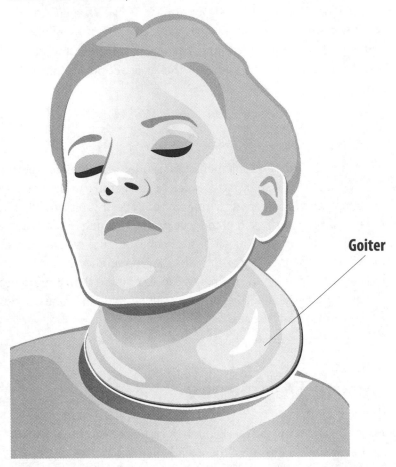

Goiter

✳ RESEARCH SPOTLIGHT

Breast and Prostate Health

Iodine may be important for breast and prostate health as well. Studies have shown that, when rats are given iodine-blocking agents, they develop fibrocystic breast disease. Researchers have also been able to increase breast cancer rates in rats simply by restricting their intake of iodine. Because of its effect on estrogen molecules, iodine protects the breast cells from turning cancerous. It has a similar effect on the prostate gland. Iodine can be used when there is excessive estrogen in the body, because it enhances the body's ability to metabolize estrogen.

Recommended Dietary Allowance for Iodine

According to the Institute of Medicine, the recommended dietary allowance (RDA) for iodine is 150 micrograms per day for adult men and women. Almost three times that amount (400 micrograms) can be found in a teaspoon (5 mL) of iodized salt.

For pregnant women, the RDA increases to 220 micrograms, and for breastfeeding women it increases to 290 micrograms. However, the World Health Organization (WHO), the United Nations Children's Fund (UNICEF) and the International Council for the Control of Iodine Deficiency Disorders (ICCIDD) suggest that pregnant women require a slightly higher intake of 250 micrograms per day.

These guidelines are based on preventing goiter, not on achieving optimal thyroid function and thyroid hormone synthesis. Consult a doctor — preferably an endocrinologist — to determine an appropriate dosage for you.

Thyroid Nodules

Thyroid nodules — abnormal growths of thyroid cells into a small lump — can be the result of iodine deficiency, inflammation or damage to thyroid tissue cells and should be examined by a skilled physician. An ultrasound provides more detailed diagnostic information.

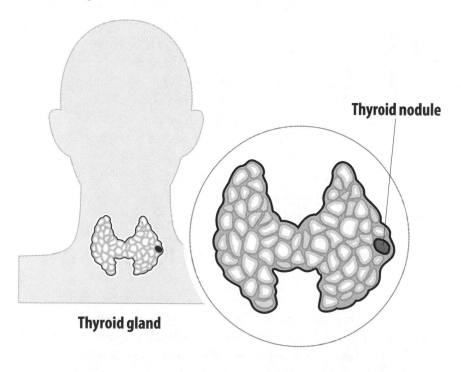

Thyroid nodule

Thyroid gland

More than 95% of thyroid nodules are benign, and 50% of people will have developed a nodule by the time they are 60. A thyroid scan can assess if the nodules are "hot" or "cold." Hot nodules are almost always benign. Decreased thyroid-stimulating hormone (TSH) levels with T4 levels above 12 micrograms per deciliter (mcg/dL) may indicate a hot nodule that is absorbing too much iodine and producing too much T4. This requires immediate medical evaluation, as it can be fatal. Cold nodules should also be thoroughly evaluated, because they are more likely to be cancerous.

Iodine supplementation has been shown to reduce the size of thyroid nodules. However, a nodule that grows while you are taking iodine supplements can indicate thyroid cancer. Nodule growth requires immediate medical evaluation and discontinuation of the iodine supplement.

If a thyroid nodule is cancerous, most or all of your thyroid gland is removed. Unless the rest of the gland grows and compensates for what was removed, you will need to take thyroid hormone replacements for the rest of your life. Most thyroid cancers are found early, though, and have an excellent prognosis.

Q What form of iodine is best?

A In nature, iodine is mainly found as iodide, which is also the form in which iodine is transported into the thyroid gland. Molecular iodine is the most effective form of iodine for breast health and for the treatment of fibrocystic breast disease. In our clinic, we use a product that combines iodine and iodide and contains 1.8 milligrams per drop.

Iodine needs to be used very carefully as a supplement. If you have autoimmune thyroiditis, iodine supplementation increases lymphocytic infiltration into the thyroid gland, which can result in inflammation and more destruction of the gland. Always consult your doctor before using iodine.

Natural Sources of Iodine

The best food source of iodine is from sea vegetables such as seaweed (kelp, nori, kombu, dulse, wakame); however, the iodine content can vary considerably depending on the type and where it is harvested. Fish and other types of seafood are also rich sources.

Fruits, vegetables and grains contain iodine, but the amount depends on the iodine content of the soil, the fertilizer used and irrigation practices. Vegans can develop iodine deficiency if the soil in which their vegetables grow has too little iodine.

Because animals feed on grains and vegetables, the meat and animal products we consume also have varying amounts of iodine. Some animal products, such as dairy products and eggs, are excellent sources, in part because the animal feed is supplemented with iodine.

Iodine does not remain in your body for long, so you must consume it regularly. However, be careful when eating foods rich in iodine to treat thyroid dysfunction, as the required intake is small.

> Vegans can develop iodine deficiency if the soil in which their vegetables grow has too little iodine.

Food Sources of Iodine

Food	Approximate micrograms (mcg) per serving
Seaweed (1 g)	16–2,984
Cranberries (4 oz/125 g)	400
Lobster (3½ oz/100 g)	100
Cod, baked (3 oz/90 g)	99
Iodized table salt (1 g)*	77
Yogurt, plain, low-fat (1 cup/250 mL)	75
Baked potato with peel (1 medium)	60
Milk, reduced-fat (1 cup/250 mL)	56
Shrimp (3 oz/90 g)	35
Baked turkey breast (3 oz/90 g)	34
Navy beans (½ cup/125 mL cooked)	32
Egg (1 large)	24
Tuna, canned in oil (3 oz/90 g)	17
Dried prunes (5)	13

* Table salt has been chemically stripped of all its natural minerals, except sodium and chloride. Iodine is added to table salt after processing. Other additives in table salt have been shown to be toxic to human health. Natural sea salt contains more than fifty minerals, which are all important for balancing blood pressure and other bodily functions, and is a better choice.

Bladderwrack Supplements

Bladderwrack (*Fucus vesiculosus*), or kelp, is a type of brown algae that has been used for food and as medicine in China, Korea and Japan for centuries. Iodine concentrations in

High Doses of Iodine

Some doctors have promoted high doses of iodine — 12.5 to 50 milligrams per day — to treat thyroid disorders, fibrocystic breast disease, fibromyalgia and chronic fatigue, and to improve prostate health and immune function. However, the research that led to these recommendations was based on the average daily iodine intake of people living in Japan, where the traditional diet is rich in seaweed. Furthermore, the studies were misquoted, with the iodine intake given as much higher than it actually is. This was corrected in a recent paper, and experts in Japan agree that the average daily iodine intake of a diet rich in seaweed is 1.2 milligrams, *not* 12 milligrams.

DID YOU KNOW?

GUGGUL EXTRACT

Guggul (*Commiphora wightii*) is an herb used in Ayurvedic medicine (the ancient Hindu science of medicine) to treat a sluggish metabolism, obesity and high cholesterol by stimulating the thyroid gland. Guggul has been shown to increase the uptake of iodine into the thyroid gland, thereby increasing the response of the enzyme thyroid peroxidase. This increased response could potentially exacerbate autoimmune thyroiditis, in which thyroid peroxidase antibodies are already high. Avoid guggul if you have autoimmune thyroiditis or a family history of thyroiditis.

bladderwrack can vary greatly, so you need to be cautious when using it as a supplement.

Bladderwrack also contains fucoxanthin, an extremely powerful antioxidant. It can lower cholesterol levels because it suppresses the enzyme trans-sialidase, which is involved in cholesterol accumulation.

Halides

The halides are a group of elements that include bromine, fluorine and iodine. Although iodine is a vital nutrient for the health of the thyroid gland, it is hypothesized that the other halides can disrupt thyroid function.

Bromine

Bromine (or its salt, bromide) is found in kelp and other seaweeds, nuts, citrus-flavored soft drinks, purified water, pesticides, fumigants, photographic film, dyes, flame retardants, carpet, upholstery, electronics, mattresses and over-the-counter antitussives. Symptoms of bromine toxicity include gastrointestinal inflammation, asthma, thyroid dysfunction, goiter, headaches, kidney inflammation, low blood pressure and inflammation of the throat.

Fluorine

Fluorine (or its salt, fluoride) is found naturally in groundwater in certain regions of the world, and in the livestock and plants that are watered from those sources. Most North Americans get their fluoride from dental products, including toothpaste, and fluoridated tap water, as well as drinks made from tap water, infant formula, cereals, non-organic grape juice, wine, beer, soft drinks, tea (especially decaffeinated tea) and fluoridated salt. Fluorine is also found in Freon, pesticides and nonstick coatings.

Many prescription drugs, such as fluorinated anesthetics, contain fluorine, but it may not necessarily be released into your system because of the strength of the chemical bond.

Acute fluorine toxicity may cause abdominal pain, nausea and vomiting, seizures and muscle spasms, and even death. Symptoms of long-term exposure to excess fluoride include intellectual impairment in children, weakened and deformed bones, calcified ligaments and tendons, bone softening, heart arrhythmias, headaches, nerve pain, vertigo, anemia, lung irritation and male reproductive system toxicity.

Iodine Testing

If iodine deficiency is suspected, your doctor may examine you for systemic inflammation that adversely affects the activity of sodium iodide symporter (NIS), which transports iodide into the thyroid. Your doctor may also test your white cell count (including the component neutrophils, lymphocytes, monocytes, eosinophils and basophils, and C-reactive protein).

Iodine spot tests and 24-hour urinary iodine tests are available to aid in diagnosing iodine deficiency; however, a good medical history is the best approach, as some of these tests have not been thoroughly evaluated for accuracy.

▷ **DOC TALK**

Iodine is an essential element not only for the thyroid but also for other body tissues. For example, breast health requires iodine, and women with fibrocystic breast disease have been shown to have low iodine levels.

Iodine supplementation is not suitable for everyone, and dosage is individualized. If you have autoimmune thyroiditis, such as Hashimoto's or Graves' disease, do not take iodine unless you are under the care of a qualified health-care practitioner. Many studies have shown that when iodine is added to the food supply to reduce iodine deficiency, the rate of autoimmune thyroiditis increases.

PART 3

Thyroid Management

CHAPTER 9

Medications and Surgery for Thyroid Dysfunction

CASE STUDY

The Best Medications

Latisha had been diagnosed with hypothyroidism and Hashimoto's thyroiditis, and had been prescribed levothyroxine. She did a lot of research and convinced her doctor to switch her medication to Armour Thyroid, because she preferred a more natural source. The levothyroxine had been working somewhat, but after switching to Armour Thyroid she began to have headaches, developed swelling in the throat and neck, and was just not "feeling right." She had tried a few different doses of Armour Thyroid, but did not feel good on any of them.

We explained to Latisha that many people with Hashimoto's thyroiditis do not do well on glandular-based thyroid hormone and actually do much better on either levothyroxine, T3 alone or a combination of both. Her doctor switched her back to levothyroxine, and Latisha began feeling much better.

This is one of many examples that shows there is no single best form of thyroid hormone for everyone. You need to find what works best for you.

Prescription Medications

Unfortunately, no single thyroid medication works best for everyone. However, we are very lucky that there are so many options available on prescription. It may take some time to learn which medication is best for you, so be sure to work with a doctor who is willing to accept that his or her go-to medication might not be the right choice for you. Some people do well on T4 alone, some on a combination of compounded T4 and T3 in varying ratios, and others on T3 alone. T3 can also be compounded in a time-released form.

Levothyroxine

Levothyroxine sodium (Synthroid), a synthetic version of T4, is the most popular prescription drug for hypothyroidism. However, levothyroxine may not help those who have compromised T4-to-T3 conversion pathways or any of the other imbalances described in this book. In addition, levothyroxine can be converted into the inactive reverse T3 (rT3). If your rT3 levels are high, prescribed T4 may further increase them and your symptoms may stay the same or even worsen.

Although, for the reasons given above, some people start to feel much worse when taking levothyroxine, it is not a "bad" drug, as some people claim. Nor does it destroy the thyroid gland. Levothyroxine is, in fact, a perfectly viable option for many people. However, if levothyroxine does not work for you, no matter what the dose, discontinue its use, under the guidance of your doctor, and substitute another medication. Keep trying various medications until you find the right one for you.

Desiccated Thyroid Tissue

Armour Thyroid and Nature-Throid are extracted from desiccated pig thyroid tissue. These naturally sourced supplements contain T4, T3 and other cofactors for thyroid hormone production. The amounts of T4 and T3 can vary in different batches. Nature-Throid may be a better choice than Armour Thyroid because it does not contain corn or other allergenic binders. Many alternative-minded medical doctors prescribe Armour Thyroid and other natural sources of thyroid tissue rather than synthetic T4 (such as levothyroxine) because these natural agents also contain T3.

A double-blind study showed that some patients prefer being treated with naturally sourced desiccated thyroid tissue despite the fact that there is no measurable clinical difference between the efficacy of desiccated thyroid tissue and levothyroxine, a synthetic T4 preparation, as thyroid hormone replacement therapy.

T3

T3 is the most active form of thyroid hormone. It is taken as a single dose, such as Cytomel, or in a time-released compounded

Thyroid Hormone Replacement

According to a paper published in the *International Journal of Clinical Practice*, thyroid hormone replacement is "...arguably the most contentious issue in clinical endocrinology."

In the early 1970s, TSH blood levels started to be used to assess the effectiveness of T4 replacement, even though TSH tests are an inadequate measure for T4. The paper states, "No studies have been published, which demonstrate that hypothyroid patients treated with thyroxine are euthyroid (normal thyroid function) when their serum TSH is within ... 'the normal range.' The use of serum TSH measurements to assess thyroid status in patients on thyroxine replacement could be considered as a classic example of the misapplication of a laboratory test."

The study reports that what has been considered an "optimal dose" of thyroxine to achieve normal thyroid function per a normal TSH does not always lead to improved symptoms. Because the pituitary has a greater affinity for T4 than for T3, and T3 is taken up by cells in the periphery, TSH levels can be suppressed to below normal levels even if T3 levels are low. In this way, lab tests may look normal in people taking thyroxine supplements despite the fact that the more active T3 is low in the cells. In addition, those taking T4 can also have a normal TSH and elevated total T4 and free T4 levels, yet normal T3 and free T3 levels.

form to "reset" a dysfunctional hypothalamic–pituitary–thyroid axis. T3 may be the only medication that works for some people. In some cases, patients need to take it for only 30 to 60 days, until the reset occurs, and then they are able to discontinue medication as their symptoms and lab tests normalize, indicating successful balancing of the HPT axis.

> In almost all patients, antithyroid drugs will normalize thyroid hormone levels, and therefore symptoms, within 4 to 8 weeks if the medication is taken regularly and in the appropriate dose.

Other Thyroid Medications

- Levothroid (contains synthetic T4)
- Levoxyl (contains synthetic T4)
- Thyrolar (contains synthetic T4 and T3)
- Tirosint (contains synthetic T4)

Antithyroid Drugs

Antithyroid drugs act chemically on the thyroid gland to slow the production of thyroid hormone and thus control hyperthyroid symptoms. Propylthiouracil and methimazole (Tapazole) are the two antithyroid drugs used in the United States and Canada. Carbimazole, which is similar to Tapazole, is used in England.

In almost all patients, antithyroid drugs will normalize thyroid hormone levels, and therefore symptoms, within 4 to 8 weeks if the medication is taken regularly and in the appropriate dose. About one-quarter of hyperthyroid patients are permanently cured if treated with regular doses of two to three antithyroid tablets a day for 6 to 12 months.

Steroids

Steroids, such as prednisone, are used for autoimmune diseases and allergies when the immune system is completely out of control. They work quickly and effectively but have many long-term health consequences, such as osteoporosis, adrenal gland dysfunction and immune system imbalances.

Absorption of Thyroid Medications

The following conditions and procedures may impair the absorption of thyroid hormones:

- achlorhydria (low stomach acid)
- biliary cirrhosis
- celiac disease
- jejunoileal bypass surgery

Certain medications also interfere with hormone absorption. Consult with your doctor about the medications you are taking, to make sure they do not work against each other.

Substances That Interfere with Absorption

Foods	Minerals	Medications
Coffee, including espresso	Aluminum hydroxide and other phosphate binders	Bile acid sequestrants
Grapefruit juice	Calcium salts	Bisphosphonates
High-fiber foods	Charcoal	Cation-exchange resins (Kayexalate/Kalexate)
Soy, infant soybean formula	Chromium picolinate	Ciprofloxacin
	Iron	H2 receptor antagonists
		Orlistat
		Proton pump inhibitors
		Raloxifene
		Sucralfate

SOURCE: ADAPTED WITH PERMISSION FROM THE AMERICAN THYROID ASSOCIATION.

Stomach Acidity

Low hydrochloric acid (HCl) levels in the stomach can hinder the breakdown and absorption of thyroid medication. Low HCl levels can be due to a number of factors:

- food sensitivities
- *Helicobacter pylori* infection
- higher cortisol levels, and the stress that often leads to these
- hypothyroidism
- vitamin B deficiency
- zinc deficiency

The liquid capsule Tirosint does not appear to be affected by changes in stomach pH. If you have low stomach HCl levels, you can request this version of thyroxine so that absorption of thyroid hormone replacement is unaffected.

Botanical and Biologic Medicines

A variety of supplements claim to support thyroid function, but too few clinical trials have been conducted to support their use. Some may, indeed, have properties that support thyroid function, and some people do report improvements when taking them, but many of these effects are uncontrolled and unsupervised, which can be dangerous.

Blue Flag

Blue flag (*Iris versicolor*) has traditionally been used to manage thyroid disorders and support the liver, spleen and lymphatic system by "enhancing movement of sluggish body fluids." Blue flag has been used mainly to manage goiter and thyroid enlargement.

Licorice

Licorice (*Glycyrrhiza glabra*) is sometimes used to improve the function of the adrenal glands. In large amounts, or if consumed over a long period of time, licorice can raise blood pressure and lower potassium levels, increase water and sodium retention, and cause weakness and paralysis, especially in people with heart or kidney disease or high blood pressure. Licorice can also lower testosterone levels in men and women.

3,5,3'-Triiodothyroacetic Acid

3,5,3'-triiodothyroacetic acid (TRIAC or tiratricol) is an active metabolite of T3 that used to be sold over the counter for weight loss. TRIAC does increase the metabolism, but some people develop hyperthyroid- or hypothyroid-like side effects. It is too difficult to use safely, so it is not recommended.

L-tyrosine

Along with iodine, L-tyrosine is one of the building blocks of thyroid hormone, but no studies have shown it to have thyromimetic properties (effects similar to thyroid hormone). Avoid taking L-tyrosine if you are taking thyroid hormone replacements.

Other Supplements That May Enhance Thyroid Function

- Asian ginseng
- capsaicin
- echinacea
- forskolin
- garlic
- ginger
- *Ginkgo biloba*
- magnesium
- manganese
- meadowsweet
- oats
- pineapple
- potassium
- saw palmetto
- valerian root
- vitamin B complex

Caution

Thyroid supplements claim to enhance thyroid function, but as yet there is no support for these claims. In fact, one study that looked at ten thyroid supplements found that nine of them had levels of T4 and T3 that could be extremely dangerous if taken without careful monitoring and a doctor's supervision. Avoid any so-called thyroid supplements that have not been proven in clinical trials, as they may actually be dangerous. Always consult an endocrinologist if you have any concerns.

Thyroid Gland Surgery

When thyroid dysfunction becomes very serious to the point of being life-threatening, surgery may be required to remove part or all of the thyroid gland.

Malignant thyroid cancers are the most common reason for thyroidectomy. Other reasons include an uncomfortably large goiter or a large nodule that is making breathing or swallowing difficult or is leading to problems with the eyes caused by increased thyroid hormone levels; failure of radioactive iodine; or continued problems with antithyroid drugs.

Surgery to remove part of the gland is called a hemithyroidectomy, while removal of the entire gland is called total thyroidectomy. Thyroid surgery is safe and effective, with a low rate of complications if performed in an experienced center.

Hemithyroidectomy

In a hemithyroidectomy, or thyroid lobectomy, part of the thyroid gland is removed and tested for malignancy. If the test indicates thyroid cancer, a follow-up total thyroidectomy removes the remainder of the gland. If only part of your thyroid is removed, your thyroid may be able to function normally after surgery.

The aftereffects of this procedure can include injury to the laryngeal nerves, which may result in a hoarse or breathy voice, voice fatigue and lack of voice projection and range. In most cases, these effects improve over time.

The risk of hypothyroidism after hemithyroidectomy varies widely. Some centers report rates as low as 1%, while others describe a 50% risk of hypothyroidism that requires thyroid hormone replacement after surgery. In most cases, the remaining thyroid tissue grows and compensates for the piece removed.

Total Thyroidectomy

Surgery is a reasonable option for some patients with hyperthyroidism, including some cases of Graves' disease. Factors that influence the decision include the size of the gland and nodule, the failure of radioactive iodine or drug treatments, the severity of symptoms, and pregnancy.

If your entire thyroid is removed, you will need lifelong daily supplements of thyroid hormone to replace your thyroid's natural function.

After total thyroidectomy, your parathyroid glands may be temporarily injured, which leads to lowered blood calcium levels, or hypocalcemia. The symptoms of hypocalcemia include tingling in the fingers and toes and around the mouth. Extremely low calcium levels can also produce muscle cramps or spasms or shortness of breath. Calcium and vitamin D supplements are used to treat hypocalcemia.

If you are pregnant and your cancer is isolated in the thyroid, you may choose to wait until after you give birth to start treatment, with few adverse consequences. Patients with larger tumors that show progressive growth may require surgery during pregnancy.

DID YOU KNOW?

THYROID CANCER

Thyroid cancers, especially papillary forms, are being diagnosed more frequently than ever before. The most effective management of aggressive thyroid cancers is surgical removal of the thyroid gland (thyroidectomy) followed by radioactive iodine ablation and TSH-suppression therapy. Five-year survival rates are 98% in the United States.

Radioactive Iodine Therapy

Radioactive iodine therapy is recognized as the safest, least expensive, most convenient and most effective treatment for hyperthyroidism. Radioactive iodine (often called radioiodine) is chemically identical to "regular" iodine, except that the nucleus of a radioactive iodine molecule has excess energy and gives off radiation that can affect the structures of cells, including cancer cells. The thyroid gland, which is the only organ in your body to store iodine, cannot distinguish between radioactive and regular iodine. Radioactive iodine that accumulates in thyroid cells radiates the gland and slows thyroid production. Excess radioactive iodine is excreted rapidly — within 2 or 3 days — primarily through the kidneys, and has little effect on the rest of your body.

Because the treatments damage or remove thyroid tissue, one effect of radioactive iodine treatment is hypothyroidism, which is often a natural consequence of hyperthyroidism anyway. The hypothyroidism, for which you will need lifelong daily supplements of thyroid hormone, may occur as soon as 2 months after treatment or as much as 20 or 30 years later.

Radioactive iodine therapy has been routinely used to treat over 1 million people in the United States alone. For more than 35 years, as many as 90% of people with hyperthyroidism have undergone this treatment with no side effects — no nausea, vomiting, hair loss or allergic reactions to iodine, and, only very rarely, a slight tenderness that lasts a day or two — or complications to either themselves or their children. In view of its safety, convenience, low cost and effectiveness, most North Americans and their doctors decide on this treatment.

Q How long does it take to treat hyperthyroidism with radioactive iodine?

A Individual radioactive iodine treatment results vary considerably. However, treatment usually has its maximum effect within 3 months of application. Most people no longer have hyperthyroidism by that time, although some cases of hyperthyroidism may take longer to resolve — even as long as 6 months — and a few people may need a second treatment. If necessary, even a third dose of radioiodine can be given without side effects.

Pregnancy Risks

Radioactive iodine therapy is not advisable during pregnancy. Iodine readily crosses the placenta from mother to baby, and radioactive iodine can be absorbed by the baby's thyroid, affecting how it functions.

Pregnant women with hyperthyroidism must seek out other methods of treatment. Women of childbearing age who are to receive radioactive iodine should be asked if they are pregnant and the date of their last menstrual period. Some doctors may ask women who fit in this category to have a routine pregnancy test before beginning radioactive iodine treatment.

Breastfeeding Risks

If you are breastfeeding, radioactive iodine can pass from you to the baby in your breast milk. The concentrated radioactivity could affect how the baby's thyroid gland function, or he or she might develop thyroid nodules or other tumors in later years.

If you must receive radioactive iodine treatment immediately, stop breastfeeding until tests show that there is no longer any radioiodine in your milk.

If you are breastfeeding, radioactive iodine can pass from you to the baby in your breast milk.

▷ **DOC TALK**

Before considering thyroid medication or surgery, you should see an endocrinologist, who can adequately assess and manage your condition. Alternative treatments have not been found to be credible replacements for conventional medical treatment. The exception is the use of T3 or a combination of T4 and T3, neither of which is recognized as a viable treatment option by conventional medicine at this time. If you have tried T4 but still feel unwell no matter what dose you take or how good your labs look, ask your doctor about trying T3 or a combination of T4 and T3 to see if one of these options may work better for you.

CHAPTER 10

Lifestyle Modifications for Thyroid Dysfunction

CASE STUDY

Simple Lifestyle Changes

Hannah had many of the symptoms of hypothyroidism: she found it difficult to lose weight, was depressed, had dry skin, aching muscles and weakness, and was losing some hair. But her thyroid numbers looked pretty good, and it just didn't seem like she was a candidate for hormone replacement therapy.

However, Hannah was drinking a lot of bromine-containing soft drinks every day, and she was eating too many processed carbohydrates and not enough protein. She had no strategies for handling the stress in her life and was staying up late, drinking a lot of coffee and working long hours.

After discussing lifestyle modification strategies with us, Hannah switched to drinking unsweetened carbonated seltzer water. She shifted her protein-to-carbohydrate ratio, with an emphasis on high-quality protein sources and lower-glycemic-index carbohydrate foods that wouldn't spike her blood sugar. She replaced coffee with green tea to stimulate fat-burning and to avoid a caffeine withdrawal crash.

She started meditating for 10 minutes a day, to help her handle stress, and started going to bed earlier. She made a list of all the tasks that she could delegate to reduce her workload. Eventually, she found that she had enough time to start taking yoga classes, which helped further reduce her stress.

Hannah is the perfect example of an overachiever and workaholic who just needed to make a few small changes to her life to garner significant gains in overall health.

Reducing Stress

Many North Americans are overworked and simply put too much unnecessary stress on their bodies. Cortisol, a glucocorticoid hormone produced by the adrenal cortex as a survival mechanism when we need to run away from a predator, slows down digestion, suppresses immune function and raises blood sugar. In the long run, cortisol can wreak havoc on your thyroid gland, as it leads to suppressed TSH levels, inhibits the conversion of T4 into T3 and disrupts thyroid hormone receptors.

Stress management can be the key to balancing your thyroid in the long run. Simple strategies, including meditation, visualization, avoiding isolation, and deep breathing, will provide significant improvements to your stress physiology.

Meditation

Meditation has been shown to alter various areas of the brain and to help people change how they react to stressful situations. Starting a daily practice of just 10 minutes of meditation can make a huge difference to your quality of life.

The free app at www.calm.com has a variety of options for beginning a meditation practice. Meditation can calm the mind, reduce stress and help you clarify what is important, so your mind is not racing.

Visualization

One simple trick is to picture a problem in your life in an extreme and exaggerated way. Blow it up in your mind to the worst possible scenario — to the point where the problem is almost comical. For example, think of an abusive boss as the gigantic Stay Puft Marshmallow Man from the movie *Ghostbusters* and imagine him exploding all over the city. Realize that abusive, angry and insulting people are actually very scared and insecure inside, and that it has nothing to do with you.

Avoiding Isolation

Keeping in touch with friends not only helps your stress hormones, but your immune system and brain chemicals as well. Even spending time with just one friend can go a long way. Join a group that stands for something you believe in or is involved in something you love. Volunteer at an animal shelter or with another cause to increase your social activity. Humans are social beings, so nurturing that part of yourself will really help you adapt to stress.

DID YOU KNOW?

STRESS REDUCTION STRATEGIES

Counseling and group therapy can help reduce stress, as can meditation, yoga, tai chi, prayer and/or exercise. Consider reducing your obligations to a minimum while trying to heal your body.

DID YOU KNOW?

CHRONIC STRESS

Chronic stress, coupled with inactivity, can lead to continually high blood sugar levels and, hence, insulin resistance.

Deep Breathing

Too much carbon dioxide in your body creates an acidic environment. If you, like many people, are a hyperventilator, or "shallow breather," you do not inhale full breaths of oxygen and/or or fully exhale carbon dioxide. To remedy this, practice deep-belly breathing for 5 minutes in the morning and 5 minutes at night. Breathe deeply into your abdomen, as if filling your stomach with air, and then passively — without effort — exhale the air. (This is how a baby breathes.) Concentrate only on your breath, without thinking about anything else. In time, this will become second nature and you will enjoy doing it twice a day. Deep breathing will help to alkalize your body and reduce stress.

You can also incorporate deep-belly breathing into any meditation practice you do. Focusing on this one task — your breathing — instead of the multitude of things you often think about is a great starting point for learning how to meditate.

✳ RESEARCH SPOTLIGHT

Sleep Deprivation

In a recent study on sleep deprivation and thyroid hormone production, the researchers concluded, "When sleep deprivation is maintained for weeks, the plasma concentrations of T4 and particularly T3 decline but TSH remains normal."

Has your doctor asked you about your sleep patterns? Sleep troubles may be behind your abnormal TSH levels. We have seen many people who suffer from insomnia and sleep problems and also have impaired thyroid function and abnormal TSH levels. As practitioners, we always take into account each patient's sleep pattern and correct it as part of our treatment plan. Sleep patterns are often abnormal due to imbalances in blood sugar and adrenal gland secretions.

Improving Sleep

Sleep is an extremely important and fundamental part of feeling great. While you sleep, your body releases a large amount of growth hormone to repair all the damage done in the day, and your brain and the rest of your body rejuvenate.

Even if you prefer to do everything holistically, you may need sleep medication. Remember that is very difficult to overcome any health problem without adequate sleep, so don't hesitate to talk to your doctor about prescription sleep medication. The benefits of achieving restful sleep outweigh the potential side effects of sleep medication.

Quick Tips for Good Sleep

- **Blood sugar:** Stabilize your blood sugar from the time you eat dinner until you go to bed. Make sure to eat a balanced meal of protein, carbohydrates and fat. Bedtime snacks are fine, but they must be balanced and free of sugar or processed carbohydrates.
- **Light:** Keep your bedroom completely dark, with no clock radios or lights of any kind. It should be pitch black, so that you cannot see your hand when you hold it in front of your face. Even with your eyes closed, your brain receives light stimuli, which can reduce melatonin levels.
- **Stimulants:** Avoid drinks and foods that contain caffeine, including chocolate, coffee, caffeinated teas, yerba mate, guarana and alcohol, from the early afternoon onward.
- **Stimulation:** Avoid watching intense television shows or movies or reading intense material before you go to bed, as these can stimulate your adrenal glands into keeping you awake.
- **Radiation:** To reduce electromagnetic radiation, turn off all electric devices in your room and power off your cell phone.
- **Schedule:** Try to keep a regular sleep schedule. Go to bed and wake up at the same time every day.
- **Magnesium:** Take 200 to 600 milligrams of magnesium before you go to bed to alkalize and calm your muscles and nervous system.

Sleep Supplements

Several hormones, nutritional supplements and herbal remedies can help support good sleep. Consult your doctor or dietitian before using these or any supplements.

Melatonin

Melatonin, a hormone produced by the pineal gland in the brain, helps control your sleep cycles. Your body works with natural circadian rhythms related to night and day and changes in season to control how much melatonin it makes. Melatonin levels increase when it gets dark in the evening and stay high throughout the night — which helps to get you to sleep and stay asleep — and then drop in the early morning.

Melatonin Synthesis

Melatonin is manufactured in your body from the amino acid tryptophan in a four-step process. The second-last step involves an enzyme, *N*-acetyl serotonin, that operates only in the dark.

The cofactors required for this process may include vitamin B$_6$, folate, magnesium, zinc, S-adenosylmethionine and iron.

Melatonin Synthesis

tryptophan

↓

5-hydroxytryptophan (5-HTP)

↓

serotonin

↓

N-acetyl serotonin

↓

melatonin

Factors Affecting Melatonin Production

Factors that reduce natural melatonin production include:

- poor sleeping habits, such as going to bed too late or at irregular times
- an insufficiently dark room due to clock radios, night lights or street lights
- insufficient sunlight during the day
- high stress levels
- caffeine or alcohol consumption close to bedtime
- a high-protein and/or low-carbohydrate diet, which results in less tryptophan in the circulation and the brain
- inadequate supply of the cofactors required for melatonin production
- medications including Aspirin, diuretics, beta blockers and benzodiazepines

Benefits of Melatonin Supplementation

Melatonin improves the quality of your sleep, as it enhances rapid eye movement (REM) sleep, your deepest and most restorative sleep — although a side effect is vivid dreams. It may also lessen the amount of time it takes you to fall asleep. It reduces jet lag and helps night-shift workers regulate sleep patterns, and it may benefit people with sleep disorders, including children, teenagers and older people. In addition, it provides many other health benefits:

- It stimulates growth hormone production.
- It may have an antioxidant effect that delays macular degeneration of your eyes and may alleviate glaucoma.
- It relieves seasonal affective disorder (SAD), also known as winter depression.
- It may improve symptoms of fibromyalgia.
- It improves recovery from stroke and delirium, and confusion after surgery.
- It may reduce migraines and chronic cluster and tension headaches.
- It may reduce blood pressure.

DID YOU KNOW?

MELATONIN CAUTIONS

Avoid melatonin if you have immune-related cancers, such as leukemia or lymphoma, as it can exacerbate these diseases. Melatonin is not recommended during pregnancy, if you are trying to get pregnant or while breastfeeding. Do not combine melatonin with corticosteroids or monoamine oxidase (MAO) inhibitors.

Sources of Melatonin

Foods high in melatonin, from highest to lowest concentration, include oats, sweet corn, rice, Japanese radish, ginger, tomatoes, bananas and barley. However, although what you eat in the daytime will affect daytime levels of melatonin, food's effect on synthesis of nocturnal melatonin is limited.

Melatonin supplements are usually prescribed in doses of 0.5 to 20 milligrams, depending on how deficient you are and your unique health history. Take the smallest dose of melatonin that will help you sleep, because melatonin can suppress other hormones, such as testosterone. Melatonin should be taken 30 minutes before you want to fall asleep. 5-hydroxytryptophan can be taken with melatonin to enhance the quality of your sleep.

5-Hydroxytryptophan

5-hydroxytryptophan (5-HTP) is a naturally occurring amino acid that is the precursor to serotonin. Double-blind clinical trials have shown 5-HTP to improve sleep quality and the time it takes to fall asleep.

5-HTP is used to relieve mild to moderate depression (though the evidence is inconclusive), anxiety, insomnia and fatigue. In combination with lithium, it has been used for bipolar (manic) depression. 5-HTP has also been shown to relieve migraine headaches. One study found that doses of 300 milligrams three times a day improved quality of sleep, depression, insomnia and muscle pain in people with fibromyalgia.

To improve sleep quality, the recommended dose of 5-HTP is 150 to 300 milligrams on an empty stomach before bed. Take vitamin B_6, niacin and magnesium on the same day, as they are required to metabolize 5-HTP.

Caution

Do not take 5-HTP with antidepressants or selective serotonin reuptake inhibitors (SSRIs). Be aware that 5-HTP may enhance the effects of St. John's wort.

Herbal Sleep Remedies

Herbal medicines can be taken in capsule form or as tinctures or teas. Dosage depends on a variety of factors. Consult your doctor about recommended doses.

Other Sleep Supplements

- **GABA:** Gamma-aminobutyric acid (GABA) is the main calming neurotransmitter in the body and central nervous system. However, ingested GABA may not be able to cross the blood–brain barrier and may exert its calming function some other way. The recommended dose is approximately 100 milligrams before bed.

- **L-theanine:** L-theanine is a non-protein amino acid found naturally in green tea (*Camellia sinensis*). Although L-theanine may reduce stress, balance mood and improve quality of sleep, the evidence suggests that these positive effects are seen mainly in unstressed people and it has no such effects on people who are anxious. The recommended dose is approximately 200 milligrams before bed.

- **Phosphatidylserine and phosphorylated serine:** These compounds are very similar in their action, but phosphorylated serine is much cheaper and just as effective. Phosphorylated serine works well for sleep problems that are due to elevated cortisol levels because it inhibits the stress response. Research has shown that after only 10 days of high doses of phosphorylated serine, excessive cortisol levels in healthy men decrease. Phosphorylated serine has also been shown to enhance brain function and memory, decrease anxiety and depression, improve mood and enhance metabolism. It is also an antioxidant. Phosphorylated serine production requires many nutrients, and supplementation is vital to optimize adrenal function.

Caution

Constituent levels in herbal medicines vary significantly depending on when and where the plants are harvested. In addition, no regulated manufacturing standards exist for many herbal compounds. Purchase herbal supplements from a reliable source to minimize variability and the risk of contamination. Always discuss herbal medicines and dosages with your doctor before beginning treatment.

Ashwagandha

Ashwagandha (*Withania somnifera*), also known as Indian ginseng, has been traditionally used as an adrenal adaptogen, sedative, anti-inflammatory, nervous system tonic, astringent, diuretic and antispasmodic. It is also used to raise low blood pressure. In Ayurvedic medicine (the ancient Hindu science of medicine), ashwagandha is used as an aphrodisiac and as a tonic for exhaustion, anxiety, depression, impaired memory and poor muscle tone. Ashwagandha is also used to support the adrenal glands, for chronic fatigue syndrome, anxiety, insomnia, stress-induced ulcers and male impotence associated with exhaustion and anxiety.

German Chamomile

German chamomile (*Matricaria recutita*) flowers have been traditionally used to reduce tension and anxiety and induce sleep, to relieve menstrual cramps and premenstrual syndrome (PMS), quiet upset stomach and heartburn, and relieve intestinal cramping, gas, diarrhea, irritable bowel syndrome and inflamed bowel.

Although there has been little research to investigate the benefits listed above, some studies have shown chamomile to benefit certain skin conditions and mouth ulcers caused by chemotherapy or radiation. It also has a hepatoprotective effect (preventing liver damage).

The alkaloids in chamomile bind to benzodiazepine receptors in the brain, which reduces anxiety and helps you sleep.

> The alkaloids in chamomile bind to benzodiazepine receptors in the brain, which reduces anxiety and helps you sleep.

Caution

Some people are allergic to chamomile, and reactions to the plant can be severe, including anaphylaxis.

Hops

Hops (*Humulus lupulus*) were traditionally used as a diuretic, placed in small pillows next to the bed to induce sleep, used as a digestive bitter for nervous stomach and digestive tract spasms, and used as a sedative for insomnia, anxiety, nervousness and tension headaches. Hops are currently used for insomnia, especially for those with difficulty falling asleep, restlessness, anxiety and stress-induced tension.

Kava

Kava (*Piper methysticum*) was traditionally used to reduce anxiety and spasms and as a sedative, a diuretic and a non-alcoholic calming drink. It is currently used to relieve anxiety, nervousness and tension. Kava works by modifying gamma-aminobutyric acid (GABA) receptors in the brain, preventing adrenaline uptake and reducing anxiety. German studies have shown that kava is as effective a treatment for anxiety disorders as tricyclic antidepressants and benzodiazepines, without the side effects. Kava enhances REM sleep without morning grogginess and relieves insomnia.

Lavender

Lavender (*Lavandula angustifolia*) flowers and essential oils have been traditionally used, along with St. John's wort and lemon balm, for depression. Lavender has also been used for insomnia, irritability, headaches, digestive disturbances and pain, and topically for burns.

Lemon Balm

Lemon balm (*Melissa officinalis*) was traditionally used for digestive disturbances. It is currently used to relieve nervousness, improve sleep and reduce overexcitability, including in people with Alzheimer's and dementia. It has a mild sedative effect. Lemon balm can be combined with St. John's wort to treat seasonal affective disorder (SAD), and also works well as a topical antiviral against the herpes virus. Lemon balm works by enhancing GABA activity, thus calming the brain and nervous system.

Passionflower

Passionflower (*Passiflora incarnata*) stems, leaves and flowers are traditionally used as a sedative for insomnia, anxiety and nervousness, including gastrointestinal upset ("nervous stomach"). Passionflower is an antispasmodic and works well for anyone who "can't turn off" his or her mind.

As with chamomile, alkaloids in passionflower bind to benzodiazepine receptors in the brain, reducing anxiety and helping you sleep. Passionflower generally does not have side effects, such as drowsiness upon awakening, impaired memory or decreased motor coordination.

Skullcap

Skullcap (*Scutellaria lateriflora*) was traditionally used to calm nerves and reduce spasms, stress headaches, and nervous exhaustion. It is currently used with chamomile, lemon balm, oats and St. John's wort for insomnia, anxiety and mild obsessive-compulsive disorder. Skullcap can also help with restless legs syndrome.

Valerian

Valerian root (*Valeriana officinalis*) has been used for hundreds of years in Europe to relieve sleep disorders, including insomnia; anxiety, stress and nervous headaches; muscle spasms and

DID YOU KNOW?

MENOPAUSE-INDUCED INSOMNIA

Black cohosh (*Actaea racemosa*) may help insomnia induced by menopausal symptoms such as hot flashes and mood swings.

cramps, and muscle and joint pain; stress-induced heart palpitations; digestive spasms; and menstrual pain. Native Americans would boil the roots into a tea used to calm nerves.

Valerian root may work by inducing the release of GABA from the nerve cells in the brain and preventing it from being taken up again or destroyed. Valerian contains GABA, as well, although this neurotransmitter may not be able to cross the blood–brain barrier. However, valerian also contains glutamine, which may be converted to GABA once it has crossed the blood–brain barrier.

Animal studies show that valerian affects levels of serotonin (associated with feelings of well-being) and of norepinephrine and dopamine (both associated with alertness) in the brain. Many studies have looked at the combination of valerian and St. John's wort for depression and anxiety. This combination was shown to be as effective as the drug amitriptyline for depression and more effective than valium for anxiety, without any side effects.

> The combination of valerian and St. John's wort was shown to be as effective as the drug amitriptyline for depression and more effective than valium for anxiety, without any side effects.

Other Calming Herbs

- wild lettuce (*Lactuca virosa*)
- Jamaican dogwood bark (*Piscidia erythrina*)
- jujube fruit (*Zizyphus spinosa*)
- California poppy (*Eschscholzia californica*).

Exercise

Exercise can significantly improve the quality of your sleep. The earlier in the day you exercise, the better, but some exercise at any time is better than none.

People often have trouble sticking with exercise for one of two reasons: they do types of exercise they don't enjoy, or they think they need to work out more than they actually do. Exercise is vital if you want to improve your health and increase your energy. It boosts your immune system, burns fat, massages your organs and improves mood.

Exercise Tips

1. What type of exercise do you really enjoy? Do you like to hike, play tennis or pump iron in the gym? Do you prefer yoga or tai chi? Would you join a gym that has a pool you can swim in? Whatever it is you like to do, start doing it.

2. Start out small. For example, walk 30 minutes a day with a companion. How much exercise do you really need? Ideally, do some kind of movement for at least 30 minutes a day. Your body was meant to move to stay flexible, burn fat and increase energy.

3. Once you have created a routine you enjoy, consider resistance training, the type of exercise that is the most beneficial for overall health.

4. Make sure you are having fun when you work out, as that will increase your chances of sticking with it.

Q What type of exercise will give me the most benefit?

A You don't have to become a bodybuilder, but resistance training provides the best overall benefit for your time. Why? Because one of the most significant factors in chronic disease is the loss of muscle mass as we age. Each year that you lose muscle mass, your health continues to deteriorate. Growth hormone levels drop, your bones lose density, your brain functions less well, your metabolic rate begins to decline, and you gain fat. So, whether through bands, weights or kettle bells, start loading your bones, muscles and joints with some weight.

You need just 30 minutes a day, 2 to 4 days a week, of resistance training. Remember, start slow, find something you love and then start maintaining your muscle mass for optimal health and well-being.

▷ DOC TALK

Some simple lifestyle modifications can play a huge role in helping you regain your health. Stress management, through one or more stress reduction strategies, will keep your body's production of cortisol under control, which may be the key to long-term thyroid balance and will lead to improved sleep, which is crucial for rejuvenating your body. Exercise also plays a role in enhancing sleep quality and comes with many side benefits that will lead to better overall health. The final piece of the puzzle is a balanced, nutritious diet that will help repair hormone imbalances and damaged tissues and gradually return you to optimal health.

CHAPTER 11

The Balanced Thyroid Diet

CASE STUDY

Healthy Carbohydrates

Sofia was really struggling with her weight and with fatigue, depression, constipation, hair loss and muscle aches — symptoms of hypothyroidism. Her thyroid numbers looked okay, except for a lower than normal free T3, despite her thyroid medication.

After a careful dietary review, it was clear to us that Sofia was eating a diet so low in carbohydrates that she was almost at the point of ketosis. A low-carbohydrate or ketogenic diet that goes on for too long can lead to decreased free T3 levels. This is an evolutionary adaptation our bodies make when food is scarce. Our bodies start burning fat but also conserve energy by lowering free T3.

Sofia added some healthy carbohydrates to each meal, including gluten-free oats, wild rice, beans, legumes, sweet potatoes and berries. These would give her some carbohydrates without significantly spiking her blood sugar. She immediately started feeling a lot better. She noticed an increase in her body temperature right away, a sure sign that her metabolism was increasing, probably due to an increase in T3 levels. It took some time for her metabolism to readjust to the carbohydrate intake, but over time, she began to feel more balanced and energetic.

Extremely low-carbohydrate and ketogenic diets are definitely helpful for some people in certain cases and for short periods of time, but the right carbohydrates are beneficial for most people. It is very difficult to stick to extreme diets of any kind, which is why we focus on balance and finding the right ratio of protein, carbohydrates and fats.

Thyroid Diet Principles

What and how you eat if you have a thyroid problem is not much different from what and how you should eat when your thyroid is functioning normally. One size does not fit all, and there is no perfect diet. Still, there are basic principles that guide a healthy diet. Some foods have greater potential to improve your health, while others are not so healthy.

A healthy diet is a balanced diet, and for people with a thyroid disorder, a healthy diet is hormone-balanced. The main goal of a thyroid diet is to remove any stress caused by hormone imbalance on the thyroid and on any systems that may be affecting the thyroid, notably the immune system and digestive system, blood sugar levels and iodine uptake, adrenal glands and reproductive organs.

1 Step 1: Determine Your Body Type

The first step in following a thyroid diet program is to determine your body type. Are you an endomorph, mesomorph or ectomorph? These common body types are dictated by your genetic predisposition, your endocrine makeup and the food you eat. You need to eat right for your body type.

Endomorphs

Endomorphs tend to be overweight, or "smooth-looking," no matter how hard they try to lose weight. They typically look "round" and gain weight everywhere. They often have sluggish thyroids and therefore a sluggish metabolism.

Endomorphs are very sensitive to carbohydrates and gain weight quickly if they eat too many. They are usually insulin-resistant and do best on a moderate- to low-carbohydrate diet, but they can typically handle a higher fat intake than the other two body types.

Ectomorphs

Ectomorphs are usually very slim, with little fat and muscle mass. They can typically eat a lot of food, even carbohydrates, without gaining much weight. Their thyroid glands usually function very well, and they consider themselves to have a "fast metabolism." They are very sensitive to stress and tend to have adrenal gland problems. Due to their adrenal sensitivities, the

DID YOU KNOW?

CHANGING BODY TYPES
It is possible for your body type to change over time if you eat and exercise correctly.

weight they do gain tends to collect around the midsection and they have difficulty gaining muscle mass.

Ectomorphs do best on a moderate to high amount of healthy carbohydrates and a lower fat intake.

Mesomorphs

Mesomorphs are in between endomorphs and ectomorphs. They have robust adrenal glands, and their thyroid function is fairly stable. Mesomorphs have a natural "athletic body" even if they are not engaging in strenuous physical activity, and they build muscle easily while their body fat stays fairly stable.

Mesomorphs do best by balancing protein, carbohydrates and fats without pushing any of the three too high or too low.

KNOW YOUR BODY TYPE

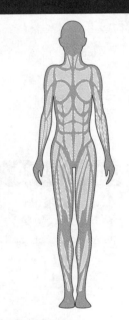 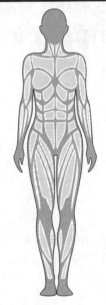 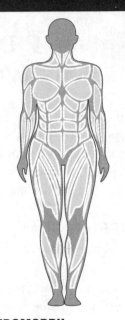

ECTOMORPH

- Typically skinny
- Small frame
- Lean muscle mass
- Doesn't gain weight easily
- Fast metabolism
- Flat chest
- Small shoulders

WORKOUT TYPE

Short and intense, focus on big muscle groups, eat before bed to prevent muscle catabolism

MESOMORPH

- Athletic and rectangular shape
- Hard body, defined muscles
- Naturally strong
- Gains muscle easily
- Gains fat more easily than ectomorphs
- Broad shoulders

WORKOUT TYPE

Cardio and resistance training, responds best to resistance training, watch calorie intake

ENDOMORPH

- Soft and round body
- Typically "short and stocky"
- Gains muscle easily
- Gains fat very easily
- Finds it hard to lose fat
- Slow metabolism
- Large shoulders

WORKOUT TYPE

Always do cardio training and resistance training, watch calorie intake

Macronutrient Proportions

After determining which body type you are, adjust your intake of the three macronutrients accordingly:

- Ectomorphs should eat more carbohydrates and less fat.
- Endomorphs should eat less carbohydrates and more fat.
- Mesomorphs should eat a balanced amount of carbohydrates and fat.
- Protein intake for all three body types is about the same.

2 Step 2: Aim for Energy Equilibrium

Food guides specify the number and size of servings you need to get enough calories, which varies according to a person's gender, age and level of activity. For example, a moderately active 50- to 70-year-old adult should consume, on average, about 2,000 calories per day. But if you have a larger body mass and are more active, you need more calories.

Some people need to avoid caloric restrictions because they become sensitive to fluctuations in blood sugar. Others, particularly those who are aging, need to maintain muscle mass. In this case, restricting calories may mean that dietary protein is used to produce energy instead of making or replacing tissues or, even worse, some of the amino acids from muscle tissue are broken down for energy. Decreasing calories by too much can signal your body to reduce thyroid hormone levels and slow down metabolism to conserve energy.

Energy Excess and Deficit

If you ingest more calories than your body expends through basal metabolic and physical activities, you will probably gain weight as your body stores the excess calories as fat — a state of energy excess. If you burn more calories than you consume, an energy deficit occurs and you will likely lose weight as your body burns those calories stored in body fat.

One pound (0.5 kg) of fat is equal to 3,500 calories, so a daily calorie deficit of 500 should result in a total loss of 3,500 calories or 1 pound (0.5 kg) of fat per week. However, our energy expenditure is not that predictable. Typically, you expend less energy as you get lighter, until you reach a plateau. The amount of food you took in that once resulted in weight loss now only allows you to maintain your weight on this plateau.

Regular Exercise

Exercise is the other side of the energy scale. Regular exercise helps to balance energy intake and improve digestion. Walking, breathing exercises, yoga and tai chi are all low-impact forms of exercise. Higher-intensity exercise includes sprinting, interval training, weightlifting with short rest periods in between sets, plyometrics and many of the various "boot camps" and CrossFit routines. Whatever you choose, pay attention to your body and keep track of your experience to help identify what exercise works for you.

> Pay attention to your body and keep track of your experience to help identify what exercise works for you.

Thyroid Equilibrium

Thyroid hormones are at the center of this process of achieving and maintaining energy equilibrium, or homeostasis. Thyroid hormones control the "burning" of protein, carbohydrates and fats inside your cells and the powerhouses known as mitochondria. Too much thyroid hormone results in excessive burning of calories; too little results in weight gain due to an inability to burn the calories you consume.

Why do we not increase thyroid hormone levels in everyone who needs to lose weight? The human body adapts to too much of any hormone, in an adaptive mechanism known as hormone receptor resistance or receptor downregulation. Whenever there is an excess of thyroid hormone, receptors become oversaturated, and they downregulate to control the excess.

Q What are good sources of energy?

A Apart from needing an adequate and consistent glucose source, you need foods that effectively and safely energize your body. Certain fats and proteins are good long-term sources of energy, but a variety of low-glycemic-index carbohydrates, mostly in their natural form, feed the thyroid most effectively.

3 Step 3: Balance Your Blood Sugar

Blood sugar swings affect the thyroid gland and also, indirectly, adrenal gland function. To avoid blood sugar swings, eat high-quality protein at every meal and fewer unhealthy carbohydrates, such as sugar and highly processed foods. Some people do best eating only "slow carbs," which include beans, lentils and peas. Slow carbs often work better for people with insulin resistance and other blood sugar issues, because they are high in fiber, have an adequate protein content and don't spike blood sugar levels.

Many people report feeling significantly better when they replace unhealthy carbohydrates with healthy carbohydrates. Their test results show a clear increase in T3 levels and a decrease in rT3 levels. For some people, this simple solution is the answer to their thyroid issues.

Q Is fruit a healthy food for the thyroid?

A Be careful. Fruits are healthy if eaten in modest portions, but fresh fruit is much larger than it was even a few years ago. Choose small fruits, such as raspberries, blackberries, blueberries and strawberries, to meet the portion requirements for your body type. Fruit contains many nutrients and fiber, but too much can affect your blood sugar levels and contribute to insulin resistance. Avoid drinking fruit juice, which is just pure plant sugar and will lead to insulin resistance.

Dietary Strategies

Carbohydrates have been demonized as unhealthy foods in general, but they may be the missing link for many people with sluggish glands. Numerous research studies have shown that low-carbohydrate diets can lead to hypothyroidism. Your body is designed for survival, and restricting carbohydrates can signal to your body that it needs to slow down its metabolism and conserve energy.

Many popular diets, such as intermittent fasting and ketogenic cycling, work on this premise. They involve fasting for long periods and only eating within a small window each day, or eating no carbohydrates for 3 to 6 days and then eating a large amount of carbohydrates 1 to 2 days a week, to kick-start the thyroid. While these diets may work well for some people, most will find them too extreme and will not stick to them. Taking a more balanced approach ensures that your adrenal glands are not stressed and your blood sugar levels remain stable.

Another strategy that works well for some people is to eat moderate to low amounts of carbohydrates for most meals but high amounts after exercise. Exercise resensitizes your insulin receptors, so you are much better able to handle the higher blood sugar levels that result from eating carbohydrates. The majority of your insulin receptors are found on skeletal muscle, so resistance training focused on building muscle will have the greatest impact on reversing insulin resistance.

> **Q** Do low-carbohydrate diets cause hypothyroidism?
>
> **A** Low-carbohydrate diets lower T3 levels and increase rT3 levels, but in most cases do not appear to affect T4 levels. This tells us that the issue is outside the thyroid gland. However, low-carb diets do not cause weight gain or an increase in the symptoms of hypothyroidism, which demonstrates that we cannot consider thyroid hormones in isolation, as other hormones — insulin and glucagon, as well as the adrenal hormones cortisol and DHEA — are also affected by dietary changes.

4 Step 4: Choose Low-GI Foods

To maintain a steady supply of glucose without spiking blood sugar levels, eat foods that are low on the glycemic index (GI) or have a low glycemic load. The glycemic index measures how much a person's blood sugar rises when a carbohydrate food is eaten. The result is ranked on a scale of 1 to 100, where pure glucose has a value of 100. Glycemic load is measured by multiplying a food's GI with the number of grams of carbohydrate in one serving, then dividing by 100. The result is an even more accurate picture of how that food will affect your blood sugar. The lower the glycemic index or glycemic load of the food, the less it affects blood sugar and insulin levels.

Organic Foods

Pesticides, herbicides, insecticides, fungicides and fumigants are used on crops to control pests and fungus. A recent study in the *American Journal of Epidemiology* reported a higher prevalence of clinical thyroid disease in women who were exposed to specific pesticides. Organic foods contain fewer thyroid-disrupting chemicals and pesticides. To see what foods have the highest pesticide content and learn more about pesticides (and to find out what foods are genetically modified), visit www.ewg.org.

Low-Glycemic-Index Foods

The following is a list of the glycemic index for more than 100 common foods. The complete list of the glycemic index and glycemic load for over 1,000 foods can be found as an appendix to the article "International tables of glycemic index and glycemic load values: 2008" by Fiona S. Atkinson, Kaye Foster-Powell and Jennie C. Brand-Miller, published in the December 2008 issue of *Diabetes Care*, volume 31, number 12: pages 2281–83. It is available at http://care.diabetesjournals.org/content/suppl/2008/09/18/dc08-1239.DC1/TableA1_1.pdf.

Type of Food	Low GI (55 or Less)	Medium GI (56–69)	High GI (70 or More)
Vegetables	• Sweet potatoes (48) • Sweet corn, frozen (47) • Carrots, boiled (41) • Green peas, frozen (39) • Yams (35) • Carrots, raw (16) • Cauliflower (15) • Green beans (15) • Eggplant (15) • Tomatoes (15) • Broccoli (10) • Cabbage (10) • Mushrooms (10) • Chile peppers (10) • Lettuce (10) • Onions (10) • Red bell peppers (10)	• Beets (64) • Potatoes, canned (61) • Baked potatoes (60) • New potatoes (54)	• Parsnips (97) • Mashed potatoes, instant (80) • French fries (75) • Pumpkin (75) • Mashed potatoes, fresh (73)
Fruit	• Kiwifruit (47) • Coconut (45) • Grapes (43) • Coconut milk (41) • Pears (41) • Oranges (40) • Strawberries (40) • Apples (34) • Dried apricots (32) • Peaches, canned in natural juice (30) • Prunes (29) • Peaches (28) • Grapefruit (25) • Plums (24) • Cherries (22)	• Pineapple (66) • Raisins (64) • Figs (61) • Mangos (60) • Papayas (60) • Bananas (58) • Sultana raisins (56)	• Dates (103) • Watermelon (80)

Type of Food	Low GI (55 or Less)	Medium GI (56–69)	High GI (70 or More)
Legumes	• Kidney beans (52) • Pinto beans (45) • Black-eyed beans (50) • Chickpeas (42) • Butter beans (36) • Yellow split peas (32) • Haricot/navy beans (31) • Green lentils (30) • Red lentils (21)	• Beans in tomato sauce (56)	
Dairy	• Soy milk (44) • Chocolate milk (42) • Custard (35) • Sugar-sweetened yogurt (33) • Skim milk (32) • Whole milk (31) • Artificially sweetened yogurt (23)	• Ice cream (62)	
Breakfast cereal	• Porridge (58) • Special K (UK/Aus) (54) • Rolled oats (51) • All-Bran (US) (50) • Oat bran (50) • Natural muesli (40) • All-Bran (UK/Aus) (30)	• Special K (US) (69) • Shredded Wheat (67) • Nutri-Grain (66) • Porridge oats (63) • Bran Buds (58) • Mini Wheats (58)	• Rice Krispies (82) • Team (82) • Cornflakes (80) • Puffed Wheat (80) • Coco Pops (77) • Total (76) • Bran Flakes (74) • Cheerios (74) • Weetabix (74) • Raisin Bran (73)
Bread	• Sourdough wheat (54) • Whole wheat (49) • Sourdough rye (48) • Whole-grain pumpernickel (46) • Heavy mixed grain (45) • Soy and flaxseed (36) • Tortilla, wheat (30)	• Taco shells (68) • Croissant (67) • Whole-grain rye (62) • Hamburger bun (61) • Pita, white (57)	• French baguette (95) • Bagel (72) • White bread (71)
Pasta	• Wheat pasta shapes (54) • Tortellini, cheese (50) • Instant noodles (47) • Meat ravioli (39) • Egg fettuccini (32) • Spaghetti (32)	• Gnocchi (68) • Chinese (rice) vermicelli (58)	

Type of Food	Low GI (55 or Less)	Medium GI (56–69)	High GI (70 or More)
Grains	• Buckwheat (51) • Brown rice (50) • Long-grain white rice (50) • Pearl barley (22)	• Cornmeal (68) • Couscous (61) • Basmati rice (58) • Wild rice (57)	
Snacks and sweet foods	• Oatmeal cookies (55) • Jam (51) • Nut and Seed Muesli Bar (49) • Sponge cake (46) • Corn chips (42) • Milk chocolate (42) • Snickers Bar, high-fat (41) • Nutella (33) • Slim-Fast meal replacement (27) • Cashews (25) • Mixed nuts and raisins (21) • Walnuts (15) • Peanuts (13) • Hummus (6)	• Ryvita (63) • Blueberry muffin (59) • Digestives (59) • Honey (58)	• Scones (92) • Rice cakes (87) • Pretzels (83) • Puffed crispbread (81) • Water crackers (78) • Doughnuts (76) • Maple syrup (68)

Processed Grain Limitations

To prevent glucose fluctuations that affect the thyroid, consider limiting or even avoiding processed grains altogether — or, at the least, all processed grains that contain gluten if you have autoimmune thyroid disease. Once processed, the grain has little food value left. The germ (the most nutritious part) has been taken out of its natural fiber and milled into white flour, alkalized, baked, and often stored for long periods.

Keep a food diary to see how often you eat grains and grain products. Many people find that they eat grains in some form or other 7 to 10 times a day!

Avoiding grains is not a hard-and-fast rule for everyone. Some people find they can tolerate a high grain intake without any ill effects. But if you have been riding the blood sugar roller coaster for a long time, or you know from experience that grains either charge you up or put you to sleep, adjust your diet accordingly.

Avoiding grains is not a hard-and-fast rule for everyone. Some people find they can tolerate a high grain intake without any ill effects.

5 Step 5: Eat High-Quality Protein

Adequate amounts of high-quality protein are fundamental to achieving optimal thyroid health because of the effect of protein and amino acids on metabolism. Of the twenty amino acids, your body is unable to synthesize eight: lysine, tryptophan, methionine, leucine, isoleucine, phenylalanine, valine and threonine. You must get these essential amino acids from food.

Calculating Optimum Protein Intake
1. Divide your weight in pounds by 2.2 to get your weight in kilograms.
2. Multiply your weight in kilograms by 0.8 to get your minimum daily protein requirement in grams.

Unfortunately, this calculation is not accurate for everyone, because we all have different activity levels, stress levels and genetic predispositions. If you are an athlete or exercise regularly, your daily protein requirements may be about 1.2 to 1.5 grams per kilogram of body weight. The scientific literature shows that people with a protein deficit must also ingest 1.2 to 1.5 grams of protein per kilogram of body weight each day.

Sometimes it is difficult to get enough protein from diet alone. This is where protein and amino acid supplements come into the picture. However, before beginning to supplement with any kind of protein, be sure that you are eating high-quality protein from food sources at every meal.

High-Quality Protein Sources
- eggs (ideally organic and free-range)
- fish that are wild-caught and known to be low in heavy metals
- chicken, turkey (ideally organic and free-range)
- non-commercial forms of red meats, such as grass-fed, locally raised beef, grass-fed buffalo and grass-fed lamb
- nuts and seeds (ideally organic)
- legumes (ideally organic), including soybeans
- dairy products (ideally organic, from locally raised dairy cows)

Dairy and Soy Products
Despite their value as sources of protein, dairy and soy should make up the lowest percentage of your daily protein intake. Dairy is an excellent but problematic source of protein. Some people

are allergic to milk or cannot tolerate lactose, and dairy products may be contaminated with antibiotics, hormones and/or toxins. Limit the amount of dairy you consume.

Allergies and sensitivities to soy are also common, and soy products tend to be highly processed. Soy is low in sulfur-based amino acids, which you need for detoxification, manufacturing glutathione (a powerful antioxidant) and tissue repair. In addition, soy has long been implicated in diet-induced goiter. Studies have shown that levels of thyroid hormones are lower in animals after they eat a diet that is exclusively soy-based. Soy-fed animals use less energy and less protein compared to animals fed milk protein. Similarly, babies with hypothyroidism need more replacement therapy if they are fed a soy-based formula. Whether this is because of an absorption problem or because of soy's interference with the action of thyroid hormone remains unclear.

If you eat a lot of soy-based foods and are concerned about your dosage of thyroid hormone replacement, have your thyroid hormone levels checked by your doctor. It's quick and easy to do and can help to optimize your thyroid management.

Protein Supplements

When it comes to protein and amino acid supplements, the variety of healthy choices is large. Whey protein is effective for those who are not sensitive or allergic to dairy, but some whey products may not have enough of the essential amino acid leucine, the most anabolic of the amino acids.

For those with impaired digestion, free-form amino acid products are useful. Some people require betaine hydrochloride or digestive enzymes to optimize digestion and absorption of amino acids.

6 Step 6: Optimize Your Omega Fats Ratio

Dietary fats preceded carbohydrates as dietary demons until the role of essential fatty acids (EFAs) in achieving good health was discovered. EFAs are, in fact, essential to our well-being.

Two kinds of polyunsaturated fatty acids (PUFAs) are essential to our health: omega-3s and omega-6s. These EFAs are involved in many vital functions, including hormone release. Without EFAs, we would not survive. Our bodies do not synthesize them, so we must obtain them from our diet.

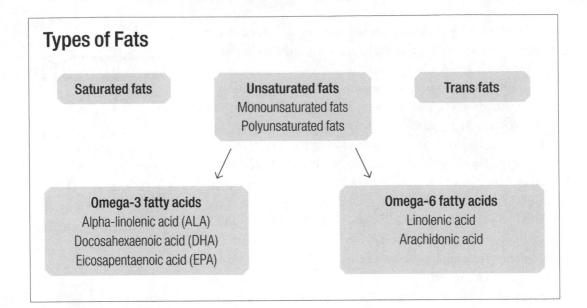

Types of Fats

Saturated fats

Unsaturated fats
Monounsaturated fats
Polyunsaturated fats

Trans fats

Omega-3 fatty acids
Alpha-linolenic acid (ALA)
Docosahexaenoic acid (DHA)
Eicosapentaenoic acid (EPA)

Omega-6 fatty acids
Linolenic acid
Arachidonic acid

For optimum health, omega-6 and omega-3 fatty acids should be ingested at a ratio of between 1:1 and 1:4. However, the ratio in the typical Western diet is between 10:1 and 30:1. This imbalance results in inflammation that can upset thyroid equilibrium and many related health issues.

DID YOU KNOW?

COOKING OIL

The best fats to cook in include coconut oil, butter, ghee, olive oil and macadamia nut oil. Use a variety of oils, rather than getting stuck in a rut of using one oil all the time.

Q Which fats should I avoid and which can I enjoy?

A Avoid trans fats, which may be labelled "hydrogenated" or "partially hydrogenated," as they increase the risk of heart disease. Saturated fat was recently vindicated by a number of scientists, who were unable to find a link between saturated fat, heart disease and high cholesterol. Trans fats are the real enemy and are a major cause of heart disease. Saturated fat and cholesterol are essential for your health, but as with anything, too much or too little can be a problem, so consume them in moderation.

Polyunsaturated fats decrease total and low-density lipoprotein (LDL) cholesterol, and certain types may protect against heart disease and sudden death, and may have positive effects on the nervous system. Foods high in omega-3 fats may help to raise HDL cholesterol, which is usually beneficial.

Ideally, balance your daily fat intake equally between polyunsaturated fatty acids, monounsaturated fats and saturated fats.

Common food sources of omega-3 EFAs include flax, hemp and various fish and seafood (though take care to eat only seafood that is low in mercury and other heavy metals). You can also increase your intake of omega-3s by taking fish oil supplements. However, do not worry about your exact intake of fatty acids: if you are eating a healthy thyroid diet, as described in this book, you will get a good balance of healthy fats.

7 Step 7: Alkalize Your Body pH

Another way to optimize thyroid function is to alkalize your body pH through diet. Your cells work best in an alkaline rather than an acidic environment. Eating foods that increase your body's acidity puts undue stress on your cells, leading to suboptimal energy production and function. High acid levels can result in metabolic acidosis, which adversely affects the thyroid.

You didn't become acidic overnight, so it will take time — possibly a few months — to reverse that state and become consistently alkaline. However, you will notice many health benefits as your alkalinity increases: an improved sense of well-being, increased energy, fat loss, improved sleep, a clearer mind, improved digestion and a reduction in allergies.

Q What is body pH?

A Potential for hydrogen, or pH, is a measure of how acid or alkaline a substance is. Body pH is controlled mainly by the kidneys and lungs, as well as buffering agents, such as bicarbonate, in the blood. On the pH scale of 1 to 14, less than 6.4 indicates acidity, higher than 7.4 indicates alkalinity, and 6.4 to 7.4 is neutral.

pH Tests

To find out if you are in an acid or alkaline state, use Hydrion pH paper strips to test the pH of your urine first thing in the morning for 5 days in a row. Eliminate the highest and the lowest of the five readings and average the other three to calculate your pH.

On the pH scale of 1 to 14, a healthy reading is 6.4 to 7.4. Below 6.4 indicates an acidic environment that could be contributing to a decrease in your metabolism. Avoid becoming too alkaline, with a pH above 7.4. This indicates a catabolic state in which your body is breaking down its tissues rapidly, due to some kind of metabolic or chemical stress.

Strategies for Improving Acid/Alkali Balance

- Start by eating at least one vegetable with every meal. Vegetables contain alkali-forming substances, including calcium, magnesium, potassium and zinc. These buffering agents help to reduce the acid by-products of metabolism. The protein content of a food will also determine its acid/alkaline status. More amino acids in a food leads to more acidity in the body because these amino acids are metabolized in the liver to form acidic by-products.

- Work up to eating at least 2 cups (500 mL) of alkalizing greens a day. Alkalizing greens include kale, mustard greens, turnip greens, Swiss chard, spinach and collard greens. If that does not increase your alkalinity, try eating the three most alkalizing grains: oats (certified gluten-free if you have Hashimoto's thyroiditis or Graves' disease), quinoa and wild rice.

- Take 15- to 20-minute-long alkalizing baths with 1 cup (250 mL) of Epsom salts and $\frac{1}{2}$ cup (125 mL) of baking soda. Epsom salts contain magnesium, a buffering mineral that helps eliminate the acid residue that results from metabolism and detoxification. Baking soda is also extremely alkaline and helps neutralize the acidic compounds that your skin is eliminating. Take these alkalizing baths frequently. If you are an athlete, take one at the end of your training day to enhance healing of your acidic muscle tissue.

- Drink a morning cocktail of $\frac{1}{4}$ to $\frac{1}{2}$ teaspoon (1 to 2 mL) unrefined Celtic sea salt, the juice of $\frac{1}{2}$ lemon or lime and a greens supplement. This cocktail will flood your system with alkalizing agents that mop up acid residues in your body. Use unrefined Celtic sea salt, which is extremely alkaline, as opposed to table salt or sodium chloride, which are extremely acidic.

- Practice deep-belly breathing (see page 113 for instructions). Acids and bases in your body are also controlled by your breath. Each time you inhale fresh oxygen, your body is preparing to exhale carbon dioxide. Too-high carbon dioxide levels in the blood lead to an acidic environment.

- Cook with culinary herbs and spices, such as turmeric, thyme and oregano, that help alkalize the body.

In general, meat, dairy and grains are acidic, while fruits, vegetables and legumes are alkaline. (A full list of alkaline and acidic foods appears on pages 137–141.) The more amino acids in a food, the more acidity in your body, as amino acids are metabolized in the liver to form acidic by-products. Nevertheless, it is extremely important to eat protein at every meal. Do not avoid it for fear of becoming too acidic! In fact, too *little* protein in your diet will also make you more acidic, because amino acids are actually buffering agents inside the cell. As long as you eat vegetables with each meal, you will become more alkaline.

> It is extremely important to eat protein at every meal. Do not avoid it for fear of becoming too acidic.

Alkalizing Supplements

If you are eating a diet that is approximately 60% to 80% alkaline foods but your pH is still acidic, try alkalizing your body by taking magnesium glycinate and potassium bicarbonate. Start with one capsule of each before bed and keep increasing by one of each capsule every night until your pH is alkaline in the morning.

Acidifying and Alkalizing Foods

This list is an easy guide to balancing the pH in your diet. Simply eat more alkaline-forming foods than acid-forming foods — about 4 alkalizing to 1 acidifying to regain health, or 3 alkalizing to 2 acidifying to maintain good health. Use this as your shopping list. Photocopy it and pin it to your bulletin board, and keep a copy in the glove compartment of your car.

Note that the acidifying property of any food may be increased by frying, deep-frying or barbecuing. Save the barbecue for special occasions, and try steaming, roasting or slow-cooking your food as a healthy change from frying.

Fruits

Alkalizing

• All dried fruits	• Cantaloupes	• Guavas
• Avocados	• Dates	• Kiwifruit

Slightly Alkalizing

• Apples	• Grapefruit	• Passion fruit
• Apricots	• Grapes	• Peaches
• Bananas	• Honeydew melons	• Pears
• Blackberries	• Lemons	• Persimmons
• Cherries	• Limes	• Pineapples
• Clementines	• Lychees	• Plums
• Coconut	• Mangos	• Raspberries
• Cranberries	• Nectarines	• Strawberries
• Currants	• Oranges	• Tangerines
• Figs	• Papayas	• Watermelon

Neutral

• Blueberries		

Vegetables

Alkalizing

- Arugula
- Beets and beet greens
- Cauliflower
- Celery
- Fennel
- Kale
- Lemongrass
- Peppers, all varieties (dried)
- Plantain
- Seaweed
- Shiitake mushrooms (dried)
- Spinach
- Sun-dried tomatoes
- Sweet potatoes
- Tomatoes and tomato products (canned)
- Turnip greens
- Wasabi
- Water chestnuts
- Watercress
- Yams

Slightly Alkalizing

- Artichokes
- Asparagus
- Bell peppers (fresh)
- Broccoli
- Brussels sprouts
- Cabbage
- Carrots
- Cauliflower
- Collard greens
- Eggplant
- Garlic
- Horseradish
- Jicama
- Leeks
- Lettuce
- Mushrooms (fresh)
- Mustard greens
- Okra
- Onions
- Parsnips
- Potatoes
- Pumpkin
- Radishes
- Rutabaga
- Shallots
- Squash
- String beans, green or yellow
- Tomatoes, all varieties (fresh)
- Turnips
- Zucchini

Slightly Acidifying

- Corn
- Peas
- Pickles
- Tomatoes (cooked)

Grains, Flours and Breads

Slightly Alkalizing

- Brown rice

Neutral

- Arrowroot flour
- Buckwheat groats and flour
- Bulgur
- Quinoa
- Rice noodles
- Tapioca
- Wild rice

Slightly Acidifying

- Amaranth grain
- Bagels
- Barley
- Corn (flour, bran, meal)
- Cornstarch
- Couscous
- Hominy
- Kamut
- Millet
- Oat bran
- Pasta (homemade, egg-free)
- Quinoa
- Rice flour
- Rye
- Rye flour (light)
- Soba noodles
- Somen noodles
- Spelt
- Teff
- Wheat bran (crude)
- White rice

Acidifying

- Barley flour or meal
- Biscuits
- Bread
- Brown rice flour
- Cake
- Cookies
- Crackers
- Doughnuts
- Egg noodles
- French toast
- Oat flour
- Pasta
- Pastry
- Rice bran
- Rye flour (dark)
- Sprouted wheat
- Wheat
- Wheat flour

Protein Foods

Alkalizing

- Fava beans
- Lima beans

Slightly Alkalizing

- Adzuki beans
- Baked beans (homemade)
- Cowpeas
- Pigeon peas
- Pink beans
- Soybeans (roasted)
- White beans

Neutral

- Black beans
- Chinese noodles (cellophane or mung)
- Egg whites
- Fish broth
- Fish oil
- Great Northern beans
- Navy beans
- Red kidney beans
- Split peas

Slightly Acidifying

- Chickpeas
- Lentils
- Mung beans
- Oysters
- Peanut butter
- Soybeans (fresh)
- Tempeh
- Tofu, extra-firm

Acidifying

- Anchovies (canned in oil)
- Bacon
- Beef
- Cod
- Chicken
- Cornish hen
- Crab
- Deli meats
- Duck
- Egg yolks
- Eggs, whole
- Goose
- Haddock
- Halibut
- Ham
- Herring
- Lamb
- Lobster
- Peanuts
- Pork
- Salmon
- Sausage
- Smoked fish
- Soybeans (dry-roasted)
- Trout (steamed)
- Tuna
- Veal

Dairy

Neutral

- Buttermilk
- Cream
- Sour cream
- Goat milk
- Ice cream
- Low-fat yogurt
- Milk
- Soy milk
- Whipped cream

Slightly Acidifying

- Cream cheese
- Cheese, full-fat soft
- Kefir

Acidifying

- Camembert cheese
- Cheese substitute
- Cheese, fresh (Quark)
- Cheese, hard
- Cottage cheese
- Processed cheese
- Ricotta cheese

Nuts and Seeds

Alkalizing

- Chestnuts
- Green pumpkin seeds (pepitas)

Slightly Acidifying

- Almonds
- Pine nuts
- Hazelnuts

Acidifying

- Cashews
- Pistachios
- Sesame seeds
- Sunflower seeds
- Walnuts

Fats and Oils

Neutral

- Almond oil
- Avocado oil
- Butter
- Canola oil
- Fish oil
- Flaxseed oil
- Ghee (clarified butter)
- Lard
- Margarine
- Olive oil
- Peanut oil
- Safflower oil
- Sunflower oil
- Vegetable oil

Flavorings, Sweeteners and Condiments

Alkalizing

- All herbs, fresh and dried
- All spices, fresh and dried
- Cocoa powder, unsweetened
- Molasses
- Tomato sauce

Slightly Alkalizing

- Carob powder
- Cider vinegar
- Maple syrup
- Marmalades
- Sea salt
- Soy sauce
- Vanilla extract

Slightly Acidifying		
• Artificial sweeteners	• Barley malt	• Gravy

Acidifying	
• Gelatin desserts	• Pudding desserts

Beverages

Alkalizing
• Instant coffee

Slightly Alkalizing		
• Alcoholic beverages • Cold chocolate beverages	• Coconut water • Fruit juices	• Mineral water • Wine, red or white

Neutral		
• Beer (draft, pale, bottled stout) • Black tea • Carbonated beverages (with caffeine)	• Coffee • Herbal teas • Hot cocoa	• Infused teas • Tap water

Slightly Acidifying
• Carob beverages

SOURCE: SAMPLED FROM USDA FOOD LISTS, HTTP://NDB.NAL.USDA.GOV/NDB/FOODS.

8 Step 8: Improve Your Eating Habits

The sympathetic nervous system is the part of the nervous system that initiates the "fight or flight" response, which makes you sweat, your pupils dilate and your heart race. Blood leaves the digestive system and is shunted to your muscles so you can escape from danger. This is not conducive to digestion (which is just not important when you are in danger).

> Put time aside each day for healthy and relaxing meals.

To support your digestion, aim to get into a parasympathetic-dominant state after eating — a "rest and digest" state — so that your digestive system is producing plenty of stomach acid and digestive enzymes. The following eating habits will help you achieve this goal:

• Put time aside each day for healthy and relaxing meals. Sit in a quiet and comfortable place, with no newspapers, books, television, phone calls or computers to distract you. Focus solely on your meal.

- "Eat food that spoils, but eat it before it does" is a simple mantra that will ensure you are eating healthy foods that are preservative-free.
- Review your carbohydrate sources and eliminate carbs that spike blood sugar too much, such as sweets, desserts, sugar, pasta, "white foods," potato chips, pretzels and other processed carbohydrates. Eat whole-food sources of carbohydrates.
- Keep your portion size for each food to the size of your fist or the palm of your hand.
- Chew your food slowly and completely before swallowing. The more liquefied your food is when it leaves your mouth, the easier it is on your digestive tract.
- Put your fork or spoon down in between mouthfuls and while chewing your food.
- Think positive thoughts and about how grateful you are to have the food.
- Avoid drinking ice water. According to traditional Chinese medicine, digestion should be a "warm" process. Ice water gives you a "cold bowel" that impairs digestion.
- Drink lemon or lime squeezed into water to aid digestion or try adding 1 teaspoon (5 mL) of cider vinegar to your water. Ginger tea, sipped with your meal, is also an excellent digestive aid that has a "warming" effect on the whole digestive system.

Q How many meals a day should I eat?

A Eating small, frequent meals was much touted in the 1990s as a weight-loss strategy. Some weak data indicated that eating several small meals rather than the traditional three meals a day enhanced metabolism. The fitness industry jumped on this idea so they could sell more energy bars, protein bars and weight-loss bars and shakes, instructing people to eat them in between meals to "rev up" their metabolism. In fact, eating three meals a day and an additional snack, if needed, works well for most people with thyroid dysfunction.

Portion Size

Eat enough at each meal so you are not hungry in between. One simple way to check whether you are eating enough is to use your hand to measure portion sizes. One "palm" of protein, one "fist" of vegetables and a small handful of carbohydrates is a great way to start. Depending on your body type, you can adjust your intake of protein, carbohydrate and fat using these simple hand measurement strategies without making things too complicated. If you are eating nuts or seeds, one to three thumb-size portions is enough, depending on how much fat you can tolerate.

This method is also an easy way to measure your food if you are eating out, as you can easily tell how much to eat without getting caught up in numbers or counting calories.

If you are hungry in between meals, try increasing your fiber and fat intake at mealtime.

Avoiding Gluten

If you have been diagnosed with Hashimoto's thyroiditis or Graves' disease, you may also have celiac disease or gluten intolerance, also known as non-celiac gluten sensitivity. There are various tests that can help you determine whether you should avoid eating gluten-containing products.

Anti-Gliadin Antibody Test

The anti-gliadin antibody test measures an immune response to gliadin, the main protein in gluten. A negative anti-gliadin antibody test in saliva, stool or blood does not rule out gluten intolerance, however. You can have gluten intolerance and have false negatives on these tests. If the test is positive in saliva, stool or blood, it is a very strong indicator that you are gluten-intolerant. In most, but not all cases, there must be some damage to the lining of the small intestine for the test to be positive in blood or saliva.

Villous Atrophy Test

Your doctor may want to order a biopsy of the small intestine to look for damage to the lining of the small intestine. This is known as villous atrophy, meaning the villi that line the gut have been damaged and are worn away because of the immune system attack on the dietary gluten intake.

The problem with this test is that you can have gluten intolerance or celiac disease but not have atrophied villi. Sixty percent of the negative effects of gluten occur outside of the intestine. You might have only mild inflammation of the intestine but extra-intestinal damage to the thyroid, bones, pancreas, brain and adrenal glands. Conversely, you can have villous atrophy but neither celiac disease nor gluten intolerance.

DID YOU KNOW?

AN ANCIENT DISEASE
Celiac disease was first documented about 10,000 years ago during the development of agriculture in the Fertile Crescent. The first symptoms recorded were chronic diarrhea, abdominal distension and muscle wasting. It was not until 1950 that a young Dutch pediatrician named Willem-Karel Dicke made the association between gluten and disease. He was the first to implement a gluten-free diet as a cure for celiac disease. In the 1960s, the genetics of gluten intolerance began to emerge in research.

Gluten Challenge Diet

You can avoid lab tests and test yourself for gluten intolerance with a gluten challenge diet. Try excluding gluten from your diet for 4 to 6 weeks. If you notice improvements in your symptoms, you should probably avoid gluten or consume it in strict moderation. If you don't note any improvements, then you are probably okay to eat gluten in moderation.

A conventional doctor might ask you to run this test in reverse by eating gluten every day for 4 to 6 weeks, and will then run a celiac disease blood panel. However, this test should be used with caution, as eating gluten regularly over such a long period of time may cause significant harm if you are, indeed, gluten-intolerant. In addition, this test has a high rate of false negative responses (negative results even though the person has celiac disease).

Gluten-Containing and Gluten-Free Grains and Starches

Gluten is a protein found in many grains, including wheat, barley, rye and spelt. Gluten can also be hidden in packaged foods, so read labels carefully. Be wary of modified food starch, dextrin, flavorings and extracts, hydrolyzed vegetable protein, imitation seafood and creamed or thickened products such as soups, stews and sauces.

Substitute gluten-free grains for grains that contain gluten.

Gluten-Containing Grains and Starches		Gluten-Free Grains and Starches	
• Barley	• Rye	• Amaranth	• Quinoa
• Bulgur	• Semolina	• Arrowroot	• Rice
• Couscous	• Spelt	• Buckwheat	• Tapioca
• Durum flour	• Triticale	• Corn	• Teff
• Kamut	• Wheat	• Millet	• Wheatgrass
		• Oats*	• Wild rice

* In nature, oats are gluten-free, but 99% of oats sold in the U.S. are processed with machinery that is also used for gluten-containing grains. Look for oats labeled "certified gluten-free."

▷ DOC TALK

The balanced thyroid diet is not a short-term fix. Make it part of a new lifestyle and stick with it. With the exception of gluten-containing foods if you have Hashimoto's thyroiditis or Graves' disease, this diet does not eliminate any types of food and doesn't have many restrictions. It allows you to eat and enjoy a wide variety of foods.

No doctor or nutritionist can tell you exactly how and what you should eat, because everyone is an individual. Start following the balanced thyroid diet and see if it works for you. If your thyroid is being treated correctly and you are not losing weight, try adjusting your carbohydrate or fat intake. Experiment and learn what works for you.

PART 4

Thyroid Meal Plans

4-Week Meal Plans

Use these 4-week meal plans as a guide to a balanced thyroid diet. "Post-workout meals" (highlighted in the meal plans) should be between 25 and 45 grams of carbohydrate; "anytime meals" (all of the other meals and snacks) should be less than 25 grams of carbohydrate. Protein should be between 15 and 30 grams for each meal. Snacks may have less protein than meals, but should still have a healthy balance of carbohydrates, protein and fat. If you are an athlete, you may need more protein to meet your metabolic needs. Tips on how to add more protein are provided with many of the recipes in this book.

Recipes from this book are indicated with an asterisk (*) in the meal plans. Feel free to sub in other recipes to suit your tastes or meet your metabolic needs. For example, you may need an "anytime" recipe for breakfast on Monday of Week 1 if you did not work out before breakfast. You can choose an "anytime"

Week 1

Meal	Sunday	Monday	Tuesday	
Breakfast	• Garden-Fresh Frittata*	<u>Post-Workout Meal</u> • 2 Buttermilk Buckwheat Pancakes* • 1 to 2 scrambled or hard-cooked eggs	<u>Post-Workout Meal</u> • Power Smoothie 1*	
Lunch	<u>Post-Workout Meal</u> • Butternut Chili*	• Pork Quinoa Salad with Indian Dressing*	• Zucchini Patties*	
Snack	• 6 raw or dry-roasted unsalted Brazil nuts	• Roasted Garlic Dip* • Cut-up raw vegetables, 2 to 3 GF crackers or 10 to 12 Beanitos	• Anti-Inflammatory Hummus* • Cut-up raw vegetables, 2 to 3 GF crackers or 10 to 12 Beanitos	
Dinner	• Fish Chowder* • Marinated Vegetable Medley*	• Meatballs for Everyday* • Steamed Vegetables with Toasted Almonds*	• Baked Salmon Patties* • Side salad or steamed non-starchy vegetables	

breakfast from another day, or you can substitute another "anytime" breakfast recipe from the list on page 154.

If you have limited time, cook enough the night before for leftovers the following day (for example, eat the same lunch on Tuesday as you had for dinner on Monday), subbing the leftovers in for the meal specified in the menu for that day. Alternatively, when you have time, you can make big batches of recipes that will store well (such as soups, chilis and curries), so that you always have options ready to take with you to work or heat up for an easy dinner when you're too exhausted to cook.

If you would like to make certain meals more alkaline, or you need more low-calorie, low-carbohydrate "fillers," add a side salad or steamed non-starchy vegetables, such as asparagus, broccoli, Brussels sprouts, carrots, cauliflower, cucumbers, green beans, kale and other greens, radishes, summer squash (such as zucchini) and tomatoes.

Wednesday	Thursday	Friday	Saturday
• Western Omelet*	• Hot Millet Amaranth Cereal* • Vanilla Almond Milk* with added protein	• Vegetable Quiche with Oat Groat Crust*	• Indian Scrambled Eggs*
• Spinach with Almonds*	• Thai-Style Pumpkin Soup* with added protein	• Beef and Quinoa Soup*	**Post-Workout Meal** • Gingery Chicken and Wild Rice Soup*
• 1 oz (30 g) almonds (dry-roasted, sprouted or raw)	• Crunchy Peanut Butter Muffin*	• 1 oz (30 g) almonds (dry-roasted, sprouted or raw)	• 10–12 raw or dry-roasted macadamia nuts
Post-Workout Meal • Thai-Inspired Peanut and Wild Rice Soup* • Roasted Asparagus*	**Post-Workout Meal** • Valencia Seafood Paella* • Steamed non-starchy vegetables	**Post-Workout Meal** • 2 slices Thin Pizza Crust* with added protein toppings (chicken, beef, shrimp, tofu) • Side salad	• Grilled Lamb Chops with Rosemary Mustard Baste* • Steamed non-starchy vegetables

Week 2

Meal	Sunday	Monday	Tuesday	
Breakfast	• 2 Coconut Pancakes* • 3 scrambled or hard-cooked egg whites	Post-Workout Meal • Breakfast Burrito*	Post-Workout Meal • Power Smoothie 2*	
Lunch	Post-Workout Meal • Lamb with Lentils and Chard*	• Baked Salmon with Ginger and Lemon* • Cumin Beets*	• Vichyssoise with Celery Root and Watercress* with added protein	
Snack	• Sardine Spread* • Cut-up raw vegetables, 2 to 3 GF crackers or 10 to 12 Beanitos	• Tomato Avocado Salsa • 10 to 12 Beanitos	• Steamed Sugar Snap Peas with Ginger*	
Dinner	• Kale and Pear Salad with Warmed Shallot Dressing* with added protein	• Tandoori Chicken with Cucumber Mint Raita* • Braised Brussels Sprouts*	• Lemon Garlic Chicken* • Baked Sweet Potato Fries* • Side salad	

Week 3

Meal	Sunday	Monday	Tuesday	
Breakfast	• Garden-Fresh Frittata*	Post-Workout Meal • 3 Buttermilk Buckwheat Pancakes* • 1 to 2 scrambled or hard-cooked eggs	Post-Workout Meal • Hot Oat Bran and Flax Porridge*	
Lunch	Post-Workout Meal • Minestrone*	• Potato, Leek and Broccoli Soup* with added protein	• Spinach Salad with Carrots and Mushrooms* with added protein • $\frac{1}{2}$ cup (125 mL) cooked lentils	
Snack	• 6 raw or dry-roasted unsalted Brazil nuts	• Oven-Baked Kale Chips*	• Chili Black Bean Dip* • Cut-up raw vegetables, 2 to 3 GF crackers or 10 to 12 Beanitos	
Dinner	• Mexican-Style Seafood Stew with Hominy* • Roasted Asparagus*	• Fish for the Sole* • Asparagus with Lemon and Garlic*	• Catalan Beef Stew* • Side salad or steamed non-starchy vegetables	

Wednesday	Thursday	Friday	Saturday
Post-Workout Meal • Cranberry Quinoa Porridge* with added protein	**Post-Workout Meal** • Black Sticky Rice Congee with Coconut* with added protein	**Post-Workout Meal** • Hot Oat Bran and Flax Porridge*	• Mango Yogurt Smoothie* with added protein
• Tofu Chop Suey*	• Fast and Easy Greek Salad* with added protein	• French Basil Chicken* • Asparagus with Lemon and Garlic*	**Post-Workout Meal** • Wild Rice Cakes* • Marinated Vegetable Medley*
• Crispy-Coated Veggie Snacks*	• Anti-Inflammatory Hummus* • Cut-up raw vegetables, 2 to 3 GF crackers or 10 to 12 Beanitos	• Spicy Cashews*	• Salty Almonds with Thyme*
• Poached Fish* • Broccoli Cilantro Pesto with Pasta*	• Catalan Beef Stew* • Sautéed Broccoli and Red Peppers*	• Grilled Salmon with Lemon Oregano Pesto* • Steamed Vegetables with Toasted Almonds*	• Indian-Style Chicken with Puréed Spinach*

Wednesday	Thursday	Friday	Saturday
Post-Workout Meal • Black Sticky Rice Congee with Coconut* with added protein	**Post-Workout Meal** • Poached Eggs on Spicy Lentils*	**Post-Workout Meal** • Power Smoothie 1*	• Vegetable Quiche with Oat Groat Crust*
• Curried Squash and Apple Soup* with added protein	• Roasted Portobello Mushroom and Fennel Salad* with added protein	• Grilled Salmon and Romaine Salad*	**Post-Workout Meal** • Indian Peas and Beans* with added protein
• Roasted Garlic Dip* • Cut-up raw vegetables, 2 to 3 GF crackers or 10 to 12 Beanitos	• Homemade Crunchy Granola Bar*	• 10–12 raw or dry-roasted macadamia nuts	• Lentil Tapenade* • Cut-up raw vegetables, 2 to 3 GF crackers or 10 to 12 Beanitos
• Bengali Fish Curry* • Thyme-Scented Carrots* • Steamed vegetables	• Mediterranean-Style Mahi-Mahi* • Side salad or steamed non-starchy vegetables	• Crunchy Almond Chicken* • Herb-Glazed Brussels Sprouts*	• 3 slices Cauliflower Pizza Crust* with vegetable and protein toppings (beef, chicken, shrimp, tofu)

Week 4

Meal	Sunday	Monday	Tuesday	
Breakfast	• Garden-Fresh Frittata	• Western Omelet	<u>Post-Workout Meal</u> • Cranberry Quinoa Porridge* with added protein	
Lunch	<u>Post-Workout Meal</u> • Lentil and Spinach Soup* with added protein	• Fish Chowder* • Marinated Vegetable Medley*	• Fast and Easy Greek Salad* with added protein	
Snack	• Steamed Sugar Snap Peas with Ginger*	• Spicy Tamari Almonds*	• Crunchy Peanut Butter Muffin*	
Dinner	• Country Supper Cabbage Rolls*	<u>Post-Workout Meal</u> • Gingery Red Lentils with Spinach and Coconut* with added protein	• Turkey Mole* • New Orleans Braised Onions*	

Post-Workout Meals (Moderate- to High-Carbohydrate)

Breakfast Options (25–40 g carbohydrate)

- Steel-Cut Oats (page 174)
- Cranberry Quinoa Porridge (page 175)
- Hot Oat Bran and Flax Porridge (page 176)
- Black Sticky Rice Congee with Coconut (page 177)
- Buttermilk Buckwheat Pancakes (page 178)
- Poached Eggs on Spicy Lentils (page 181)
- Breakfast Burritos (page 188)
- Lemon Blueberry Almond Muffins (page 356)
- Pumpkin Millet Muffins (page 358)
- Power Smoothie 1 (page 191)
- Power Smoothie 2 (page 192)

Lunch and Dinner Options (25–40 g carbohydrate)

- Thai-Inspired Peanut and Wild Rice Soup (page 203)
- Old-Fashioned Split Pea Soup (page 208)
- Mushroom Lentil Soup (page 209)
- Lentil and Spinach Soup (page 210)
- Minestrone (page 211)
- Fassolada (Greek Bean Soup) (page 212)
- Gingery Chicken and Wild Rice Soup (page 214)
- Quinoa Salad (page 231)
- Wild Rice Cakes (page 254)

Wednesday	Thursday	Friday	Saturday
• Mango Yogurt Smoothie* with added protein	**Post-Workout Meal** • Poached Eggs on Spicy Lentils*	**Post-Workout Meal** • Power Smoothie 1*	• 2 Coconut Pancakes* served with 3 scrambled or hard-cooked egg whites
• Beet Soup with Lemongrass and Lime* • Crunchy Almond Chicken*	• Potato, Leek, and Broccoli Soup* with added protein	• Catalan Beef Stew* • Marinated Vegetable Medley*	**Post-Workout Meal** • Mushroom Lentil Soup*
• Tomato Avocado Salsa* • 10 to 12 Beanitos	• Grain-Free Granola* • Vanilla Almond Milk*	• Salty Almonds with Thyme*	• Lentil Tapenade* • Cut-up raw vegetables, 2 to 3 GF crackers or 10 to 12 Beanitos
Post-Workout Meal • Celery Root and Mushroom Lasagna*	• Pan-Roasted Trout with Fresh Tomato Basil Sauce* • Thyme-Scented Carrots*	• Miso Mushroom Chicken with Chinese Cabbage*	• Salmon and Wild Rice Cakes with Avocado-Chili Topping*

- Basic Beans (page 255)
- Gingery Red Lentils with Spinach and Coconut (page 256)
- Indian Peas and Beans (page 258)
- Butternut Chili (page 260)
- Celery Root and Mushroom Lasagna (page 262)
- Thin Pizza Crust (page 264)

- Shrimp and Vegetable Spring Rolls (page 288)
- Valencia Seafood Paella (page 292)
- Italian-Style Chicken in White Wine with Olives and Polenta (page 298)
- Turkey Ratatouille Chili (page 309)
- Spicy Lamb with Chickpeas (page 320)
- Lamb with Lentils and Chard (page 322)

Side Dish Options (15–30 g carbohydrate)

- Spanish Orange and Avocado Salad (page 221)
- Cactus Salad (page 230)
- Lentil Squash Salad (page 232)
- Stuffed Artichokes (page 324)
- Herb-Glazed Brussels Sprouts (page 331)
- Roasted Butternut Squash with Onion and Sage (page 340)

- Baked Sweet Potato Fries (page 341)
- Creamy Mashed Potatoes with Cauliflower (page 342)
- Savory Vegetarian Quinoa Pilaf (page 343)
- Red Beans and Greens (page 344)
- Creamy Polenta (page 346)

Anytime Meals and Snacks (Lower-Carbohydrate)

Breakfast Options (less than 25 g carbohydrate)

- Grain-Free Granola (page 172)
- Hot Millet Amaranth Cereal (page 173)
- Coconut Pancakes (page 179)
- Crêpes (page 180)
- Indian Scrambled Eggs (page 182)
- Western Omelet (page 183)
- Garden-Fresh Frittata (page 184)
- Buckwheat Walnut Bread (page 186)
- Mango Yogurt Smoothie (page 190)

Lunch and Dinner Options (less than 25 g carbohydrate)

- Moroccan-Spiced Carrot Soup (page 197)
- Beet Soup with Lemongrass and Lime (page 198)
- Vichyssoise with Celery Root and Watercress (page 200)
- Potato, Leek and Broccoli Soup (page 202)
- Thai-Style Pumpkin Soup (page 204)
- Curried Squash and Apple Soup (page 206)
- Beef and Quinoa Soup (page 216)
- Fish Chowder (page 218)
- Fast and Easy Greek Salad (page 220)
- Kale and Pear Salad with Warmed Shallot Dressing (page 222)
- Spinach Salad with Carrots and Mushrooms (page 223)
- Warm Spinach and Mushroom Salad (page 224)
- Roasted Portobello Mushroom and Fennel Salad (page 226)
- Kasha and Beet Salad with Celery and Feta (page 228)
- Grilled Salmon and Romaine Salad (page 234)
- Pork Quinoa Salad with Indian Dressing (page 236)
- Spinach with Almonds (page 252)
- Zucchini Patties (page 253)
- Quinoa-Stuffed Tomatoes (page 267)
- Cauliflower Pizza Crust (page 266); toppings may increase carbohydrate count
- Spinach and Tofu Curry (page 268)
- Tofu Chop Suey (page 270)
- Tofu Vegetable Quiche (page 271)
- Vegetable Quiche with Oat Groat Crust (page 272)
- Crustless Dill Spinach Quiche with Mushrooms and Cheese (page 274)
- Poached Fish (page 276)
- Fish Fillets with Corn and Red Pepper Salsa (page 277)
- Peruvian Ceviche (page 278)
- Bengali Fish Curry (page 279)
- Mediterranean-Style Mahi-Mahi (page 280)
- Salmon and Wild Rice Cakes with Avocado-Chili Topping (page 281)
- Baked Salmon Patties (page 282)
- Baked Salmon with Ginger and Lemon (page 283)
- Grilled Salmon with Lemon Oregano Pesto (page 284)
- Fish for the Sole (page 285)
- Pan-Roasted Trout with Fresh Tomato Basil Sauce (page 286)
- Sweet Potato Coconut Curry with Shrimp (page 287)
- Mexican-Style Seafood Stew with Hominy (page 290)
- Onion-Braised Shrimp (page 294)
- Crunchy Almond Chicken (page 296)
- French Basil Chicken (page 297)
- Lemon Garlic Chicken (page 300)
- Jerk Chicken (page 301)
- Indian-Style Grilled Chicken Breasts (page 302)
- Tandoori Chicken with Cucumber Mint Raita (page 304)

- Miso Mushroom Chicken with Chinese Cabbage (page 305)
- Indian-Style Chicken with Puréed Spinach (page 306)
- Spicy Peanut Chicken (page 308)
- Turkey Mole (page 310)
- Pork Vindaloo (page 312)
- Catalan Beef Stew (page 313)
- Zesty Braised Beef with New Potatoes (page 314)
- Meatballs for Everyday (page 316)
- Country Supper Cabbage Rolls (page 317)
- Grilled Lamb Chops with Rosemary Mustard Baste (page 318)
- Segovia-Style Lamb (page 319)

Side Dish Options (less than 15 g carbohydrate)

- Marinated Vegetable Medley (page 225)
- Roasted Asparagus (page 325)
- Asparagus with Lemon and Garlic (page 326)
- Cumin Beets (page 327)
- Sautéed Broccoli and Red Peppers (page 328)
- Broccoli Cilantro Pesto with Pasta (page 329)
- Braised Brussels Sprouts (page 330)
- Thyme-Scented Carrots (page 332)
- Lemon Almond Sautéed Greens (page 333)
- New Orleans Braised Onions (page 334)
- Lentil-Stuffed Tomatoes (page 335)
- Cherry Tomato and Zucchini Sauté (page 336)
- Mix 'n' Mash Vegetables (page 337)
- Steamed Vegetables with Toasted Almonds (page 338)

Stocks, Sauces and Salad Dressings (5 g of carbohydrate or less)

- Basic Vegetable Stock (page 194)
- Homemade Chicken Stock (page 195)
- Hearty Beef Stock (page 196)
- Green Goddess Salad Dressing (page 237)
- Roasted Garlic and Sun-Dried Tomato Dressing (page 238)
- Basic Pesto (page 246)
- Creamy Basil Pesto (page 247)
- Parsley Pesto Sauce (page 248)
- Cucumber Mint Raita (page 248)
- Basic Tomato Sauce (page 250)

Low-Carbohydrate Snacks (25 g of carbohydrate or less)

- Vanilla Almond Milk (page 189)
- Roasted Garlic Dip (page 240)
- Chili Black Bean Dip (page 241)
- Artichoke and White Bean Spread (page 242)
- Anti-Inflammatory Hummus (page 243)
- Lentil Tapenade (page 244)
- Sardine Spread (page 245)
- Tomato Avocado Salsa (page 249)
- Crispy-Coated Veggie Snacks (page 348)
- Steamed Sugar Snap Peas with Ginger (page 349)
- Oven-Baked Kale Chips (page 350)
- Spicy Cashews (page 351)
- Salty Almonds with Thyme (page 352)
- Spicy Tamari Almonds (page 353)
- Crunchy Peanut Butter Muffins (page 354)
- Homemade Crunchy Granola Bars (page 361)

Low-Carbohydrate Desserts (15 g of carbohydrate or less)

- Almond Sponge Cake (page 359)
- Pumpkin Date Bars (page 360)
- Peanut Butter Cookies (page 362)
- Cinnamon Crisps (page 363)

PART 5

Thyroid Recipes

Introduction to the Recipes

Wholesome food is a cornerstone of good health and thyroid function. We have provided a 4-week meal plan, recipes and health-enhancing tips to make it easier for you to achieve great health. Below are a few general recommendations to keep in mind when choosing what foods to purchase and how to prepare them.

1. **Eat real, fresh food!** If you need to use packaged foods, look for foods with five or fewer ingredients and make sure you recognize them all.

2. **Use low to medium heat to cook your food.** When you cook on a high heat, as with barbecuing, grilling, frying or broiling above 390°F (199°C), it creates heterocyclic amines, which damage our cells when ingested. In addition, when the flame of a grill touches the food, it produces polycyclic aromatic hydrocarbons, which are carcinogenic (cancer-causing). Cooking on high temperatures also increases the formation of advanced glycation end products (AGEs), which cause tissue damage and inflammation when the foods are eaten. Finally, cooking with high heat increases nutrient loss from our foods. All of these changes can impact our general health and our thyroid function. The best cooking methods are boiling, steaming, slow cooking and baking at 350°F (180°C) or lower. When cooking on the stovetop, use medium heat or lower. You may need to increase the cooking time to achieve the desired doneness. If you do barbecue, use a lower heat and do not let the flame touch the foods. It will also help to eat some dark green vegetables with your barbecued foods.

3. **Purchase organic foods when possible.** Pesticides are used on crops to control pests and fungi. Examples of pesticides include herbicides, insecticides, fungicides and fumigants. A 2009 study in the *American Journal of Epidemiology* reported a higher prevalence of clinical thyroid disease in women who were exposed to certain pesticides. Eating organic foods can lower your exposure to the pesticides routinely sprayed on crops. To see what foods have the highest pesticide content, and to learn more about pesticides, visit www.ewg.org.

4. **Avoid genetically modified foods (GMOs).** GMOs have been genetically modified in the laboratory to enhance certain

A 2009 study in the *American Journal of Epidemiology* reported a higher prevalence of clinical thyroid disease in women who were exposed to certain pesticides.

traits, such as resistance to herbicides or improved nutritional content. A few examples include insect-resistant corn and the altered fatty acid content in canola oil. The impact of GMOs on our health has not been clearly established in humans; however, several animal studies suggest adverse effects. There is also some evidence that consuming GMO foods may increase food allergies and alter our immune response, increasing the potential to develop autoimmune diseases, such as Graves' disease and Hashimoto's thyroiditis. To learn more about what foods are genetically modified and how to avoid them, visit www.ewg.org.

5. **Choose high-quality animal protein.** Good options include wild fish, organic chicken and turkey, and grass-fed beef and lamb. Avoid protein from animals that have been given antibiotics or hormones, or have been fed grains. When you consume the flesh of animals that were fed antibiotics or hormones, it is like taking a low dose of antibiotics or hormones yourself. And grain-fed animals have more inflammatory fats in their tissues, which will increase the inflammation in your body when you eat their flesh. In addition to being fed grains and given antibiotics and hormones, farm-raised fish may be exposed to chemicals that leach into the waters where they are raised.

> When you consume the flesh of animals that were fed antibiotics or hormones, it is like taking a low dose of antibiotics or hormones yourself.

6. **Avoid cans lined with bisphenol A (BPA).** BPA has been shown to lower T4. Eating unprocessed foods can help you lower your BPA exposure. If you must consume canned goods, look for BPA-free cans. In addition, avoid plastic water bottles and food storage containers.

7. **Choose healthy fats.** The best fats for thyroid disease include avocados, avocado oil, coconut oil, macadamia nuts, macadamia nut butter, macadamia nut oil, organic butter, organic ghee (clarified butter) and olive oil.

8. **Add protein powder to your baked goods.** For added protein in baked goods, you can add 1 to 2 scoops of unflavored protein powder (organic rice, organic pea, organic hemp or whey from grass-fed cows not given antibiotics or hormones). You may need to add 1 to 2 tbsp (15 to 30 mL) more liquid to your batter.

9. **Increase your fiber intake.** Add 1 to 3 tbsp (15 to 45 mL) of ground flax seeds (flaxseed meal) or chia seeds to smoothies, oatmeal and baked goods. How much you add depends on the desired consistency; chia seeds tend to thicken the mix more than flax seeds.

10. **Use unrefined Celtic sea salt.** Processed table salt has many added chemicals and is deficient in nutrients. Unrefined Celtic sea salt contains over 50 different minerals that are important for health and thyroid function.

11. **Add flavor and nutrition with fresh and dried herbs.** Rosemary, for example, adds wonderful flavor to meats, roasted vegetables and soups. In addition, it has been found to positively impact the immune system, support vitamin D receptors and support liver function.

12. **Incorporate healing ingredients into your cooking.** See the list of Common Ingredients for Healing Your Body, below, for some great options that will help improve your health and thyroid function with every bite. These ingredients are already included in many of the recipes in this book.

> Rosemary has been found to positively impact the immune system, support vitamin D receptors, and support liver function.

Common Ingredients for Healing Your Body

Almonds are a good source of protein, fiber, calcium and iron. They are a fantastic source of biotin, vitamin E (an antioxidant), manganese, copper, vitamin B_{12}, phosphorus, magnesium and molybdenum. Many of these nutrients are heart-protective, assist with weight loss, increase energy and are essential for good thyroid function. Almonds also contain the important flavonoids quercetin and kaempferol, which help to decrease inflammation and protect cells. Almonds, almond butter and almond flour can be found in Grain-Free Granola (page 172), Black Sticky Rice Congee with Coconut (page 177), Vanilla Almond Milk (page 189), Power Smoothie 1 (page 191), Power Smoothie 2 (page 192), Spinach with Almonds (page 252), Sweet Potato Coconut Curry with Shrimp (page 287), Crunchy Almond Chicken (page 296), Lemon Almond Sautéed Greens (page 333), Steamed Vegetables with Toasted Almonds (page 338), Salty Almonds with Thyme (page 352), Spicy Tamari Almonds (page 353), Lemon Blueberry Almond Muffins (page 356) and Almond Sponge Cake (page 359).

Amaranth, a gluten-free grain, contains the most protein of all the grains. It is high in the essential amino acid lysine (which is important for fighting viruses, including Epstein-Barr) and fiber, and is a good source of calcium, magnesium and folate.

Amaranth and amaranth flour can be found in Hot Millet Amaranth Cereal (page 173), Lemon Blueberry Almond Muffins (page 356) and Almond Sponge Cake (page 359).

Asparagus is an excellent source of folate and a good source of vitamin C, thiamine and vitamin B_6. It is high in rutin (a flavonoid that helps lower inflammation, strengthen blood vessels and protect cells from damage) and glutathione (a potent antioxidant, critical for detoxification). It contains protodioscin, which has been shown to reduce bone loss, improve libido and help defend against cancer. Asparagus can be found in Roasted Asparagus (page 325) and Asparagus with Lemon and Garlic (page 326).

Basil has strong antioxidant properties and provides important phytochemicals, such as orientin and vicerin, that help lower inflammation and protect cells from damage. It also contains antibacterial volatile oils, such as camphor and eucalyptol. Basil can be found in large amounts in Minestrone (page 211), Basic Pesto (page 246), Creamy Basil Pesto (page 247), Parsley Pesto Sauce (page 248), French Basil Chicken (page 297), Broccoli Cilantro Pesto with Pasta (page 329) and Herb-Glazed Brussels Sprouts (page 331), and in smaller amounts in a number of other recipes.

Beans and lentils are rich in fiber and protein. They are also excellent sources of potassium, folate and magnesium, and good sources of manganese, molybdenum and thiamine. Lentils are especially alkalizing, which can help your enzymes work more efficiently. (People with chronic health conditions tend to be more acidic.) Beans and lentils can be found in Poached Eggs on Spicy Lentils (page 181), Breakfast Burritos (page 188), Old-Fashioned Split Pea Soup (page 208), Mushroom Lentil Soup (page 209), Lentil and Spinach Soup (page 210), Minestrone (page 211), Fassolada (page 212), Lentil Squash Salad (page 232), Roasted Garlic Dip (page 240), Chili Black Bean Dip (page 241), Artichoke and White Bean Spread (page 242), Anti-Inflammatory Hummus (page 243), Lentil Tapenade (page 244), Basic Beans (page 255), Gingery Red Lentils with Spinach and Coconut (page 256), Indian Peas and Beans (page 258), Butternut Chili (page 260), Turkey Ratatouille Chili (page 309), Spicy Lamb with Chickpeas (page 320), Lentil-Stuffed Tomatoes (page 335) and Red Beans and Greens (page 344).

> Lentils are especially alkalizing, which can help your enzymes work more efficiently. (People with chronic health conditions tend to be more acidic.)

Blueberries are rich in phytochemicals that are very protective to the body, such as phenolic acid, anthocyanins (the pigment that makes them blue) and ellagic acid. They also contain a large quantity of the potent antioxidant vitamin C. Blueberries can be found in Power Smoothie 1 (page 191) and Lemon Blueberry Almond Muffins (page 356).

Brazil nuts are a great source of monounsaturated fats, which help to protect our heart. They are also one of the highest concentrated sources of selenium, which is critical for thyroid health and works as a strong antioxidant in the body. Just one Brazil nut contains 137% of the RDA for selenium! They are also a good source of phosphorus, magnesium, manganese, copper, vitamin E, thiamine and zinc. However, these nutritious nuts are high in calories, so keep your portion sizes to a minimum. Brazil nuts are included as snacks in the 4-week meal plans (pages 148–153).

> Brazil nuts are one of the highest concentrated sources of selenium, which is critical for thyroid health and works as a strong antioxidant in the body. Just one Brazil nut contains 137% of the RDA for selenium!

Broccoli contains many important nutrients, including vitamin C, beta-carotene, folate, calcium and chromium, and is rich in cancer-fighting compounds, such as indoles and isothiocyanates. It also contains large amounts of sulforaphane glucosinolate, a potent antioxidant. Broccoli can be found in Garden-Fresh Frittata (page 184), Potato, Leek and Broccoli Soup (page 202), Marinated Vegetable Medley (page 225), Sautéed Broccoli and Red Peppers (page 328), Broccoli Cilantro Pesto with Pasta (page 329) and Steamed Vegetables with Toasted Almonds (page 338).

Buckwheat, a gluten-free grain, is high in fiber, magnesium, B vitamins and manganese. It also contains beneficial antioxidants, such as vitamin E, selenium and phenolic acids, which help protect the body's cells. Buckwheat is a great source of lignans and flavonoids, which can help to protect against certain cancers and heart disease. In addition, buckwheat may help you maintain satiety (fullness) longer than other grains. Buckwheat groats and buckwheat flour can be found in Buttermilk Buckwheat Pancakes (page 178), Buckwheat Walnut Bread (page 186) and Kasha and Beet Salad with Celery and Feta (page 228).

Celery was used in the Middle Ages to treat conditions such as anxiety, insomnia, gout and arthritis. It is a good source of vitamin A, which is important for a healthy immune system and for fighting viruses. Celery is also a source of vitamin C, thiamin, riboflavin, calcium, iron, magnesium, phosphorus and potassium, and has antibacterial, antifungal and anti-inflammatory properties. Celery can be found in a large number of recipes in this book.

Cilantro is a powerful antioxidant and a source of iron, magnesium and manganese. It helps remove heavy metals, such as mercury, from the body. Cilantro is also antibacterial and can aid in digestion by enhancing pancreatic enzyme activity and stimulating bile flow and secretions. Cilantro can be found in large amounts in Cactus Salad (page 230), Indian Peas and Beans (page 258), Butternut Chili (page 260), Mexican-Style Seafood Stew with Hominy (page 290), Spicy Peanut Chicken (page 308), Turkey Mole (page 310) and Broccoli Cilantro Pesto with Pasta (page 329), and in smaller amounts in a number of other recipes.

> Cilantro is a powerful antioxidant and a source of iron, magnesium and manganese. It helps remove heavy metals, such as mercury, from the body.

Cinnamon is a good source of manganese, iron, calcium and antioxidants, and can help lower blood sugar and reduce inflammation. Cinnamon can be found in Grain-Free Granola (page 172), Hot Oat Bran and Flax Porridge (page 176), Coconut Pancakes (page 179), Moroccan-Spiced Carrot Soup (page 197), Butternut Chili (page 260), Bengali Fish Curry (page 279), Jerk Chicken (page 301), Turkey Mole (page 310), Pork Vindaloo (page 312), Catalan Beef Stew (page 313), Spicy Lamb with Chickpeas (page 320), Spicy Cashews (page 351), Pumpkin Millet Muffins (page 358), Pumpkin Date Bars (page 360), Homemade Crunchy Granola Bars (page 361) and Cinnamon Crisps (page 363).

Coconut is a source of fiber, medium-chain triglycerides, B vitamins, manganese, copper, iron, phosphorus, magnesium, potassium, zinc and selenium. Its medicinal benefits include fighting fungi, bacteria and viruses. Coconut, coconut milk and coconut flour can be found in Grain-Free Granola (page 172), Black Sticky Rice Congee with Coconut (page 177), Coconut Pancakes (page 179), Poached Eggs on Spicy Lentils (page 181), Thai-Style Pumpkin Soup (page 204), Gingery Red Lentils with Spinach and Coconut (page 256), Indian Peas and Beans (page 258), Sweet Potato Coconut Curry with Shrimp (page 287) and Spicy Peanut Chicken (page 308).

Fennel is a good source of fiber, folate, vitamin C and potassium. It is anti-inflammatory and contains a phytochemical called anethole, which helps inhibit spasms in the intestinal tract, relieving gas pain and cramping. Since many people with thyroid disease also have gastrointestinal issues, fennel may be a helpful food to add to your diet. Fennel can be found in Roasted Portobello Mushroom and Fennel Salad (page 226).

Garlic contains a phytochemical called allicin, which has strong antibacterial, antifungal and antiviral properties. Garlic is also a strong anti-inflammatory and antioxidant. Garlic can be found in a large number of recipes in this book, with significant amounts used in Hearty Beef Stock (page 196), Roasted Garlic and Sun-Dried Tomato Dressing (page 238), Roasted Garlic Dip (page 240), Spinach and Tofu Curry (page 268), Miso Mushroom Chicken with Chinese Cabbage (page 305) and Pork Vindaloo (page 312).

Ginger contains powerful antioxidants, such as gingerol, shogaols and zingerone. Ginger is a strong anti-inflammatory and can help settle an upset stomach. Ginger can be found in large amounts in Beet Soup with Lemongrass and Lime (page 198), Thai-Inspired Peanut and Wild Rice Soup (page 203), Thai-Style Pumpkin Soup (page 204), Curried Squash and Apple Soup (page 206), Gingery Chicken and Wild Rice Soup (page 214), Gingery Red Lentils with Spinach and Coconut (page 256), Spinach and Tofu Curry (page 268) and Spicy Lamb with Chickpeas (page 320), and in smaller amounts in many other recipes.

Kale is one of the healthiest foods you can eat. It is packed with vitamin A, vitamin C and potassium, and is a good source of calcium, iron and folate. It also contains lutein, a phytochemical that enhances eye health and helps fight cancer. There is some controversy over whether cruciferous vegetables (such as kale, broccoli and cauliflower) might cause hypothyroidism, as they contain goitrogens (substances that suppress thyroid function by interfering with the uptake of iodine), but there is little research to support this, especially among those with adequate iodine stores. If you prefer to be on the safe side, cooking your cruciferous vegetables reduces the goitrogens. Kale can be found in Power Smoothie 1 (page 191), Power Smoothie 2 (page 192), Kale and Pear Salad with Warmed Shallot Dressing (page 222) and Oven-Baked Kale Chips (page 350).

Macadamia nuts are a great source of monounsaturated fats, which help to protect our heart. They are also high in omega-7 fats, which can help with weight loss by increasing the amount of fat burned and decreasing appetite. In addition, macadamia nuts are rich in flavonoids, which help to protect our cells from damage and environmental toxins. They are also a great source of vitamin A, iron and B vitamins, which are important for thyroid health. However, these nutritious nuts are high in calories, so keep your portion sizes to a minimum. Macadamia nuts are included as snacks in the 4-week meal plans (pages 148–153).

Millet, a gluten-free grain, is a good source of fiber, protein, thiamine, niacin, magnesium phosphorus, zinc, copper and manganese. Millet can be found in Hot Millet Amaranth Cereal (page 173) and Pumpkin Millet Muffins (page 358).

Mushrooms are considered a superfood and are particularly helpful for thyroid health. They are one of the best vegetable sources of selenium and vitamin D, and are good sources of riboflavin and pantothenic acid, which are important for thyroid and adrenal health. Mushrooms also have strong antioxidant activity and can help with healthy estrogen metabolism. Mushrooms are found in large amounts in Garden-Fresh Frittata (page 184), Mushroom Lentil Soup (page 209), Spinach Salad with Carrots and Mushrooms (page 223), Warm Spinach and Mushroom Salad (page 224), Roasted Portobello Mushroom and Fennel Salad (page 226), Celery Root and Mushroom Lasagna (page 262), Miso Mushroom Chicken with Chinese Cabbage (page 305) and Turkey Ratatouille Chili (page 309), and in smaller amounts in several other recipes.

> Mushrooms are considered a superfood and are particularly helpful for thyroid health. They are one of the best vegetable sources of selenium and vitamin D, and are good sources of riboflavin and pantothenic acid, which are important for thyroid and adrenal health.

Oats are a gluten-free grain, but may be contaminated with gluten during processing. Be sure to look for "certified gluten-free" oats, which have been processed in a gluten-free facility. Oats contain healthy amounts of vitamin E, several B vitamins, calcium, magnesium, potassium, selenium, copper, zinc, iron and manganese. They are also a good source of fiber. Oats and oat bran can be found in Steel-Cut Oats (page 174), Hot Oat Bran and Flax Porridge (page 176), Vegetable Quiche with Oat Groat Crust (page 272) and Homemade Crunchy Granola Bars (page 361).

Olives and extra virgin olive oil contain potent antioxidants, which protect cells. Olive oil also has antibacterial activity and contains a compound called oleocanthal, which has strong anti-inflammatory properties. Olives can be found in Fast and Easy Greek Salad (page 220), Lentil Tapenade (page 244), Mediterranean-Style Mahi-Mahi (page 280) and Italian-Style Chicken in White Wine with Olives and Polenta (page 298). Olive oil can be found in a large number of recipes in this book.

Onions are a great source of quercetin, which helps decrease inflammation and protect cells. Quercetin is also helpful with allergies, including food allergies and sensitivities. Onions contain ample inulin, which helps feed healthy bacteria in the gut. Onions can be found in a large number of recipes in this book.

Oregano has potent antibacterial, antifungal, antiparasitic and antiviral properties, and contains potent antioxidants, such as beta-carotene. It is high in vitamin K, which is important for bone health and blood clotting. Oregano is also high in beta-caryophyllene, which has strong anti-inflammatory properties. Fresh oregano can be found in Grilled Salmon with Lemon Oregano Pesto (page 284), Catalan Beef Stew (page 313) and Meatballs for Everyday (page 316). Dried oregano can be found in many other recipes in this book.

> Oregano has potent antibacterial, antifungal, antiparasitic and antiviral properties, and contains potent antioxidants, such as beta-carotene.

Peanuts are full of antioxidants, including polyphenols, resveratrol and beta-sitosterol. They are also a good source of protein. Peanuts and peanut butter can be found in Thai-Inspired Peanut and Wild Rice Soup (page 203), Shrimp and Vegetable Spring Rolls (page 288), Spicy Peanut Chicken (page 308), Crunchy Peanut Butter Muffins (page 354) and Peanut Butter Cookies (page 362).

Potatoes are a rich source of vitamin C and potassium (if the skin is left on). Potatoes with red or purple skin are high in antioxidants, which protect your cells. Potatoes can be found in Potato, Leek and Broccoli Soup (page 202), Fish Chowder (page 218), Gingery Red Lentils with Spinach and Coconut (page 256), Turkey Ratatouille Chili (page 309), Zesty Braised Beef with New Potatoes (page 314), Mix 'n' Mash Vegetables (page 337) and Creamy Mashed Potatoes with Cauliflower (page 342).

Quinoa is a gluten-free grain. Some varieties are up to 20% protein, and that protein contains all of the essential amino acids, making it equal to animal protein in the nutrition it provides. Quinoa is also a rich source of iron, potassium, several B vitamins, magnesium, zinc, copper and manganese. Quinoa can be found in Cranberry Quinoa Porridge (page 175), Beef and Quinoa Soup (page 216), Quinoa Salad (page 231), Pork Quinoa Salad with Indian Dressing (page 236), Quinoa-Stuffed Tomatoes (page 267) and Savory Vegetarian Quinoa Pilaf (page 343).

Rosemary is a strong antioxidant and inhibits bacterial growth. It is also helpful for supporting the vitamin D receptor, which helps maintain healthy vitamin D levels, critical for a healthy immune system. Rosemary can be found in Fassolada (page 212), Celery Root and Mushroom Lasagna (page 262), Cauliflower Pizza Crust (page 266), Vegetable Quiche with Oat Groat Crust (page 272), Crunchy Almond Chicken (page 296), Grilled Lamb Chops with Rosemary Mustard Baste (page 318) and Crispy-Coated Veggie Snacks (page 348).

Rosemary is a strong antioxidant and inhibits bacterial growth. It is also helpful for supporting the vitamin D receptor, which helps maintain healthy vitamin D levels, critical for a healthy immune system.

Salmon is a rich source of anti-inflammatory omega-3 fatty acids, protein, vitamin A, calcium, phosphorus, potassium, iron, magnesium, selenium and zinc. It contains an important carotenoid, astaxanthin, a potent antioxidant that gives salmon its natural orange-red coloring. Wild salmon is lower in heavy metals, such as mercury, than many other large fish. Salmon can be found in Grilled Salmon and Romaine Salad (page 234), Salmon and Wild Rice Cakes with Avocado-Chili Topping (page 281), Baked Salmon Patties (page 282), Baked Salmon with Ginger and Lemon (page 283) and Grilled Salmon with Lemon Oregano Pesto (page 284).

Sardines are a great source of anti-inflammatory omega-3 fatty acids and are high in protein and calcium. In fact, a 3-oz (90 g) serving of sardines provides as much calcium as 1 cup (250 mL) of milk. Sardines are lower in heavy metals, such as mercury, than many other fish. Sardines can be found in Sardine Spread (page 245).

Sorghum, a gluten-free grain, is a good source of niacin, riboflavin, thiamine, calcium, iron, phosphorus and potassium. It is rich in various phytochemicals, such as proanthocyanidins, phenolic acid, phytosterols and policosanols, that protect our cells from damage. Sorghum is also a great source of fiber. Sorghum flour can be found in Crêpes (page 180), Zucchini Patties (page 253), Thin Pizza Crust (page 264), Lemon

Blueberry Almond Muffins (page 356) and Pumpkin Millet Muffins (page 358).

Spinach contains high amounts of fiber, vitamin K, beta-carotene, folate, calcium, iron, magnesium and manganese. It is one of the richest sources of lutein, which is important for eye health. Lutein has also been shown to protect against several cancers and to be neuroprotective. Spinach can be found in Lentil and Spinach Soup (page 210), Minestrone (page 211), Spinach Salad with Carrots and Mushrooms (page 223), Warm Spinach and Mushroom Salad (page 224), Spinach with Almonds (page 252), Gingery Red Lentils with Spinach and Coconut (page 256), Spinach and Tofu Curry (page 268), Crustless Dill Spinach Quiche with Mushrooms and Cheese (page 274) and Indian-Style Chicken with Puréed Spinach (page 306).

Eight strawberries contain more vitamin C than an orange, with less sugar.

Strawberries are rich in antioxidants. Eight strawberries contain more vitamin C than an orange, with less sugar. Strawberries are also high in anthocyanins, ellagic acid, quercetin, catechin and kaempferol, which help protect cells from damage. Strawberries can be found in Power Smoothie 2 (page 192).

Sunflower seeds are a good source of vitamin E, folate, magnesium, selenium and copper. They are also high in phytosterols, which may help with healthy cholesterol metabolism. Sunflower seeds can be found in Hot Oat Bran and Flax Porridge (page 176).

Tomatoes are a great source of vitamin C and potassium, and an excellent source of the phytochemical lycopene, which is anti-inflammatory and anticarcinogenic (it fights cancer). Tomatoes can be found in a large number of recipes in this book.

Turmeric contains important vitamins and minerals, such as iron, manganese, potassium, vitamin B_6 and vitamin C. It is also high in the phytochemical curcumin, which strengthens the immune system, lowers inflammation, improves digestion and helps fight viruses, such as Epstein-Barr. Turmeric can be found in Indian Scrambled Eggs (page 182), Moroccan-Spiced Carrot Soup (page 197), Anti-Inflammatory Hummus (page 243), Gingery Red Lentils with Spinach and Coconut (page 256), Indian Peas and Beans (page 258), Bengali Fish Curry (page 279), Onion-Braised Shrimp (page 294), Tandoori Chicken with Cucumber Mint Raita (page 304), Indian-Style Chicken with Puréed Spinach (page 306) and Spicy Lamb with Chickpeas (page 320).

Walnuts are a rich source of anti-inflammatory omega-3 fatty acids, B vitamins, vitamin E, phosphorus, magnesium and copper. They are also rich in ellagitannins, a type of polyphenol, which have strong antioxidant and cancer-fighting properties. Walnuts can be found in Buckwheat Walnut Bread (page 186), Vichyssoise with Celery Root and Watercress (page 200), Kale and Pear Salad with Warmed Shallot Dressing (page 222), Warm Spinach and Mushroom Salad (page 224) and Pumpkin Date Bars (page 360).

Yogurt is a rich source of calcium and probiotics (healthy bacteria for the gut). Making your own yogurt and fermenting it for 24 hours will help increase the healthy bacteria count and reduce the lactose content for those who are lactose-intolerant (because the bacteria eats the lactose). Yogurt can be found in Mango Yogurt Smoothie (page 190), Pork Quinoa Salad with Indian Dressing (page 236), Green Goddess Salad Dressing (page 237), Roasted Garlic and Sun-Dried Tomato Dressing (page 238), Creamy Basil Pesto (page 247), Cucumber Mint Raita (page 248), Wild Rice Cakes (page 254), Bengali Fish Curry (page 279), Onion-Braised Shrimp (page 294), Crunchy Almond Chicken (page 296), Indian-Style Grilled Chicken Breasts (page 302), Tandoori Chicken with Cucumber Mint Raita (page 304) and Crispy-Coated Veggie Snacks (page 348).

Making your own yogurt and fermenting it for 24 hours will help increase the healthy bacteria count and reduce the lactose content for those who are lactose-intolerant

About the Nutrient Analysis

The nutrient analysis done on the recipes in this book was derived from the Food Processor SQL Nutrition Analysis Software, version 10.9, ESHA Research (2011). Where necessary, data were supplemented using the following references:

1. USDA National Nutrient Database for Standard Reference, Release #27 (2014). Retrieved January 2015, from www.nal.usda.gov/fnic/foodcomp/search.
2. Vitacost (2015). Nutrition Facts Pea Protein Vanilla. Retrieved January 2015, from www.vitacost.com/vitacost-pea-protein-vanilla-28-4-oz-1-lb-12-4-oz-805-g-non-gmo-4.

Recipes were evaluated as follows:

- The larger number of servings was used where there is a range.
- The smaller quantity of an ingredient was used there is a range.
- Where alternatives are given, the first ingredient and amount listed were used.
- Optional ingredients and ingredients that are not quantified were not included.
- Calculations were based on imperial measures and weights.
- Nutrient values for fat, carbohydrate, fiber, protein, vitamin A and magnesium were rounded to the nearest whole number. Nutrient values for iron, zinc and selenium were rounded to one decimal point.
- Calculations involving meat and poultry used lean portions without skin.
- Recipes were analyzed prior to cooking.

It is important to note that the cooking method used to prepare the recipe may alter the nutrient content per serving, as may ingredient substitutions and differences among brand-name products.

Breakfasts

Grain-Free Granola 172

Hot Millet Amaranth Cereal 173

Steel-Cut Oats 174

Cranberry Quinoa Porridge 175

Hot Oat Bran and Flax Porridge 176

Black Sticky Rice Congee with Coconut. 177

Buttermilk Buckwheat Pancakes. 178

Coconut Pancakes. 179

Crêpes 180

Poached Eggs on Spicy Lentils 181

Indian Scrambled Eggs 182

Western Omelet 183

Garden-Fresh Frittata 184

Buckwheat Walnut Bread 186

Breakfast Burritos 188

Vanilla Almond Milk 189

Mango Yogurt Smoothie. 190

Power Smoothie 1 191

Power Smoothie 2 192

Grain-Free Granola

Because this granola is grain-free, it is a great gluten-free alternative to store-bought granolas. It is also higher in protein and healthy fats.

Makes about 2½ cups (625 mL)

TIP

This granola is great with homemade Vanilla Almond Milk (page 189) or yogurt, or on its own as a crunchy snack!

- **Preheat oven to 300°F (150°C)**
- **Baking sheet, lightly greased**

1 cup	raw almonds, finely chopped	250 mL
½ cup	raw cashews, finely chopped	125 mL
½ cup	raw green pumpkin seeds (pepitas)	125 mL
½ cup	unsweetened flaked coconut	125 mL
¼ cup	liquid honey	60 mL
¼ cup	virgin coconut oil	60 mL
2 tsp	ground cinnamon	10 mL
½ tsp	salt	2 mL
½ tsp	GF vanilla extract	2 mL

1. In a large bowl, combine almonds, cashews, pumpkin seeds and coconut.

2. In a small saucepan, melt honey and coconut oil over medium heat. Stir in cinnamon, salt and vanilla; bring to a boil.

3. Slowly pour honey mixture over nut mixture, stirring until well combined. Spread into a thin layer on prepared baking sheet.

4. Bake in preheated oven for 25 minutes, stirring every 5 to 10 minutes to keep mixture from burning, until golden brown. Let cool completely on a wire rack. As it cools, the mixture will harden. Once cool, break apart into smaller clusters. Store in an airtight container at room temperature for up to 2 weeks.

Nutrients per ¼ cup (60 mL)

Calories	236
Fat	19 g
Carbohydrate	14 g
Fiber	3 g
Protein	5 g
Vitamin A	2 IU
Iron	1.5 mg
Magnesium	83 mg
Zinc	1.3 mg
Selenium	2.5 mcg

Health-Enhancing Tip

For easier digestion, soak and dry the nuts and seeds before starting the recipe. Place the nuts and seeds in a pot and add enough purified drinking water to cover them by about 2 inches (5 cm). Cover the pot and let stand at room temperature for 12 to 24 hours. Drain and transfer nuts and seeds to a baking sheet, spreading them out in a single layer. Dry in a 150°F (70°C) oven for 12 to 24 hours. When nuts are dry, proceed with step 1.

Hot Millet Amaranth Cereal

Here's a great way to start your day and add variety to your diet. Both millet and amaranth are relatively quick and easy to cook — so long as you keep the temperature low, they don't need to be stirred. Use a sweetener of your choice and add fruit and nuts as you please.

Makes 6 servings

TIPS

For best results, toast the millet and amaranth before cooking. Stir the grains in a dry skillet over medium heat until they crackle and release their aroma, about 5 minutes.

If you're having trouble digesting grains, try soaking them overnight in warm non-chlorinated water (about 2 parts water to 1 part grain) with a spoonful or so of cider vinegar. Drain, rinse and cook in the morning.

2½ cups	water	625 mL
½ cup	millet, toasted (see tips, at left)	125 mL
½ cup	amaranth	125 mL
	Liquid honey, pure maple syrup or raw cane sugar	
	Milk or non-dairy alternative	
	Dried cranberries, cherries or raisins (optional)	
	Toasted chopped nuts (optional)	

1. In a saucepan over medium heat, bring water to a boil. Add millet and amaranth in a steady stream, stirring constantly. Return to a boil. Reduce heat to low (see tip, page 175). Cover and simmer until grains are tender and liquid is absorbed, about 25 minutes. Serve hot, sweetened to taste and with milk or non-dairy alternative. Sprinkle with dried fruit and nuts, if desired.

Health-Enhancing Tips

To increase the protein content per serving, add 1 to 2 scoops of protein powder (organic rice, organic pea, hemp or whey from grass-fed cows not given antibiotics or hormones) just before serving. You may need to add 1 to 2 tbsp (15 to 30 mL) more milk to achieve your desired consistency.

Add the optional nuts and/or 1 tbsp (15 mL) chia seeds or ground flax seeds (flaxseed meal) per serving.

Because the amount of sweetener is not specified in this recipe, it is not included in the nutrient analysis. Be aware that the sugar and carbohydrate content will increase based on the amount of sweetener you add. Adding the optional dried fruit will increase them even more.

Nutrients per serving

Calories	123
Fat	2 g
Carbohydrate	23 g
Fiber	3 g
Protein	4 g
Vitamin A	0 IU
Iron	1.7 mg
Magnesium	60 mg
Zinc	0.8 mg
Selenium	3.5 mcg

Steel-Cut Oats

Steel-cut oats, often sold under the name "Irish Oatmeal," have more flavor than rolled oats and an appealing crunchy texture. They also have much more fiber, which will have a positive impact on post-meal blood sugars, improve digestion and increase fullness.

Makes 4 servings

TIPS

You can halve this recipe, but be sure to use a small (1½- to 2-quart) slow cooker.

If you prefer a creamier version of this cereal, make it using half 2% evaporated milk and half water. If using half evaporated milk (2 cups/500 mL), the nutrient content increases dramatically. For only an extra 100 calories, you get 15 g carb, 10 g protein, 504 IU vitamin A, 35 mg magnesium and 1.2 mg of zinc per serving.

- **Small to medium (1½- to 3½-quart) slow cooker, stoneware lightly greased**

1 cup	certified GF steel-cut oats	250 mL
½ tsp	sea salt	2 mL
4 cups	water	1 L
	Raisins, chopped bananas or pitted dates (optional)	
	Toasted nuts or seeds (optional)	
	Milk (optional)	

1. In prepared slow cooker, combine oats and salt. Add water. Cover and cook on High for 4 hours or on Low for 8 hours or overnight. Stir well. If desired, stir in fruit to taste, garnish with nuts or seeds, or add milk.

Health-Enhancing Tips

To increase the protein content per serving, stir in 1 scoop of protein power (organic rice, organic pea, hemp or whey from grass-fed cows not given antibiotics or hormones) and/or 1 tbsp (15 mL) ground flax seeds (flaxseed meal) just before serving. You may need to add more water or milk to achieve your desired consistency. Or add the optional nuts or seeds.

Be careful when adding dried fruits and banana, as these will increase the carbohydrate content significantly. The best fruit to add would be ¼ cup (60 mL) fresh or thawed frozen organic berries per serving.

Nutrients per serving

Calories	170
Fat	3 g
Carbohydrate	29 g
Fiber	5 g
Protein	7 g
Vitamin A	0 IU
Iron	1.8 mg
Magnesium	2 mg
Zinc	0.0 mg
Selenium	0.0 mcg

Cranberry Quinoa Porridge

If you're not organized enough to make hot cereal ahead of time, here's one you can enjoy in less than 30 minutes, start to finish, and that doesn't require any attention while it's cooking. Quinoa is a truly amazing grain. Some varieties are up to 20% protein, and that protein contains all of the essential amino acids, making it equal to animal protein in the nutrition it provides.

Makes 6 servings

3 cups	water	750 mL
1 cup	quinoa, rinsed	250 mL
½ cup	dried cranberries	125 mL
	Pure maple syrup or liquid honey	
	Milk or non-dairy alternative (optional)	

TIP

Unless you have a stove with a true simmer, after reducing the heat to low, place a heat diffuser under the pot to prevent the mixture from boiling. This also helps ensure the grains cook evenly and prevents hot spots, which might cause scorching, from forming. Heat diffusers are available at kitchen supply and hardware stores and are made to work on gas or electric stoves.

1. In a saucepan over medium heat, bring water to a boil. Stir in quinoa and cranberries and return to a boil. Reduce heat to low. Cover and simmer until quinoa is cooked (look for a white line around the seeds), about 15 minutes. Remove from heat and let stand, covered, about 5 minutes. Serve with maple syrup and, if desired, milk or non-dairy alternative.

Variations

Substitute dried cherries or blueberries or raisins for the cranberries.

Use red quinoa for a change.

Nutrients per serving

Calories	137
Fat	2 g
Carbohydrate	27 g
Fiber	2 g
Protein	4 g
Vitamin A	0 IU
Iron	1.4 mg
Magnesium	56 mg
Zinc	0.9 mg
Selenium	2.5 mcg

Health-Enhancing Tips

To decrease the sugar and carbohydrate content of this recipe, replace the dried cranberries with ⅓ cup (75 mL) fresh or thawed frozen blueberries. The sweetener (maple syrup or honey) is not included in the nutrient analysis, so omit it to avoid adding even more sugar and carbohydrate. If you want to add some sweetness, try organic stevia leaf, which will not add carbs. Stevia is very sweet, so start with just a small amount and add more if needed.

To increase the protein content per serving, add 1 scoop of protein powder just before serving. You may need to add additional water, milk or non-dairy alternative to achieve your desired consistency.

Add ¼ cup (60 mL) nuts or seeds per serving for extra protein, healthy fat and fiber.

Hot Oat Bran and Flax Porridge

If you're not fond of oatmeal made with quick-cooking rolled oats, try this deliciously creamy porridge instead. It has a sweet oats flavor and smooth texture, takes no time to prepare — and it's nourishing, too!

Makes 1 serving

TIPS

Ground flax seeds (flaxseed meal), hemp seeds and chia seeds contain oil, so store them in airtight containers in the refrigerator or freezer.

Microwave Method: Combine milk and bran in a 4-cup (1 L) glass measuring cup or heatproof bowl and microwave on High, stirring once, for 3 minutes or until mixture comes to a boil and thickens. Continue with step 2.

⅓ cup	certified GF oat bran	75 mL
1 cup	low-fat (1%) milk or plain soy milk	250 mL
1 tbsp	ground flax seeds (flaxseed meal)	15 mL
1 tbsp	dried cranberries	15 mL
1 tbsp	toasted unsalted sunflower seeds	15 mL
¼ tsp	ground cinnamon	1 mL

1. In a small saucepan, combine oat bran and milk. Bring to a boil over medium-high heat. Reduce heat and simmer, stirring, for 1 to 2 minutes or until thickened. Remove from heat.

2. Stir in flax seeds, cranberries and sunflower seeds; sprinkle with cinnamon. Serve immediately.

Health-Enhancing Tips

To reduce the carbohydrate content of this recipe, omit the dried cranberries.

To increase the protein content, add 1 to 2 scoops of protein powder (organic rice, organic pea, hemp or whey from grass-fed cows not given antibiotics or hormones) with the flax seeds. You may need to add more milk to achieve your desired consistency.

Nutrients per serving

Calories	289
Fat	12 g
Carbohydrate	44 g
Fiber	8 g
Protein	17 g
Vitamin A	481 IU
Iron	2.6 mg
Magnesium	139 mg
Zinc	2.8 mg
Selenium	30.4 mcg

Black Sticky Rice Congee with Coconut

This is a substantial serving (about 1 cup/250 mL), so it will certainly keep you satisfied throughout the morning. Congee is typically described as porridge, but it's actually more like soup.

Makes 6 servings

TIPS

You can halve this recipe, but be sure to use a small (1½- to 2-quart) slow cooker.

The carbs and fats in this recipe are almost equally balanced (51.4% and 49.6% respectively). That means the fat also balances any potential blood sugar impact of the carbohydrates, provided mainly by the rice, coconut sugar and bananas.

• **Small to medium (1½- to 3½-quart) slow cooker, stoneware lightly greased**

3 cups	water	750 mL
⅓ cup	black sticky rice	75 mL
½ cup	coconut sugar	125 mL
1 tsp	GF almond extract	5 mL
Pinch	sea salt	Pinch
1	can (14 oz/400 mL) coconut milk	1
2	bananas, sliced	2
¼ cup	chopped toasted almonds	60 mL

1. In a small saucepan over high heat, bring water and black sticky rice to a vigorous boil. Boil for 2 minutes. Stir in coconut sugar, almond extract and salt, then transfer to slow cooker stoneware.

2. Cover and cook on Low for 8 hours or overnight, or on High for 4 hours. Stir well, then stir in coconut milk.

3. Ladle congee into bowls and top with bananas and almonds, dividing equally. Refrigerate any leftovers. This reheats beautifully on the stovetop or in a microwave.

Nutrients per serving

Calories	300
Fat	17 g
Carbohydrate	39 g
Fiber	2 g
Protein	3 g
Vitamin A	22 IU
Iron	3.6 mg
Magnesium	55 mg
Zinc	0.7 mg
Selenium	2.1 mcg

Health-Enhancing Tips

To reduce the carbohydrate content of this recipe, use an equal amount of xylitol or puréed fruit in place of the coconut sugar and replace the banana with 1⅓ cups (325 mL) blueberries. To add flavor, add ½ to 1 tsp (2 to 5 mL) ground cinnamon, which can help lower blood sugar and decrease inflammation.

To increase the protein content per serving, stir in 1 scoop of protein powder (organic rice, organic pea, hemp or whey from grass-fed cows not given antibiotics or hormones) before eating. You may need to add 1 to 2 tbsp (15 to 30 mL) more coconut milk or other fluid, to desired consistency.

Buttermilk Buckwheat Pancakes

Pancakes are many people's favorite breakfast, and finding a healthy, tasty gluten-free option can be a challenge. This delicious option is a perfect treat for a post-workout meal.

Makes 12 pancakes

TIP

Buckwheat flour is available in natural foods stores. If you don't have it, you can make your own by processing toasted buckwheat groats (kasha) in a food processor until finely ground.

MAKE AHEAD

You can make this batter ahead and keep, covered, in the refrigerator for up to 2 days. The batter will thicken a bit, so you may need to add a little buttermilk to thin it out.

Nutrients per 2 pancakes

Calories	214
Fat	4 g
Carbohydrate	37 g
Fiber	4 g
Protein	10 g
Vitamin A	104 IU
Iron	2.1 mg
Magnesium	123 mg
Zinc	1.6 mg
Selenium	7.8 mcg

- **Food processor**

2½ cups	buttermilk	625 mL
2 tsp	GF baking powder	10 mL
1 tsp	baking soda	5 mL
½ tsp	salt	2 mL
1 tbsp	light (fancy) molasses	15 mL
1	large egg	1
2 cups	buckwheat flour (see tip, at left)	500 mL

1. In food processor, combine buttermilk, baking powder, baking soda and salt. Pulse to blend. Add molasses and egg and pulse to blend. Add buckwheat flour and pulse just until combined. Set aside for 5 minutes. Mixture should be of a pourable consistency. If necessary, add more flour or buttermilk and pulse until blended.

2. Heat a lightly greased nonstick skillet over medium heat until water dropped on the surface bounces before evaporating. Add about ¼ cup (60 mL) batter at a time and cook until bubbles appear all over the top surface, then flip and cook until bottom side is browned, about 1 minute per side. Keep warm. Continue with the remaining batter.

Health-Enhancing Tips

To increase the protein content of this recipe, add 1 to 2 scoops of protein powder (organic rice, organic pea, hemp or whey from grass-fed cows not given antibiotics or hormones) to the batter. You may need to add 1 to 2 tbsp (15 to 30 mL) more buttermilk to achieve a pourable consistency.

If you enjoy moist pancakes, you can add ¾ cup (175 mL) organic cottage cheese to the batter for added protein. The pancakes will be a bit heavier.

Coconut Pancakes

Coconut pancakes are a great grain-free, lower-carbohydrate alternative to traditional pancakes. They also provide easily digested medium-chain triglycerides and fiber, which will keep you full for longer. Serve with your choice of topping.

Makes about 14 small pancakes

TIP

Ghee is a type of clarified butter highly valued in Indian cooking as it can be heated to a very high temperature. It is available in grocery stores specializing in Indian ingredients and will keep, refrigerated, for as long as a year.

½ cup	coconut flour	125 mL
1 tsp	baking soda	5 mL
1 tsp	ground cinnamon	5 mL
4	large eggs	4
1 cup	well-stirred coconut milk	250 mL
1 tbsp	dark (cooking) molasses	15 mL
1 tsp	GF vanilla extract	5 mL
	Ghee (see tip, at left) or virgin coconut oil	

1. In a small bowl, whisk together flour, baking soda and cinnamon.

2. In a large bowl, beat eggs, coconut milk, molasses and vanilla. Stir in flour mixture until well blended.

3. Heat a griddle or nonstick skillet greased well with ghee or coconut oil over medium heat. For each pancake, pour in a heaping tbsp (15 mL) batter. Cook until bubbles start to form and edges are firm. Flip over and cook until bottom is golden brown. Transfer to a plate and keep warm. Repeat with the remaining batter, greasing griddle and adjusting heat between batches as needed.

Nutrients per 2 pancakes

Calories	153
Fat	13 g
Carbohydrate	5 g
Fiber	1 g
Protein	5 g
Vitamin A	155 IU
Iron	1.9 mg
Magnesium	31 mg
Zinc	0.7 mg
Selenium	10.4 mcg

Crêpes

These crêpes are a great alternative to traditional wheat flour crêpes. In addition to being gluten-free, the sorghum flour adds health benefits, such as increased fiber.

Makes 10 crêpes

TIP

Choose your favorite GF non-dairy milk, such as soy, rice, almond or potato-based milk or, if you tolerate lactose, use regular 1% lactose-free milk.

MAKE AHEAD

Crêpes can be prepared ahead of time, cooled, layered between sheets of parchment paper and stored in an airtight container in the refrigerator for up to 3 days. Just before serving, reheat each crêpe on a plate in the microwave on High for about 20 seconds.

- **9-inch (23 cm) skillet**

½ cup	sorghum flour	125 mL
½ cup	potato starch	125 mL
½ tsp	granulated raw cane sugar	2 mL
2	large eggs	2
½ cup	lactose-free 1% milk or fortified GF non-dairy milk	125 mL
2 tbsp	butter or vegan hard margarine, melted	30 mL
	Butter or vegan hard margarine	

1. In a large bowl, using a whisk, combine sorghum flour, potato starch and sugar.

2. In another bowl, beat eggs, milk, melted butter and ½ cup (125 mL) water. Stir into flour mixture until well blended.

3. In skillet, melt ½ tsp (2 mL) butter over medium heat, making sure to coat the bottom of the skillet. For each crêpe, pour in a scant ¼ cup (60 mL) batter and swirl so that the batter covers the whole surface. Cook for about 1 minute or until edges start to curl up. Flip over and cook for 1 minute or until bottom is golden. Transfer to a plate and keep warm. Repeat with the remaining batter, adjusting heat and melting ½ tsp (2 mL) butter between each batch as needed.

Health-Enhancing Tip

For a healthier, less inflammatory fat, use organic butter or ghee (see tip, page 179).

Nutrients per crêpe

Calories	105
Fat	4 g
Carbohydrate	16 g
Fiber	1 g
Protein	3 g
Vitamin A	150 IU
Iron	0.6 mg
Magnesium	3 mg
Zinc	0.2 mg
Selenium	3.3 mcg

Poached Eggs on Spicy Lentils

This delicious combination is a great cold-weather dish. The Egg and Lentil Curry (see variation, below) is a high-protein option. This dish is also packed with health-promoting ingredients to help you regain your health.

Makes 6 servings

TIPS

You can halve this recipe, but be sure to use a small (1½- to 3-quart) slow cooker.

To poach eggs, in a deep skillet, bring about 2 inches (5 cm) lightly salted water to a boil over medium heat. Reduce heat to low. Break eggs into a measuring cup and, holding the cup close to the surface of the water, slip the eggs into the pan. Cook until whites are set and centers are still soft, 3 to 4 minutes. Remove with a slotted spoon.

Nutrients per serving

Calories	321
Fat	16 g
Carbohydrate	30 g
Fiber	6 g
Protein	17 g
Vitamin A	825 IU
Iron	6.2 mg
Magnesium	66 mg
Zinc	2.4 mg
Selenium	18.3 mcg

- **Medium (about 4-quart) slow cooker**

1 tbsp	olive oil	15 mL
2	onions, finely chopped	2
1 tbsp	minced garlic	15 mL
1 tbsp	minced gingerroot	15 mL
1 tsp	ground coriander	5 mL
1 tsp	ground cumin	5 mL
1 tsp	cracked black peppercorns	5 mL
1 cup	dried red lentils, rinsed	250 mL
1	can (28 oz/796 mL) no-salt-added tomatoes, with juice, coarsely chopped	1
2 cups	ready-to-use GF vegetable broth	500 mL
1 cup	coconut milk	250 mL
	Salt	
1	long green chile pepper (or 2 Thai bird's-eye chiles), finely chopped (optional)	1
6	poached eggs (see tip, at left)	6
¼ cup	finely chopped fresh parsley leaves	60 mL

1. In a large skillet, heat oil over medium heat. Add onions and cook, stirring, until softened, about 3 minutes. Add garlic, ginger, coriander, cumin and peppercorns and cook, stirring, for 1 minute. Add lentils, tomatoes and broth and bring to a boil. Transfer to slow cooker stoneware.

2. Cover and cook on Low for 6 hours or on High for 4 hours, until lentils are tender and mixture is bubbly. Stir in coconut milk, salt to taste and chile pepper (if using). Cover and cook for 20 to 30 minutes, until heated through.

3. Ladle into soup bowls and top each serving with a poached egg. Garnish with parsley.

Variation

Egg and Lentil Curry: Substitute 4 to 6 hard-cooked eggs for the poached. Peel them and cut into halves. Ladle the curry into a serving dish, arrange the eggs on top and garnish.

Indian Scrambled Eggs

This dish is an exciting alternative to regular scrambled eggs, and is packed with health-promoting ingredients.

Makes 2 to 3 servings

VARIATION

Sauté chopped non-starchy vegetables (broccoli, cauliflower, spinach, zucchini, kale, collard greens, sea vegetables) with the onion, increasing the cooking time as needed.

8	large eggs	8
1 tsp	salt (or to taste)	5 mL
¼ tsp	freshly ground black pepper	1 mL
3 tbsp	vegetable oil	45 mL
1 tsp	cumin seeds	5 mL
1 cup	chopped onion	250 mL
2 tsp	finely chopped green chile peppers (preferably serranos)	10 mL
1 cup	chopped tomato	250 mL
½ tsp	cayenne pepper	2 mL
¼ tsp	ground turmeric	1 mL
¼ cup	fresh cilantro leaves, chopped	60 mL
	Tomato wedges and fresh cilantro sprigs	

1. In a bowl, gently whisk eggs, salt and black pepper. Do not beat.

2. In a large skillet, heat oil over medium-high heat and add cumin seeds. Stir in onion and green chiles and sauté until golden, 3 to 4 minutes.

3. Add tomato and sauté, stirring continuously, for 1 minute. Stir in cayenne, turmeric and cilantro. Cook for 1 minute. Reduce heat to medium-low and slowly add egg mixture. Cook, stirring gently, until eggs are soft and creamy, 3 to 4 minutes. Do not overcook.

4. Serve garnished with tomato wedges and cilantro sprigs.

Nutrients per serving (1 of 3)

Calories	352
Fat	27 g
Carbohydrate	9 g
Fiber	2 g
Protein	18 g
Vitamin A	1365 IU
Iron	3.2 mg
Magnesium	32 mg
Zinc	2.0 mg
Selenium	41.3 mcg

Health-Enhancing Tips

For a healthier fat, substitute ghee (see tip, page 179) for the vegetable oil.

To decrease the fat content, use 16 large egg whites in place of the 8 whole eggs and decrease the cooking time to 2 to 3 minutes.

Western Omelet

This omelet is delicious tucked between slices of GF toast or wrapped in a steamed collard green and accompanied by avocado, tomato slices, spinach and sprouts.

Makes 1 serving

TIP

Use the cooking method in this recipe to create a simple omelet with or without the vegetables. Serve with a toasted GF English muffin.

2	large egg whites	2
1	large egg	1
1 tbsp	freshly grated Parmesan cheese	15 mL
	Freshly ground black pepper	
1 tsp	extra virgin olive oil	1 mL
2 tbsp	finely chopped green onion or yellow onion	30 mL
¼ cup	finely chopped green or red bell pepper	60 mL
¼ cup	chopped mushrooms	60 mL

1. In a bowl, whisk together egg whites, egg and Parmesan. Season with pepper.

2. In small nonstick skillet, heat oil over medium heat. Add green onion, green pepper and mushrooms; cook, stirring, for about 2 minutes or until softened.

3. Pour in egg mixture and stir briefly with a heatproof rubber spatula. Cook for about 1 minute, using spatula to lift cooked edges to allow uncooked egg to flow underneath, until underside is golden and top is set. Fold omelet in half.

Health-Enhancing Tip

To make this recipe more alkaline, sauté an additional ½ cup (125 mL) fresh or thawed frozen vegetables with the onion, pepper and mushrooms, increasing the cooking time as needed.

Nutrients per serving

Calories	183
Fat	11 g
Carbohydrate	5 g
Fiber	1 g
Protein	16 g
Vitamin A	576 IU
Iron	1.4 mg
Magnesium	21 mg
Zinc	1.1 mg
Selenium	33.5 mcg

Garden-Fresh Frittata

A frittata can be described as a Spanish-Italian omelet or a crustless quiche and makes a quick and easy any-time-of-day meal. This recipe is packed full of health-promoting nutrition.

Makes 4 to 6 servings

TIP

To clean leeks, trim roots and wilted green ends. Peel off tough outer layer. Cut leeks in half lengthwise and rinse under cold running water, separating the leaves so the water gets between the layers. Trim individual leaves at the point where they start to become dark in color and coarse in texture — this will be higher up on the plant the closer you get to the center.

Nutrients per serving (1 of 6)

Calories	239
Fat	13 g
Carbohydrate	12 g
Fiber	3 g
Protein	19 g
Vitamin A	1815 IU
Iron	1.8 mg
Magnesium	31 mg
Zinc	1.7 mg
Selenium	23.2 mcg

- **Preheat broiler**
- **9- to 10-inch (23 to 25 cm) ovenproof nonstick or cast-iron skillet**

1 tbsp	extra virgin olive oil	15 mL
2	leeks (white and light green parts only), coarsely chopped	2
2	cloves garlic, minced	2
½	red bell pepper, cut into ½-inch (1 cm) cubes	½
2 cups	thickly sliced mushrooms	500 mL
1	small zucchini, cut into ¼-inch (0.5 cm) slices	1
8	large egg whites (1 cup/250 mL)	8
4	large eggs	4
1 tsp	Dijon mustard	5 mL
¼ cup	snipped fresh chives	60 mL
2 tbsp	snipped fresh parsley	30 mL
2 tsp	dried tarragon	10 mL
½ tsp	salt	2 mL
Pinch	freshly ground white pepper	Pinch
1 cup	broccoli florets, cooked	500 mL
1½ cups	shredded Swiss cheese	375 mL

1. In skillet, heat olive oil over medium heat. Add leeks, garlic, red pepper and mushrooms. Cook, stirring frequently, for 5 minutes or until tender. Add zucchini and cook, stirring, for 2 to 3 minutes or until vegetables are softened. Remove skillet from heat and reduce heat to medium-low.

2. In a large bowl, whisk together egg whites, eggs, Dijon mustard, chives, parsley, tarragon, salt and pepper. Add broccoli and Swiss cheese, stirring to combine.

3. Pour into skillet over vegetables. Cook, without stirring, for 9 to 11 minutes or until bottom and sides are firm yet top is still slightly runny.

If you are using pre-shredded cheese, check the label to make sure the manufacturer has not added a product containing gluten to prevent sticking.

4. Place under preheated broiler, 3 inches (7.5 cm) from the element, until golden brown and set, 2 to 5 minutes.

5. Cut into wedges and serve hot from the oven or at room temperature. Refrigerate, covered, for up to 2 days. Reheat individual wedges, uncovered, in microwave on Medium (50%) for $1\frac{1}{2}$ to 2 minutes, just until hot, if desired.

Variations

For a change from a vegetarian frittata, add cooked chicken, smoked salmon or crisp bacon and use only 1 cup (250 mL) of mushrooms and 1 leek.

Use different varieties of mushrooms for a more intense flavor.

Health-Enhancing Tip

To make this recipe more alkaline, add more snipped fresh herbs, such as cilantro, rosemary, thyme or basil.

Buckwheat Walnut Bread

This is the bread for those who love to combine strong, robust flavors — buckwheat, whole bean flour and cardamom, which also add incredible health benefits to your bread.

Makes 12 slices

TIPS

Buckwheat flour is very fine, with a unique strong, musty, slightly nutty, slightly sour flavor.

Be sure to use potato starch, not potato flour, to make this bread.

Nutrients per slice

Calories	195
Fat	10 g
Carbohydrate	23 g
Fiber	3 g
Protein	6 g
Vitamin A	48 IU
Iron	1.3 mg
Magnesium	26 mg
Zinc	0.5 mg
Selenium	4.1 mcg

- 9- by 5-inch (23 by 12.5 cm) loaf pan, lightly greased

1 cup	whole bean flour	250 mL
1/3 cup	buckwheat flour	75 mL
1/2 cup	potato starch	125 mL
1/4 cup	tapioca starch	60 mL
1/4 cup	packed brown sugar	60 mL
2 tsp	xanthan gum	10 mL
1 tbsp	bread machine or instant yeast	15 mL
1 tsp	salt	5 mL
3/4 tsp	ground cardamom	3 mL
3/4 cup	chopped walnuts	175 mL
1 1/4 cups	water	300 mL
1 tsp	cider vinegar	5 mL
3 tbsp	vegetable oil	45 mL
2	large eggs	2

1. In a large bowl or plastic bag, combine whole bean flour, buckwheat flour, potato starch, tapioca starch, brown sugar, xanthan gum, yeast, salt, cardamom and walnuts. Mix well and set aside.

2. In a separate bowl, using a heavy-duty electric mixer with paddle attachment, combine water, vinegar, oil and eggs until well blended.

3. With the mixer on lowest speed, slowly add the dry ingredients until combined. With a rubber spatula, scrape the bottom and sides of the bowl. With the mixer on medium speed, beat for 4 minutes.

VARIATIONS

Substitute brown rice flour for the buckwheat flour.

Substitute fresh, dried or frozen blueberries for the walnuts. Fold the fruit in just before spooning into pan.

Substitute an equal amount of nutmeg for the cardamom.

4. Spoon into prepared pan. Let rise, uncovered, in a warm, draft-free place for 60 to 75 minutes or until the dough has risen to the top of the pan. Meanwhile, preheat oven to 350°F (180°C). Bake for 35 to 45 minutes or until the loaf sounds hollow when tapped on the bottom.

Health-Enhancing Tips

For a healthier, less inflammatory fat, use ghee (see tip, page 179), organic butter or olive oil in place of the vegetable oil.

Serve with a poached egg, tomato, sprouts and avocado, or salmon lox with tomato, sprouts and avocado.

Breakfast Burritos

These burritos are fantastic for breakfast — or any meal, for that matter. Like most burritos, they contain beans, which are rich in fiber and protein and are naturally alkalizing. Serve with sliced avocado, tomato and mango.

Makes 6 servings

TIPS

You can substitute GF Cheddar-style rice cheese for the Cheddar cheese.

If you already have crêpes made, be sure to microwave them on High for 20 seconds before assembling.

If you are using pre-shredded cheese, check the label to make sure the manufacturer has not added a product containing gluten to prevent sticking.

1 tsp	grapeseed oil	5 mL
1½ cups	rinsed drained canned black beans	375 mL
½ cup	salsa	125 mL
¼ cup	chopped drained pickled hot peppers	60 mL
4	large eggs, beaten	4
1 cup	shredded Cheddar cheese, divided	250 mL
6	Crêpes (page 180)	6

1. In a skillet, heat oil over medium-high heat. Sauté black beans for 3 to 5 minutes or until heated through. Add salsa and hot peppers; sauté for 3 to 5 minutes or until heated through. Add eggs and cook, stirring, until set. Remove from heat and stir in half the cheese.

2. Spoon one-sixth of the egg mixture along the center of each crêpe. Top with the remaining cheese and roll up.

Health-Enhancing Tips

To make this recipe more alkaline, add up to 1 cup (250 mL) of sautéed vegetables (broccoli, cauliflower, spinach, zucchini, kale, collard greens, sea vegetables, tomato).

Substitute small GF tortillas for the crêpes.

Nutrients per serving

Calories	255
Fat	9 g
Carbohydrate	28 g
Fiber	5 g
Protein	15 g
Vitamin A	512 IU
Iron	2.5 mg
Magnesium	32.5 mg
Zinc	1.3 mg
Selenium	17.1 mcg

Vanilla Almond Milk

This is a delicious dairy-free option to cow's milk, a problematic food for many people with thyroid disease. It is also easy to make, tastes better and is less expensive than store-bought almond milk.

Makes about 8 cups (2 L)

TIP

The leftover almond meal that is strained out in step 2 can be used for baking or added to smoothies.

● **Blender**

1 cup	raw almonds	250 mL
7 cups	filtered water	1.75 L
1 tsp	vanilla extract	5 mL
5 to 6	drops liquid stevia	5 to 6

1. Place almonds and water in an airtight glass container. Soak for 12 to 24 hours.
2. Transfer almond mixture to the blender and blend until thoroughly combined and frothy. Strain through cheesecloth, a fine-mesh strainer or a nut-milk bag into a jug. Stir in vanilla and stevia to taste.
3. Store in the refrigerator for up to 3 days. Shake or stir each time before pouring.

Health-Enhancing Tips

To increase the protein content of this recipe, add 1 scoop of protein powder (organic rice, organic pea, hemp or whey from grass-fed cows not given antibiotics or hormones) with the stevia.

Nutrients per 1 cup (250 mL)

Calories	104
Fat	9 g
Carbohydrate	4 g
Fiber	2 g
Protein	4 g
Vitamin A	0 IU
Iron	0.7 mg
Magnesium	50 mg
Zinc	0.6 mg
Selenium	0.5 mcg

Mango Yogurt Smoothie

Lassi is a yogurt-based cold drink that is popular in India and Pakistan. Traditionally, it is made with a large amount of added sugar, but fully ripe or frozen mangos provide a naturally sweet flavor, so there's no need to add more than a small touch of honey.

Makes about 4 cups (1 L)

TIPS

The best way to tell whether a mango is ripe is to smell it. If the fruit has a distinctive aroma, it is ready for eating. Another good sign is if the fruit yields slightly to gentle pressure.

It is best to use fresh, ripe mangos, but frozen will work if fresh are not available.

To keep this recipe low in fat, make sure to use nonfat yogurt and skim milk.

• Blender

4 cups	chopped fresh or frozen mangos	1 L
1 cup	nonfat plain yogurt	250 mL
1 cup	skim milk	250 mL
1 tbsp	liquid honey	15 mL
Pinch	ground cardamom (optional)	Pinch

1. In blender, combine mangos, yogurt, milk and honey; blend until smooth.

2. Pour into glasses and sprinkle with cardamom, if desired.

Variation

Substitute chopped fresh or frozen peaches for the mangos.

Health-Enhancing Tips

To reduce the carbohydrate content of this recipe, replace the honey with liquid or powdered stevia. Stevia is very sweet, so start with just a few drops or $\frac{1}{8}$ tsp (0.5 mL) and gradually add more until you attain the desired sweetness.

To increase the protein content of this recipe, add 3 to 4 scoops of protein powder (organic rice, organic pea, hemp or whey from grass-fed cows not given antibiotics or hormones) to the mixture before blending.

Nutrients per ¾ cup (175 mL)

Calories	116
Fat	1 g
Carbohydrate	24 g
Fiber	2 g
Protein	4 g
Vitamin A	1294 IU
Iron	0.2 mg
Magnesium	23 mg
Zinc	0.6 mg
Selenium	3.3 mcg

Power Smoothie 1

This quick and easy smoothie provides long-lasting energy for a busy morning, as well as several nutrients to enhance your health.

Makes 1 serving

TIPS

The nutrient analysis for this recipe is based on the use of Prescribed Choice Pea Protein, natural vanilla flavor, for the protein powder.

Choose an almond butter that has almonds as the only ingredient.

If your smoothie is too thick, add filtered water until you achieve the desired consistency.

- **Blender**

1 to 10	ice cubes (depending on desired thickness)	1 to 10
1 to 2	large kale leaves	1 to 2
1	scoop protein powder (see tip, at left)	1
½ cup	fresh or frozen blueberries	125 mL
1 tbsp	ground flax seeds (flaxseed meal)	15 mL
1 tbsp	natural almond butter	15 mL
1 cup	unsweetened almond milk	250 mL

1. In blender, combine ice cubes, kale, protein powder, blueberries, flax seeds, almond butter and almond milk; blend until smooth.

Health-Enhancing Tip

Increase the alkalinity of this recipe by adding more vegetables. You could also use juiced vegetables (beets, carrots, celery, kale, parsley, etc.) in place of the almond milk or use ½ cup (125 mL) almond milk and ½ cup (125 mL) juiced vegetables.

Nutrients per serving

Calories	389
Fat	17 g
Carbohydrate	32 g
Fiber	8 g
Protein	32 g
Vitamin A	5193 IU
Iron	8.9 mg
Magnesium	103 mg
Zinc	3.4 mg
Selenium	30.5 mcg

Power Smoothie 2

When you feel like shaking things up, here's another quick and easy smoothie with health-enhancing, thyroid-strengthening nutrients.

Makes 1 serving

TIPS

The nutrient analysis for this recipe is based on the use of Prescribed Choice Pea Protein, natural vanilla flavor, for the protein powder.

Choose a nut butter that has nuts as the only ingredient.

If your smoothie is too thick, add filtered water until you achieve the desired consistency.

● **Blender**

1 to 10	ice cubes (depending on desired thickness)	1 to 10
1 to 2	large kale leaves	1 to 2
1	scoop protein powder (see tip, at left)	1
½ cup	fresh or frozen strawberries	125 mL
1½ tbsp	chia seeds	22 mL
1 tbsp	natural almond butter or other nut butter	15 mL
1 cup	unsweetened hemp or almond milk	250 mL

1. In blender, combine ice cubes, kale, protein powder, strawberries, chia seeds, almond butter and hemp milk; blend until smooth.

Health-Enhancing Tips

Increase the alkalinity of this recipe by adding more vegetables. You could also use juiced vegetables (beets, carrots, celery, kale, parsley, etc.) in place of the hemp milk or use ½ cup (125 mL) hemp milk and ½ cup (125 mL) juiced vegetables.

To lower the fat content, you can omit the almond butter and/or use filtered water in place of the hemp milk.

Nutrients per serving

Calories	485
Fat	19 g
Carbohydrate	44 g
Fiber	13 g
Protein	36 g
Vitamin A	5563 IU
Iron	11.3 mg
Magnesium	158 mg
Zinc	5.0 mg
Selenium	29.0 mcg

Soups

Basic Vegetable Stock 194

Homemade Chicken Stock 195

Hearty Beef Stock 196

Moroccan-Spiced Carrot Soup. 197

Beet Soup with Lemongrass and Lime. 198

Vichyssoise with Celery Root and Watercress 200

Potato, Leek and Broccoli Soup 202

Thai-Inspired Peanut and Wild Rice Soup 203

Thai-Style Pumpkin Soup 204

Curried Squash and Apple Soup 206

Old-Fashioned Split Pea Soup 208

Mushroom Lentil Soup 209

Lentil and Spinach Soup 210

Minestrone. 211

Fassolada (Greek Bean Soup) 212

Gingery Chicken and Wild Rice Soup 214

Beef and Quinoa Soup 216

Fish Chowder 218

Basic Vegetable Stock

All the stock recipes in this book (Basic Vegetable Stock, Homemade Chicken Stock and Hearty Beef Stock) make enough for two average soup recipes. They can be made ahead and frozen. For convenience, cook them overnight in the slow cooker. If your slow cooker is not large enough to make a full batch, you can halve the recipes. Vegetable stocks are packed with health-promoting nutrients, such as vitamin A, potassium, iodine, iron and many other minerals and antioxidants.

Makes about 12 cups (3 L)

TIP

To freeze this stock and all others, transfer to airtight containers in small, measured portions (2 cups/500 mL or 4 cups/ 1 L are handy), leaving at least 1-inch (2.5 cm) headspace for expansion. Refrigerate until chilled, cover and freeze for up to 3 months. Thaw in refrigerator before using.

• Large (about 5-quart) slow cooker

8	carrots, scrubbed and coarsely chopped	8
6	stalks celery, coarsely chopped	6
3	onions, coarsely chopped	3
3	cloves garlic, coarsely chopped	3
6	sprigs parsley	6
3	bay leaves	3
10	whole black peppercorns	10
¼ cup	dried alfalfa leaves (optional)	60 mL
1 tsp	dried thyme	5 mL
	Sea salt (optional)	
12 cups	water	3 L

1. In slow cooker stoneware, combine carrots, celery, onions, garlic, parsley, bay leaves, peppercorns, alfalfa leaves (if using), thyme, salt to taste (if using) and water. Cover and cook on Low for 8 hours or on High for 4 hours.

2. Strain and discard solids. Cover and refrigerate for up to 5 days or freeze in an airtight container.

Variation

Enhanced Vegetable Stock: To enhance 8 cups (2 L) Basic Vegetable or prepared stock, combine in a large saucepan over medium heat with 2 carrots, coarsely chopped, 1 tbsp (15 mL) tomato paste, 1 tsp (5 mL) celery seeds, 1 tsp (5 mL) cracked black peppercorns, ½ tsp (2 mL) dried thyme leaves, 4 parsley sprigs, 1 bay leaf and 1 cup (250 mL) white wine. Bring to a boil. Reduce heat to low and simmer, covered, for 30 minutes, then strain and discard solids.

Nutrients per 1 cup (250 mL)

Calories	1
Fat	0 g
Carbohydrate	0 g
Fiber	0 g
Protein	0 g
Vitamin A	6933 IU
Iron	0.4 mg
Magnesium	12 mg
Zinc	0.2 mg
Selenium	0.3 mcg

Homemade Chicken Stock

There's nothing like the flavor of homemade chicken stock, which is very easy to make and wonderfully nourishing. Homemade chicken stock can boost your immune system, improve bone density, help to heal a damaged gut, improve sleep and reduce inflammation. Not bad for a simple, tasty food!

Makes about 12 cups (3 L)

TIPS

The more economical parts of the chicken, such as necks, backs and wings, make the best stock.

The acid in the vinegar helps to draw nutrients from the bones and intensifies the flavor of the stock.

• **Large (about 5-quart) slow cooker**

4 lbs	bone-in skin-on chicken parts (see tip, at left)	2 kg
4	carrots, scrubbed and coarsely chopped	4
4	stalks celery, coarsely chopped	4
3	onions, coarsely chopped	3
6	sprigs parsley	6
3	bay leaves	3
10	whole black peppercorns	10
¼ cup	dried alfalfa leaves (optional)	60 mL
1 tsp	dried thyme	5 mL
12 cups	water	3 L
3 tbsp	cider vinegar	45 mL

1. In slow cooker stoneware, combine chicken, carrots, celery, onions, parsley, bay leaves, peppercorns, alfalfa, thyme, water and vinegar. Cover and cook on High for 8 hours.

2. Strain into a large bowl, discarding solids. Cover and refrigerate for up to 5 days.

Health-Enhancing Tip

Look for organic bone-in chicken parts. Conventional chickens may be given hormones and antibiotics, and may be fed genetically modified, arsenic-enhanced, inflammatory grains. All of these factors may negatively impact your thyroid and general health.

Nutrients per 1 cup (250 mL)

Calories	1
Fat	0 g
Carbohydrate	1 g
Fiber	0 g
Protein	0 g
Vitamin A	3503 IU
Iron	0.2 mg
Magnesium	9 mg
Zinc	0.1 mg
Selenium	0.2 mcg

Hearty Beef Stock

Like chicken stock, homemade beef stock can boost your immune system, improve bone density, help to heal a damaged gut, improve sleep and reduce inflammation.

Makes about 12 cups (3 L)

TIP

Demi-glace is intensely flavored concentrated stock that is useful for adding a burst of flavor to dishes. After making stock, transfer 2 cups (500 mL) to a saucepan. Bring to a boil, then reduce heat and simmer for $1\frac{1}{2}$ hours, until syrupy. Let cool, then transfer to a shallow dish and refrigerate until solid. Transfer to a cutting board, then cut into 8 squares. Wrap individually in plastic wrap and freeze.

- **Large (about 6-quart) slow cooker**
- **Preheat oven to 375°F (190°C)**
- **Sieve, lined with a double layer of cheesecloth**

3	each onions, quartered, and carrots, cut into chunks	3
3	stalks celery	3
6	cloves garlic	6
2 tbsp	extra virgin olive oil or melted butter	30 mL
3 lbs	beef bones	1.5 kg
4	sprigs parsley	4
3	sprigs fresh thyme	3
10	whole black peppercorns	10
1/4 cup	dried alfalfa leaves (optional)	60 mL
3 tbsp	red wine vinegar	45 mL
12 cups	filtered water	3 L

1. Place onions, carrots, celery and garlic in a roasting pan and toss well with oil. Add bones and toss again. Arrange in a single layer (as much as possible) in pan and roast in preheated oven until ingredients are browning nicely, about 1 hour. Transfer to stoneware, along with juices.

2. Add parsley, thyme, peppercorns, alfalfa leaves (if using), vinegar and water. Cover and cook on Low for 12 hours or on High for 6 hours, until stock is brown and flavorful.

3. Strain through prepared sieve and discard solids. Cool slightly. Refrigerate for up to 5 days or freeze in portions in airtight containers.

Nutrients per 1 cup (250 mL)

Calories	21
Fat	2 g
Carbohydrate	0 g
Fiber	0 g
Protein	0 g
Vitamin A	2174 IU
Iron	0.2 mg
Magnesium	7 mg
Zinc	0.1 mg
Selenium	0.1 mcg

Health-Enhancing Tip

Try to use bones from grass-fed or grass-finished cows. Grass-fed cows have been raised on grasses for the majority of their life; grass-finished cows have never been fed grains. Conventionally raised cows may be given antibiotics and hormones, and may be fed genetically modified, inflammatory grains.

Moroccan-Spiced Carrot Soup

The combination of cinnamon and turmeric provides a pleasantly sweet accent to the carrots and sweet potato. This recipe is full of health-enhancing, thyroid-strengthening ingredients, such as garlic, turmeric and cinnamon.

Makes 6 servings

TIP

If you have time to make Homemade Chicken Stock (page 195) or Basic Vegetable Stock (page 194), use it in place of the ready-to-use broth.

- **Blender, food processor or immersion blender**

1 tbsp	canola oil	15 mL
2	onions, chopped	2
2	cloves garlic, finely chopped	2
1½ tsp	ground cumin	7 mL
1 tsp	ground turmeric	5 mL
1 tsp	ground cinnamon	5 mL
½ tsp	freshly ground black pepper	2 mL
3 cups	sliced carrots (4 to 5 medium)	750 mL
1½ cups	diced peeled sweet potato	375 mL
5 cups	ready-to-use GF chicken or vegetable broth	1.25 L
¼ tsp	salt	1 mL
¼ cup	chopped fresh chives or cilantro	60 mL

1. In a large saucepan, heat oil over medium heat. Add onions, garlic, cumin, turmeric, cinnamon and pepper; cook, stirring often, for 4 minutes or until onions are softened.

2. Stir in carrots, sweet potato and broth; bring to a boil over high heat. Reduce heat to medium-low, cover and simmer for 25 minutes or until vegetables are very tender. Let cool slightly.

3. Working in batches, transfer soup to blender (or use immersion blender in pan) and purée until smooth. Return to saucepan, if necessary, and stir in salt. Heat over medium heat, stirring often, until piping hot.

4. Ladle soup into warm bowls and sprinkle with chives.

Nutrients per serving

Calories	124
Fat	4 g
Carbohydrate	19 g
Fiber	4 g
Protein	6 g
Vitamin A	15,501 IU
Iron	1.3 mg
Magnesium	23 mg
Zinc	0.5 mg
Selenium	0.6 mcg

Health-Enhancing Tips

To increase the protein content of this recipe, add cooked chicken or tofu after puréeing the soup and simmer until heated through.

For a healthier, less inflammatory fat, use virgin coconut oil or olive oil in place of the canola oil.

Beet Soup with Lemongrass and Lime

This Thai-inspired soup, which is served cold, is elegant and refreshing. Its jewel-like appearance and intriguing flavors make it a perfect prelude to any meal, but especially summer dinners in the garden. It is packed with many health-enhancing ingredients, including garlic, ginger and cilantro.

Makes 8 servings

TIPS

You can halve this recipe, but be sure to use a small (1½- to 3½-quart) slow cooker.

Coconut oil's pleasantly nutty taste complements the Thai flavors in this soup. Moreover, in recent years significant health benefits have been identified in this food.

- **Medium to large (3½- to 5-quart) slow cooker**
- **Food processor, blender or immersion blender**

1 tbsp	olive oil or virgin coconut oil	15 mL
1	onion, chopped	1
4	cloves garlic, minced	4
2 tbsp	minced gingerroot	30 mL
2	stalks lemongrass, trimmed, smashed and cut in half crosswise	2
2 tsp	cracked black peppercorns	10 mL
6	beets (about 2½ lbs/1.25 kg), peeled and chopped	6
6 cups	ready-to-use GF vegetable broth	1.5 L
1	red bell pepper, finely chopped	1
1	long red chile pepper, seeded and finely chopped	1
	Grated zest and juice of 1 lime	
	Sea salt (optional)	
	Coconut cream (optional)	
	Finely chopped cilantro	

1. In a skillet, heat oil over medium heat. Add onion and cook, stirring, until softened, about 3 minutes. Add garlic, ginger, lemongrass and peppercorns and cook, stirring, for 1 minute. Transfer to slow cooker stoneware.

2. Add beets and broth. Cover and cook on Low for 6 to 8 hours or on High for 3 to 4 hours, until beets are tender. Add red pepper and chile pepper (if using). Cover and cook on High for 30 minutes, until peppers are tender. Remove lemongrass and discard.

Nutrients per serving

Calories	67
Fat	2 g
Carbohydrate	12 g
Fiber	2 g
Protein	2 g
Vitamin A	916 IU
Iron	0.9 mg
Magnesium	21 mg
Zinc	0.4 mg
Selenium	0.8 mcg

Ideally, make this soup the day before you intend to serve it so it can chill overnight in the refrigerator.

3. Working in batches, purée soup in food processor or blender. (You can also do this in the stoneware using an immersion blender.) Transfer to a large bowl. Stir in lime zest and lime juice. Season to taste with salt (if using). Chill thoroughly, preferably overnight.

4. When ready to serve, spoon into individual bowls, drizzle with coconut cream (if using), and garnish with cilantro.

Health-Enhancing Tip

To increase the protein content of this recipe, add cold cooked tofu or chicken to the bowls, then spoon the soup on top.

Vichyssoise with Celery Root and Watercress

This refreshing soup is delicious, easy to make and can be a prelude to the most sophisticated meal. Its pleasing nutty flavor is nutritionally enhanced with several health-promoting ingredients.

Makes 8 servings

TIPS

You can halve this recipe, but be sure to use a small (about 2-quart) slow cooker.

Since celery root oxidizes quickly on contact with air, be sure to use as soon as you have peeled and chopped it, or toss with 1 tbsp (15 mL) lemon juice to prevent discoloration.

To cool the soup more quickly, transfer it to a large bowl before refrigerating.

Nutrients per serving

Calories	192
Fat	13 g
Carbohydrate	14 g
Fiber	2 g
Protein	7 g
Vitamin A	1683 IU
Iron	1.8 mg
Magnesium	41 mg
Zinc	0.7 mg
Selenium	1.5 mcg

- **Large (about 5-quart) slow cooker**
- **Food processor, blender or immersion blender**

1 tbsp	olive oil	15 mL
3	leeks, white and light green parts only, cleaned and coarsely chopped (see tip, page 202)	3
2	cloves garlic, minced	2
½ tsp	cracked black peppercorns	2 mL
6 cups	ready-to-use GF chicken or vegetable broth	1.5 L
1	large celery root (about 1 lb/500 g), peeled and sliced	1
2	bunches (each about 4 oz/125 g) watercress, tough parts of the stems removed	2
	Sea salt (optional)	
½ cup	heavy or whipping (35%) cream or soy milk	125 mL
½ cup	toasted chopped walnuts	125 mL
	Watercress sprigs (optional)	

1. In a skillet, heat oil over medium heat. Add leeks and cook, stirring, until softened, about 5 minutes. Add garlic and peppercorns and cook, stirring, for 1 minute. Add broth and stir well.

2. Transfer to slow cooker stoneware. Stir in celery root. Cover and cook on Low for 6 hours or on High for 3 hours, until celery root is tender. Stir in watercress until wilted.

Complete step 1. Cover and refrigerate overnight or for up to 2 days. When you're ready to cook, continue with steps 2 and 3.

3. Working in batches, purée mixture in food processor or blender. (You can also do this in the stoneware using an immersion blender. Season to taste with salt (if using). Stir in cream and refrigerate until thoroughly chilled, about 4 hours (see tip, page 200).

4. Ladle soup into bowls and garnish with toasted walnuts and watercress sprigs (if using).

Health-Enhancing Tips

To increase the protein content of this recipe, add cold cooked chicken, shrimp or tofu to the bowls, then ladle the soup on top.

To increase both carbohydrate and protein, add $\frac{1}{2}$ cup (125 mL) quinoa to the slow cooker for the last hour of cooking.

Try using hemp or rice milk in place of the cream or soy milk.

Potato, Leek and Broccoli Soup

This yummy, nutritious soup can be either chunky or smooth, depending on how your family likes it.

Makes 6 to 8 servings

TIPS

Leeks hold a lot of dirt in their layers and must be rinsed thoroughly under cold running water before they are sliced.

If you have time to make Basic Vegetable Stock (page 194), use it in place of the ready-to-use broth.

If you have an immersion blender, you can purée the soup right in the pot.

- **Food processor or blender**

2 tbsp	grapeseed oil	30 mL
2	leeks (white and light green parts only), sliced	2
4 cups	ready-to-use GF vegetable broth	1 L
2	potatoes, peeled and chopped	2
2 cups	chopped fresh or frozen broccoli	500 mL
1 tsp	salt	5 mL
¼ tsp	freshly ground black pepper	1 mL

1. In a large pot, heat oil over medium-high heat. Sauté leeks for 4 to 5 minutes or until wilted. Add broth and 4 cups (1 L) water; bring to a boil. Add potatoes, broccoli, salt and pepper; return to a boil. Reduce heat and simmer for 15 minutes or until potatoes are tender.

2. Serve chunky or, to serve smooth, transfer soup in batches to a food processor or blender and purée to desired consistency.

Health-Enhancing Tips

To increase the protein content of this recipe, add cooked chicken or tofu. Stir it in at the end of step 1 if serving chunky or after puréeing the soup if serving smooth. Return the soup to the pot (if necessary) and cook over medium heat for 5 to 10 minutes or until heated through.

Sauté the leeks over medium heat instead of medium-high, adjusting the cooking time as necessary.

Nutrients per serving (1 of 8)

Calories	98
Fat	4 g
Carbohydrate	15 g
Fiber	2 g
Protein	2 g
Vitamin A	760 IU
Iron	1.1 mg
Iodine	0.4 mcg
Magnesium	23.2 mg
Zinc	0.3 mg
Selenium	0.9 mcg

Thai-Inspired Peanut and Wild Rice Soup

If your taste buds have grown tired of the same old thing, here's a delightfully different soup, packed with health-promoting ingredients, to wake them up. It makes a great lunch, or even a light dinner accompanied by a platter of stir-fried bok choy.

Makes 6 servings

TIPS

Tamari is a type of soy sauce that shouldn't contain wheat. However, check the label.

Although this soup is relatively high in fat, it is very low in saturated fat. Virtually all of the fat comes from the peanuts and most is the heart-healthy unsaturated kind. Moreover, peanuts have a very high antioxidant content.

Nutrients per serving

Calories	391
Fat	25 g
Carbohydrate	34 g
Fiber	6 g
Protein	15 g
Vitamin A	800 IU
Iron	2.2 mg
Magnesium	116 mg
Zinc	2.6 mg
Selenium	4.9 mcg

- **Food processor or blender**

2 cups	cooked wild rice	500 mL
2	stalks lemongrass, smashed and chopped	2
4	cloves garlic, minced	4
2 tbsp	minced gingerroot	30 mL
3	dried red chile peppers, crumbled	3
2 tbsp	tomato paste	30 mL
6 cups	ready-to-use GF vegetable or chicken broth	1.5 L
2 cups	unsalted roasted peanuts	500 mL
3 tbsp	rice vinegar	45 mL
2 tbsp	GF soy sauce or tamari (see tip, at left)	30 mL
1 tbsp	liquid honey	15 mL
	Finely grated zest and juice of 1 lime	
	Finely chopped cilantro	
	Finely chopped fresh chile peppers (optional)	

1. In a large saucepan or stockpot, combine lemongrass, garlic, ginger, dried chile peppers, tomato paste and stock. Bring to a boil over medium heat. Reduce heat to low. Cover and simmer for 30 minutes. Strain, discarding solids. Return liquid to pot.

2. In food processor, combine peanuts, rice vinegar, soy sauce, honey and lime zest. Process until mixture is the consistency of chunky peanut butter. Stir into liquid. Add wild rice and bring to a boil over medium heat. Reduce heat to low. Cover and simmer to allow flavors to meld, about 20 minutes. Stir in lime juice. Ladle into bowls and garnish with cilantro and chile peppers (if using).

Thai-Style Pumpkin Soup

This soup is versatile, delicious and loaded with health-enhancing ingredients. It has an exotic combination of flavors and works well as a prelude to a meal. If you prefer a more substantial soup, add some protein (see the health-enhancing tip, opposite).

Makes 8 servings

TIPS

You can halve this recipe, but be sure to use a small (2- to 3½-quart) slow cooker.

For best results, toast and grind cumin seeds yourself. Place in a dry skillet over medium heat and cook, stirring, until fragrant, about 3 minutes. Immediately transfer to a spice grinder or mortar and grind finely.

Check the label to make sure your curry paste does not contain gluten.

- **Large (about 5-quart) slow cooker**
- **Food processor, blender or immersion blender**

1 tbsp	olive oil or virgin coconut oil	15 mL
2	onions, finely chopped	2
4	cloves garlic, minced	4
2 tbsp	minced gingerroot	30 mL
1 tsp	cracked black peppercorns	5 mL
2	stalks lemongrass, trimmed, smashed and cut in half crosswise	2
1 tbsp	ground cumin (see tip, at left)	15 mL
6 cups	ready-to-use GF vegetable or chicken broth, divided	1.5 L
8 cups	cubed peeled pumpkin or other orange squash (2-inch/5 cm cubes)	2 L
1 cup	coconut milk	250 mL
1 tsp	Thai red curry paste (see tip, at left)	5 mL
	Finely grated zest and juice of 1 lime	
¼ cup	toasted green pumpkin seeds (optional)	60 mL
	Cherry tomatoes, halved (optional)	
	Finely chopped cilantro	

1. In a skillet, heat oil over medium heat. Add onions and cook, stirring, until softened, about 3 minutes. Add garlic, ginger, peppercorns, lemongrass and cumin and cook, stirring, for 1 minute. Add 1 cup (250 mL) broth and stir well.

2. Transfer to slow cooker stoneware. Add pumpkin and the remaining broth. Cover and cook on Low for 6 hours or on High for 3 hours, until pumpkin is tender. Skim off 1 tbsp (15 mL) coconut milk. In a small bowl, combine with curry paste and blend well. Add to slow cooker along with the remaining coconut milk, lime zest and lime juice. Cover and cook on High until heated through, about 20 minutes. Discard lemongrass.

Nutrients per serving

Calories	126
Fat	8 g
Carbohydrate	14 g
Fiber	2 g
Protein	2 g
Vitamin A	8956 IU
Iron	2.4 mg
Magnesium	31 mg
Zinc	0.6 mg
Selenium	0.7 mcg

MAKE AHEAD

This soup can be partially prepared before it is cooked. Complete step 1. Cover and refrigerate overnight or for up to 2 days. When you're ready to cook, complete the recipe.

3. Working in batches, purée soup in food processor or blender. (You can also do this in the stoneware using an immersion blender.)

4. Ladle soup into bowls and garnish with pumpkin seeds and tomatoes (if using) and cilantro.

Health-Enhancing Tip

To increase the protein content of this recipe, add 2 to 3 oz (60 to 90 g) hot cooked shrimp, scallops or chicken to each serving of soup. If you are a vegetarian, add $\frac{1}{2}$ cup (125 mL) hot cooked quinoa or tofu to each serving. (Note that if you add quinoa, the soup becomes a post-workout recipe.)

Curried Squash and Apple Soup

Take advantage of economical squash, sold at farmers' markets in the fall. Steam or bake the squash, purée it, pack it into airtight containers and freeze for up to 3 months.

Makes 8 servings

TIPS

There are many varieties of winter squash and pumpkin, and any of them can be turned into a thick purée to use as a base for this delicious soup.

If you have time to make Homemade Chicken Stock (page 195) or Basic Vegetable Stock (page 194), use it in place of the ready-to-use broth.

• Blender, food processor or immersion blender

1 tbsp	canola oil	15 mL
3	stalks celery, diced	3
1	large onion, chopped	1
3	cloves garlic, minced	3
1½ cups	diced peeled apples	375 mL
2 tbsp	minced gingerroot	30 mL
1 tbsp	curry powder	15 mL
1 tsp	ground cumin	5 mL
1 tsp	ground coriander	5 mL
Pinch	cayenne pepper	Pinch
2 cups	thick winter squash or pumpkin purée (see box, opposite)	500 mL
5 cups	ready-to-use GF chicken or vegetable broth	1.25 L
¼ tsp	salt	1 mL
¼ tsp	freshly ground black pepper	1 mL
⅓ cup	chopped fresh cilantro, parsley or chives	75 mL

1. In a large saucepan, heat oil over medium heat. Add celery, onion, garlic, apples, ginger, curry powder, cumin, coriander and cayenne; cook, stirring often, for 5 minutes or until vegetables are softened.

2. Stir in squash purée and stock; bring to a boil over high heat. Reduce heat to medium-low, cover and simmer for 20 minutes or until vegetables are very tender. Let cool slightly.

3. Working in batches, transfer soup to blender (or use immersion blender in pan) and purée until smooth. Return to saucepan, if necessary, and stir in salt and black pepper. Heat over medium heat, stirring often, until piping hot.

4. Ladle soup into warm bowls and sprinkle with cilantro.

Nutrients per serving

Calories	78
Fat	3 g
Carbohydrate	11 g
Fiber	2 g
Protein	4 g
Vitamin A	491 IU
Iron	0.9 mg
Magnesium	13 mg
Zinc	0.3 mg
Selenium	0.6 mcg

TIP

To increase the protein content of this health-enhancing recipe, add cooked chicken, red meat, shrimp or tofu after puréeing the soup and simmer until heated through.

Winter Squash or Pumpkin Purée

Cut squash into halves or quarters and remove seeds. For large pumpkins, cut into chunks. Place in a large casserole dish or roasting pan. Add 1 cup (250 mL) water. Cover and bake in a preheated 350°F (180°C) oven for 1 to 1¼ hours or until tender when pierced with a fork. (Or place squash in a large casserole dish with ½ cup/125 mL water, cover and microwave on High for 15 to 25 minutes or until tender when tested with a knife in several places.) Cooking time will vary according to the amount and type of squash or pumpkin. Let cool. Scoop out pulp, discarding skin, and purée in a food processor or blender. If required, place purée in a fine-mesh strainer for several hours, stirring occasionally, to drain off excess moisture. The purée should be thick enough to mound on a spoon without dripping off. Save liquid to add to soups and broths.

Old-Fashioned Split Pea Soup

Split pea soup is typically made with ham or salt pork, but this lower-sodium version relies on vegetables that are first sautéed to bring out their sweet flavor. This comfort food is incredibly nutritious and healing.

Makes 8 servings

TIPS

Leftover soup thickens when cool; when reheating, thin with water to desired consistency.

Slow Cooker Method: Complete step 1, then transfer sautéed vegetables to a 5-quart or larger slow cooker. Add split peas and broth. Cover and cook on Low for 8 to 10 hours or on High for 4 to 5 hours, until split peas are tender.

1 tbsp	canola oil	15 mL
3	carrots, diced	3
3	cloves garlic, minced	3
2	stalks celery, including leaves, chopped	2
1	leek (white and light green parts only), chopped	1
1	large onion, chopped	1
2	bay leaves	2
2 tsp	dried marjoram	10 mL
½ tsp	freshly ground black pepper	2 mL
1¼ cups	dried green or yellow split peas, rinsed	300 mL
8 cups	ready-to-use GF chicken broth	2 L
¼ cup	chopped fresh parsley	60 mL

1. In a stockpot, heat oil over medium-high heat. Add carrots, garlic, celery, leek, onion, bay leaves, marjoram and pepper; cook, stirring often, for 8 minutes or until vegetables are softened and lightly colored (reduce heat to medium if vegetables are browning).

2. Stir in split peas and broth; bring to a boil over high heat. Reduce heat to medium-low, cover and simmer, stirring occasionally, for 1½ to 2 hours or until peas are tender. Discard bay leaves and stir in parsley. Ladle into warm bowls.

Variation

Curried Split Pea Soup: Add 2 tsp (10 mL) curry powder and a generous pinch of cayenne pepper along with the marjoram. Garnish bowls of soup with chopped fresh cilantro instead of stirring in parsley.

Health-Enhancing Tip

To increase the protein content of this recipe, add chopped cooked chicken, ham or tofu about 5 minutes before the end of cooking time and simmer until heated through.

Nutrients per serving

Calories	187
Fat	4 g
Carbohydrate	28 g
Fiber	9 g
Protein	13 g
Vitamin A	4274 IU
Iron	2.5 mg
Magnesium	49 mg
Zinc	1.3 mg
Selenium	0.9 mcg

Mushroom Lentil Soup

Dried lentils are so fast and easy to cook — and healthy, too! Just bring the broth to a boil, add the lentils and vegetables, and you'll soon enjoy a homey aroma as the soup simmers on the stovetop. In about 40 minutes, you'll be ladling out bowlfuls of wholesome soup.

Makes 6 servings

TIPS

To save time, chop the mushrooms, carrots, celery and onion in batches in a food processor.

If you have time to make Homemade Chicken Stock (page 195), use it in place of the ready-to-use broth.

8 oz	mushrooms, chopped	250 g
3	carrots, chopped	3
2	stalks celery, including leaves, chopped	2
1	large onion, chopped	1
2	cloves garlic, minced	2
1 cup	dried brown or green lentils, rinsed	250 mL
1 tsp	dried thyme or marjoram	5 mL
1/4 tsp	freshly ground black pepper	1 mL
8 cups	ready-to-use GF chicken broth	2 L
1/4 cup	chopped fresh dill or parsley	60 mL

1. In a stockpot, combine mushrooms, carrots, celery, onion, garlic, lentils, thyme, pepper and broth. Bring to a boil over high heat. Reduce heat to medium-low, cover and simmer for 35 to 40 minutes or until lentils are tender. Stir in dill. Ladle into warm bowls.

Health-Enhancing Tip

To add extra bulk to fill you up, add up to 2 cups (500 mL) chopped non-starchy vegetables (broccoli, spinach, zucchini, kale, collard greens, sea vegetables, tomato) in the last 10 to 15 minutes of cooking.

Nutrients per serving

Calories	197
Fat	3 g
Carbohydrate	30 g
Fiber	5 g
Protein	16 g
Vitamin A	5210 IU
Iron	3.7 mg
Magnesium	38 mg
Zinc	1.9 mg
Selenium	6.5 mcg

Lentil and Spinach Soup

This recipe is not only filling and easy to make, but is also packed with healing nutrition. It's the perfect meal to refuel your body after a good workout.

Makes 4 servings

TIPS

A 19-oz (540 mL) can of lentils will yield about 2 cups (500 mL) once the lentils are drained and rinsed. If you have smaller or larger cans, you can use the volume called for or just add the amount from your can(s).

Look for bags of spinach that have been frozen in small cubes rather than in a large block. You can measure the cubes and add them to the pot without thawing them. If you can't find them, use ½ cup (125 mL) drained thawed chopped spinach.

2 tbsp	olive oil	30 mL
2	cloves garlic, minced	2
¼ cup	chopped onion	60 mL
¼ cup	chopped celery	60 mL
½ cup	chopped carrots	125 mL
2 cups	rinsed drained canned lentils (see tip, at left)	500 mL
1 cup	frozen spinach cubes (see tip, at left)	250 mL
4 cups	ready-to-use GF chicken or vegetable broth	1 L
	Salt and freshly ground black pepper	

1. In a large saucepan, heat oil over medium heat. Sauté garlic, onion, celery and carrots for 3 to 4 minutes or until softened.

2. Stir in lentils, spinach and broth; bring to a boil over high heat. Cover, leaving lid ajar, reduce heat to low and simmer, stirring occasionally, for 30 minutes or until vegetables are tender (or for up to 1 hour if you prefer a very soft texture). Season to taste with salt and pepper.

Health-Enhancing Tip

To increase the protein content of this recipe, add cooked chicken, tofu or red meat about 5 minutes before the end of cooking time and simmer until heated through.

Nutrients per serving

Calories	223
Fat	9 g
Carbohydrate	25 g
Fiber	11 g
Protein	15 g
Vitamin A	7275 IU
Iron	1.4 mg
Magnesium	36 mg
Zinc	0.5 mg
Selenium	2.6 mcg

Minestrone

A steaming bowl of minestrone is as comforting as it gets! This inexpensive, filling soup is also packed full of health-promoting and healing ingredients.

Makes 5 servings

TIPS

Use the shape of pasta you prefer, from small shells to small elbows. Follow package directions to be sure pasta is not overcooked. Rinse the cooked pasta with cold water to stop the cooking process and remove excess starch.

Soup can be divided into 2-cup (500 mL) portions and frozen for up to 1 month. Reheat in the microwave on High for 5 to 7 minutes or until steaming.

Look for BPA-free cans of tomatoes, beans and tomato paste.

2 tsp	extra virgin olive oil	10 mL
2	carrots, chopped	2
1	stalk celery, chopped	1
1	clove garlic, minced	1
1	small onion, chopped	1
1	small zucchini, diced	1
1	can (28 oz/796 mL) diced tomatoes, with juice	1
1	can (14 to 19 oz/398 to 540 mL) kidney beans, drained and rinsed	1
1 cup	diced cooked GF ham	250 mL
1 cup	ready-to-use GF chicken or vegetable broth	250 mL
2 tbsp	tomato paste	30 mL
1 cup	packed spinach, trimmed and coarsely chopped	250 mL
1 cup	cooked small GF pasta	250 mL
¼ cup	snipped fresh basil	60 mL
	Salt and freshly ground black pepper	

1. In a large saucepan, heat oil over medium-low heat. Add carrots, celery, garlic and onion; cover and cook, stirring occasionally, for about 20 minutes or until tender but not brown.

2. Add zucchini, tomatoes, beans, ham, broth and tomato paste; bring to a boil over medium-high heat. Reduce heat to low and simmer for 10 minutes or until soup is hot. Stir in spinach, pasta and basil; heat until spinach is wilted. Season to taste with salt and pepper.

Variations

Substitute an equal amount of shredded cabbage or cooked green beans for the spinach.

Substitute 6 slices GF bacon, chopped and cooked crisp, or 1 cup (250 mL) diced cooked chicken, beef or turkey for the ham.

For a spicier soup, substitute GF pepperoni for the ham.

Sprinkle with freshly grated Parmesan cheese.

Nutrients per serving

Calories	256
Fat	6 g
Carbohydrate	37 g
Fiber	9 g
Protein	17 g
Vitamin A	5323 IU
Iron	4.4 mg
Magnesium	75 mg
Zinc	2.4 mg
Selenium	12.0 mcg

Fassolada (Greek Bean Soup)

This easy-to-prepare, filling meal turns the ordinary bean into a delicious, healing superstar!

Makes 8 servings

TIP

This soup is meant to be fairly thick; if too thick, add 1 to 2 cups (250 to 500 mL) water, stir and bring back to boil.

2½ cups	dried white kidney beans	625 mL
1 tbsp	baking soda	15 mL
12 cups	water	3 L
1	onion, diced	1
1	large carrot, diced	1
½ cup	chopped fresh celery leaves, packed down (or 2 celery stalks, finely chopped)	125 mL
2 tbsp	tomato paste	30 mL
1 tsp	freshly squeezed lemon juice	5 mL
1	tomato, blanched, peeled and chopped	1
1 tsp	dried rosemary, basil or oregano	5 mL
1 tsp	salt (optional)	5 mL
½ tsp	freshly ground black pepper	2 mL
¼ cup	chopped fresh parsley, packed down	60 mL
¼ cup	olive oil	60 mL
	Extra virgin olive oil, olive bits, diced red onion and crumbled feta cheese	

1. In a large bowl, cover beans with plenty of warm water. Add baking soda and mix well. (The water will foam and remove some of the gas from the beans.) Let soak for at least 3 hours, preferably overnight, unrefrigerated.

2. Drain beans and transfer to a soup pot. Add plenty of water and bring to a boil. Reduce heat to medium-low and simmer for 30 minutes, occasionally skimming froth that rises to the top.

3. Drain beans; rinse and drain again. Scrub pot, cleaning off foam stuck to the sides. Return the beans to the pot; add the 12 cups (3 L) water and place over high heat. Add onion, carrot, celery, tomato paste, lemon juice and tomato. Bring to boil, stirring; reduce heat to medium-low. Cook for 1½ hours at a rolling bubble, stirring very occasionally, until the beans and vegetables are very tender.

Nutrients per serving	
Calories	250
Fat	8 g
Carbohydrate	35 g
Fiber	10 g
Protein	13 g
Vitamin A	1905 IU
Iron	3.5 mg
Magnesium	69 mg
Zinc	1.5 mg
Selenium	1.8 mcg

This recipe can be easily halved, but leftovers freeze well and can be reheated with minimal loss of flavor.

4. Add rosemary, salt (if using), pepper, parsley and olive oil. Cook for another 5 minutes, stirring occasionally, and take off heat. Cover soup and let rest for 5 to 10 minutes. Season to taste with salt and pepper. Serve with any or all of suggested garnishes.

Health-Enhancing Tips

To increase the protein content of this recipe, add cooked chicken or tofu about 5 minutes before the end of cooking time and simmer until heated through.

Use tomato paste from a BPA-free can.

Gingery Chicken and Wild Rice Soup

The addition of a flavorful whole grain, leeks and a hint of ginger is a particularly delicious spin on classic chicken and rice soup. Make the stock a day ahead so it can be refrigerated, which makes easy work of skimming off the fat. This makes a great light dinner accompanied by a tossed salad.

Makes 6 servings

TIPS

Lundberg makes a brown and wild rice mixture, which works well in this soup. If you prefer, combine equal quantities of plain brown and wild rice.

Rinsing rice reduces stickiness. Place the rice in a strainer and rinse under cold running water. Drain thoroughly before using.

1	whole chicken (about 3 lbs/1.5 kg), cut into pieces	1
1	onion, coarsely chopped	1
2	carrots, diced	2
2	stalks celery, diced	2
4	sprigs parsley	4
1	clove garlic	1
1	bay leaf	1
1/2 tsp	salt	2 mL
1/2 tsp	cracked black peppercorns	2 mL
12 cups	water	3 L
1 tbsp	olive oil	15 mL
2	large leeks (white part only), cleaned (see tip, page 202) and sliced	2
2	cloves garlic, minced	2
2 tbsp	minced gingerroot	30 mL
1 cup	brown and wild rice mixture, rinsed (see tips, at left)	250 mL

1. In a stockpot, combine chicken, onion, carrots, celery, parsley, whole garlic, bay leaf, salt, peppercorns and water. Bring to a boil over high heat. Using a slotted spoon, skim off foam. Reduce heat to medium-low and simmer, uncovered, until chicken is falling off the bone, about 1 1/2 hours. Drain, reserving chicken and liquid separately. Let cool. Cut the chicken into bite-size pieces, discarding skin and bones. Skim off fat from the stock (see tip, opposite).

Nutrients per serving

Calories	269
Fat	8 g
Carbohydrate	27 g
Fiber	2 g
Protein	22 g
Vitamin A	4067 IU
Iron	2.0 mg
Magnesium	61 mg
Zinc	2.1 mg
Selenium	21.1 mcg

For best results, make the stock and cook the chicken the day before you plan to serve the soup. Cover and refrigerate stock and chicken separately. The fat will rise to the surface of the stock and can be easily removed. It will be easy to remove the skin and chop the cold chicken. Save the excess chicken to make sandwiches or a salad.

2. Measure 2 cups (500 mL) of chicken and set aside in the refrigerator. (Refrigerate remainder for other uses; see tip, at left.) In a large saucepan or stockpot, heat oil over medium heat for 30 seconds. Add leeks and cook, stirring, until softened, about 5 minutes. Add minced garlic and ginger and cook, stirring, for 1 minute. Add rice and toss to coat. Add reserved stock and bring to a boil. Reduce heat and simmer, uncovered, until rice is quite tender, about 1 hour. Add reserved chicken. Cover and simmer until chicken is heated through, about 15 minutes.

Variation

Substitute an equal quantity of rinsed wild rice for the mixture. You may need to increase the cooking time, depending upon the size of the grains.

Health-Enhancing Tips

For additional protein and a more alkaline soup, you can substitute an equal amount of quinoa, amaranth or millet for the brown and wild rice mixture. After adding the quinoa and reserved stock and bringing to a boil, reduce heat to low, cover and simmer for 15 to 20 minutes or until quinoa is very tender, then add the reserved chicken and continue as directed.

To further increase the alkalinity of your soup, add some leafy greens, such as chopped kale (tough stems and center ribs removed) or watercress, and/or chopped fresh herbs, such as cilantro, basil or rosemary. Add leafy greens 5 to 10 minutes before the end of cooking time and cook, stirring, until wilted. Stir in fresh herbs 5 minutes before the end of cooking time or just before serving, or sprinkle them on top of the soup as garnish.

To decrease the carbohydrate content, use less of the brown and wild rice mixture.

Beef and Quinoa Soup

This hearty, rich soup is a meal in a bowl. Replacing the more typical pasta, quinoa provides enhanced nutrition and a unique texture.

Makes 7 servings

TIPS

This recipe can be halved or quartered.

Browning the beef in small batches before adding the broth results in a richer beef flavor.

2 tbsp	extra virgin olive oil (approx.)	30 mL
1½ lbs	stewing beef, cut into ¾-inch (2 cm) cubes	750 g
1	large onion, coarsely chopped	1
4 cups	ready-to-use GF beef broth	1 L
3	carrots, coarsely chopped	3
2	stalks celery, coarsely chopped	2
¼ cup	quinoa, rinsed	60 mL
1	can (28 oz/796 mL) diced tomatoes, with juice	1
1 tbsp	snipped fresh thyme	15 mL
	Salt and freshly ground black pepper	

1. In a large saucepan, heat 1 tbsp (15 mL) of the oil over medium heat. Working in small batches, sauté beef and onion for 20 minutes or until beef is browned on all sides, adding oil as needed between batches. Transfer each batch as completed to a plate lined with paper towels. Drain off fat.

2. Add broth and scrape up any brown bits from bottom of pan. Return the beef mixture to the pan. Reduce heat to low and simmer for 35 minutes or until beef is tender.

3. Add carrots, celery and quinoa; simmer for 30 minutes or until vegetables are tender and quinoa is transparent and the tiny, spiral-like germ is separated.

4. Add tomatoes and thyme, increase heat to medium-high and heat until steaming. Season to taste with salt and pepper.

Nutrients per serving

Calories	357
Fat	22 g
Carbohydrate	16 g
Fiber	3 g
Protein	23 g
Vitamin A	4631 IU
Iron	4.2 mg
Magnesium	53 mg
Zinc	4.3 mg
Selenium	15.0 mcg

TIP

Soup can be divided into 2-cup (500 mL) portions and frozen for up to 1 month. Reheat in the microwave on High for 5 to 7 minutes or until steaming.

Variation

After step 1, transfer beef mixture to the stoneware of a large (minimum 5-quart) slow cooker. Add broth, carrots, celery, tomatoes and thyme. Cover and cook on Low for 8 to 10 hours. Meanwhile, cook quinoa. Fifteen minutes before you're ready to serve, add the quinoa to the slow cooker.

Health-Enhancing Tips

Look for a BPA-free can of diced tomatoes.

To make this recipe more alkaline, add up to 2 cups (500 mL) chopped vegetables with the celery and/ or add leafy greens, such as chopped kale (tough stems and center ribs removed) or collard greens, 5 to 10 minutes before the end of cooking time and cook, stirring, until wilted.

Fish Chowder

The word "chowder" comes from the French word *chaudière*, which was the name for the pot French fishermen cooked their seafood stews in.

Makes 4 servings

TIPS

If good fresh fish is hard to come by in your area, you can use partially thawed frozen fish fillets or even smoked fish fillets.

Heat milk-based soups just to a simmer. If they are allowed to boil, they may curdle.

1 tbsp	butter or margarine	15 mL
1 cup	chopped onion	250 mL
1/2 cup	chopped celery	125 mL
1 1/2 cups	cubed potatoes	375 mL
1/2 cup	coarsely chopped carrot	125 mL
1/2 tsp	dried summer savory or thyme	2 mL
1/2 tsp	salt	2 mL
1/4 tsp	freshly ground black pepper	1 mL
1 lb	skinless fish fillets, cut into bite-size pieces	500 g
2 cups	2% milk	500 mL

1. In a heavy saucepan, melt butter over medium heat. Sauté onion and celery for 5 minutes or until softened.

2. Stir in potatoes, carrot, savory, salt, pepper and 2 cups (500 mL) water; bring to a boil. Reduce heat to low, cover and simmer for 20 minutes or until vegetables are tender.

3. Stir in fish, cover and simmer for 10 minutes or until fish is opaque and flakes easily when tested with a fork. Stir in milk and return to a simmer (do not let boil).

Health-Enhancing Tips

To create a more alkaline meal, serve this chowder with a side salad or steamed vegetables.

For a healthier fat, use organic butter or ghee (see tip, page 179).

If you are lactose-intolerant or sensitive to dairy, use rice or hemp milk in place of the cow's milk.

Nutrients per serving

Calories	233
Fat	6 g
Carbohydrate	20 g
Fiber	3 g
Protein	24 g
Vitamin A	3073 IU
Iron	0.7 mg
Magnesium	56 mg
Zinc	1.2 mg
Selenium	32.9 mcg

Salads and Dressings

Fast and Easy Greek Salad 220

Spanish Orange and Avocado Salad 221

Kale and Pear Salad with Warmed Shallot Dressing 222

Spinach Salad with Carrots and Mushrooms 223

Warm Spinach and Mushroom Salad 224

Marinated Vegetable Medley 225

Roasted Portobello Mushroom and Fennel Salad 226

Kasha and Beet Salad with Celery and Feta 228

Cactus Salad 230

Quinoa Salad 231

Lentil Squash Salad 232

Grilled Salmon and Romaine Salad 234

Pork Quinoa Salad with Indian Dressing 236

Green Goddess Salad Dressing 237

Roasted Garlic and Sun-Dried Tomato Dressing 238

Fast and Easy Greek Salad

Here's a simple salad that is also incredibly healthy and healing. It's especially good when tomatoes are in season.

Makes 4 servings

TIPS

If desired, substitute 1 tbsp (15 mL) chopped fresh basil for the dried.

This salad is higher in fat, so it is best served with lower-fat dishes. If you don't have time to make the dressing, use a bottled oil-and-vinegar-type dressing. Choose a dressing that contains less than 3 g of fat per 1 tbsp (15 mL) to help cut the fat.

2 cups	diced tomatoes	500 mL
2 cups	diced cucumbers	500 mL
1 cup	cubed feta cheese (about 8 oz/250 g)	250 mL
½ cup	thinly sliced onions	125 mL
¼ cup	sliced black olives (optional)	60 mL
2 tbsp	white wine vinegar	30 mL
2 tbsp	olive oil	30 mL
½ tsp	minced garlic	2 mL
½ tsp	dried basil	2 mL
½ tsp	dried oregano	2 mL
	Freshly ground black pepper	

1. In a large bowl, combine tomatoes, cucumbers, cheese, onions and olives (if using). Set aside.

2. In a small bowl or measuring cup, whisk together vinegar, oil, garlic, basil, oregano and pepper to taste. Add to tomato mixture; toss gently to combine. Chill before serving.

Health-Enhancing Tips

To reduce the fat content of this recipe, use less feta cheese.

To increase the protein, top the salad with cooked shrimp, chicken, beef or tofu.

Nutrients per serving

Calories	192
Fat	15 g
Carbohydrate	8 g
Fiber	2 g
Protein	7 g
Vitamin A	954 IU
Iron	0.8 mg
Magnesium	27 mg
Zinc	1.4 mg
Selenium	5.8 mcg

Spanish Orange and Avocado Salad

This delightfully refreshing, nutritious, easy salad includes many important healing ingredients. In Spain, it is eaten during the winter months, when tomatoes are not at their prime, but it is also wonderful on a hot summer day. The use of avocado is a Mexican influence on Spanish cuisine.

Makes 8 servings

TIPS

This salad is best eaten soon after it is made.

Grainy Dijon mustard (also called old-fashioned or whole Dijon mustard) is preferred in this recipe because it has a milder flavor. If it's not available, you can use regular Dijon, but use half as much, as the flavor is very strong.

It is important to buy seedless oranges, such as navel or Valencia oranges, for this salad. Navel and Valencia oranges are available almost year-round.

Nutrients per serving

Calories	178
Fat	13 g
Carbohydrate	17 g
Fiber	6 g
Protein	3 g
Vitamin A	4137 IU
Iron	0.9 mg
Magnesium	31 mg
Zinc	0.5 mg
Selenium	0.5 mcg

DRESSING

3 tbsp	extra virgin olive oil	45 mL
1 tbsp	sherry vinegar	15 mL
1½ tsp	freshly squeezed lemon juice	7 mL
1 tsp	grainy Dijon mustard	5 mL
¼ tsp	salt	1 mL

SALAD

½	head romaine lettuce (green part only), finely chopped (about 4 cups/1 L)	½
4	large navel or Valencia oranges, cut into ½-inch (1 cm) thick slices	4
2	large avocados, thinly sliced	2
1	roasted red bell pepper (see tip, page 245), julienned	1
1 cup	thinly sliced red onion	250 mL
2 tbsp	finely chopped fresh mint	30 mL

1. *Dressing:* In a small bowl, whisk together oil, vinegar, lemon juice, mustard and salt.

2. *Salad:* Arrange lettuce on a large platter. Arrange oranges decoratively on top, then avocados, roasted peppers and onion.

3. Just before serving, drizzle dressing over salad and sprinkle with mint.

Kale and Pear Salad with Warmed Shallot Dressing

This salad is great on a hot summer day when you don't want to cook or as a side at an elegant dinner party.

Makes 6 servings

TIPS

Baby kale leaves are a new addition to the prewashed packaged salads available in supermarkets. If unavailable, use regular bunched kale. Remove tough stems and center ribs, and finely shred the leaves.

To toast walnuts, place on a rimmed baking sheet in 350°F (180°C) oven for 8 to 10 minutes or until light golden and fragrant.

8 cups	lightly packed baby kale leaves	2 L
2	small pears or apples, cut lengthwise into thin slices, then halved diagonally	2
1/4 cup	minced shallots	60 mL
1/4 tsp	salt	1 mL
1/4 tsp	freshly ground black pepper	1 mL
2 tbsp	pomegranate, cider or other fruit vinegar	30 mL
2 tsp	grainy Dijon mustard	10 mL
2 tsp	liquid honey	10 mL
4 tsp	walnut, hazelnut or extra virgin olive oil	20 mL
3 tbsp	chopped toasted walnuts or hazelnuts (see tip, at left)	45 mL

1. Place kale in a salad bowl and top with pear slices.

2. In a small saucepan, combine shallots, salt, pepper, vinegar, mustard and honey. Bring to a boil over medium-low heat, whisking. Remove from heat and whisk in oil.

3. Pour dressing over salad and toss to coat. Sprinkle with walnuts. Serve immediately.

Variations

Replace one of the pears with 1/4 cup (60 mL) fresh pomegranate seeds.

Any assertive green, such as dandelion, curly endive or arugula, will work in this tasty salad. Or use more mellow leaves, such as Swiss chard, watercress or romaine.

Health-Enhancing Tips

To reduce the carbohydrate, omit the honey.

Check the label when buying fruit vinegars and avoid any with added sugars or other sweetners.

To increase the protein, top the salad with cooked shrimp, chicken, hard-boiled eggs, tofu or another concentrated protein source.

Nutrients per serving	
Calories	139
Fat	6 g
Carbohydrate	20 g
Fiber	4 g
Protein	4 g
Vitamin A	13,829 IU
Iron	1.8 mg
Magnesium	44 mg
Zinc	0.6 mg
Selenium	1.6 mcg

Spinach Salad with Carrots and Mushrooms

The tangy dressing, accented with cumin, nicely balances the sweetness of the raisins and carrots in this colorful salad that is easy to assemble.

Makes 6 servings

MAKE AHEAD

Assemble salad up to 4 hours ahead, cover and refrigerate. Add dressing and toss just before serving.

VARIATION

Use 1 tsp (5 mL) dried fines herbes instead of cumin.

8 cups	loosely packed fresh baby spinach	2 L
1½ cups	sliced mushrooms	375 mL
1½ cups	shredded or matchstick carrots	375 mL
1	small red onion, thinly sliced	1
¼ cup	dark raisins or dried cranberries	60 mL
2 tbsp	unsalted roasted green pumpkin seeds (pepitas)	30 mL

DRESSING

1	clove garlic, minced	1
¾ tsp	ground cumin	3 mL
¼ tsp	salt	1 mL
¼ tsp	freshly ground black pepper	1 mL
2 tbsp	pumpkin seed oil or extra virgin olive oil	30 mL
2 tbsp	red wine vinegar	30 mL
1 tbsp	liquid honey	15 mL
2 tsp	Dijon mustard	10 mL

1. In a serving bowl, layer one-third of the spinach, all of the mushrooms, another third of the spinach, all of the carrots, then the remaining spinach. Arrange onion, raisins and pumpkin seeds on top.

2. *Dressing:* In a small bowl, whisk together garlic, cumin, salt, pepper, oil, vinegar, honey and mustard.

3. Drizzle dressing over salad and toss to coat.

Nutrients per serving

Calories	116
Fat	6 g
Carbohydrate	14 g
Fiber	3 g
Protein	3 g
Vitamin A	8347 IU
Iron	1.8 mg
Magnesium	54 mg
Zinc	0.6 mg
Selenium	2.5 mcg

Health-Enhancing Tips

To reduce the carbohydrate content of this recipe, omit the raisins or cranberries, or replace them with sliced fresh strawberries.

For more protein, top this salad with cooked chicken, tofu, shrimp, hard-cooked eggs or beef.

To increase both alkalinity and protein, top each serving with ½ cup (125 mL) cooked lentils. This will also increase the carbohydrate.

Warm Spinach and Mushroom Salad

This mouth-watering warm salad is a great alternative to more mundane spinach salads. Each bite provides an explosion of flavor and healing magic.

Makes 2 to 3 servings

TIPS

To soften sun-dried tomatoes, cover with boiling water and let soak for 15 minutes. Drain and chop.

Try this recipe with different mushrooms — such as cremini or, for a decadent evening, shiitake or chanterelles. Button mushrooms will also work well.

DRESSING

3 tbsp	balsamic vinegar	45 mL
4 tsp	olive oil	20 mL
1 tsp	minced garlic	5 mL

SALAD

6 cups	torn spinach leaves	1.5 L
½ cup	chopped softened sun-dried tomatoes (see tip, at left)	125 mL
¼ cup	toasted chopped walnuts (see tip, page 222)	60 mL
2 tsp	vegetable oil	10 mL
1 tsp	minced garlic	5 mL
2 cups	sliced oyster mushrooms	500 mL
¾ cup	sliced red onions	175 mL

1. *Dressing:* In a small bowl, whisk together vinegar, olive oil and garlic. Set aside.

2. *Salad:* Put spinach, sun-dried tomatoes and walnuts in a large serving bowl.

3. In a large nonstick frying pan, heat vegetable oil over high heat. Add garlic, mushrooms and red onions; cook for 6 minutes or until mushrooms are browned and any excess liquid is absorbed. Quickly add hot vegetables and dressing to spinach and toss. Serve immediately.

Nutrients per serving (1 of 3)

Calories	236
Fat	16 g
Carbohydrate	18 g
Fiber	5 g
Protein	8 g
Vitamin A	5737 IU
Iron	3.7 mg
Magnesium	101 mg
Zinc	1.4 mg
Selenium	4.5 mcg

Health-Enhancing Tips

To increase the protein content of this recipe, top the salad with cooked shrimp, chicken, beef or tofu.

For a healthier fat, substitute ghee (see tip, page 179) for the vegetable oil. In step 3, cook the vegetables over medium-high heat instead of high heat, adjusting the cooking time as necessary.

Marinated Vegetable Medley

In this relish salad, marinating gives the garden vegetables a lightly pickled taste. The longer you refrigerate the salad, the better the flavor will be.

Makes 6 servings

TIPS

Choose the flavor of vinegar you enjoy most. If you like a mild vinegar, choose white wine vinegar, distilled white vinegar or cider vinegar. For a bolder flavor, use red wine vinegar, balsamic vinegar or malt vinegar. Herb-flavored vinegar would add a nice flavor too.

You can also shake the dressing ingredients together in a small jar.

1	carrot, sliced	1
½	cucumber, sliced	½
1 cup	cauliflower florets	250 mL
1 cup	broccoli florets	250 mL
1 cup	sliced celery	250 mL
¼ cup	vinegar (see tip, at left)	60 mL
1 tbsp	vegetable oil	15 mL
½ tsp	onion salt	2 mL
½ tsp	freshly ground black pepper	2 mL
1	firm tomato, cut into 8 wedges	1

1. In a large bowl, combine carrot, cucumber, cauliflower, broccoli and celery.

2. In a small bowl, whisk together vinegar, oil, onion salt and pepper. Pour over salad and toss to coat. Cover and refrigerate for at least 3 hours or for up to 3 days to marinate. Add tomato wedges just before serving.

Health-Enhancing Tip

For a healthier, less inflammatory fat, use olive oil in place of the vegetable oil.

Nutrients per serving

Calories	41
Fat	3 g
Carbohydrate	4 g
Fiber	2 g
Protein	1 g
Vitamin A	2301 IU
Iron	0.3 mg
Magnesium	11.4 mg
Zinc	0.2 mg
Selenium	0.6 mcg

Roasted Portobello Mushroom and Fennel Salad

Portobello mushrooms appear in soups, salads, side dishes and main courses. Although not a complete protein, they are often the mainstay of vegetarian menus, perhaps because of their meaty texture.

Makes 6 servings

TIPS

If you wish, you can use a spoon to scrape away the dark gills on the underside of the mushrooms.

To toast nuts and seeds, place in a small baking dish. Convection bake in a preheated 300°F (150°C) oven for 5 to 10 minutes or until golden.

- **Preheat convection oven to 400°F (200°C)**
- **2 baking sheets, lined with parchment paper**

MUSHROOMS AND FENNEL

⅓ cup	olive oil	75 mL
4	cloves garlic, minced	4
2 tsp	chopped fresh tarragon (or ¾ tsp/3 mL dried)	10 mL
½ tsp	salt	2 mL
¼ tsp	freshly ground black pepper	1 mL
6	portobello mushrooms (about 1½ lbs/750 g total), stems removed	6
1	large bulb fennel (about 1½ lbs/750 g), trimmed and cut into 12 wedges	1

BALSAMIC VINAIGRETTE

2 tbsp	balsamic vinegar	30 mL
1 tbsp	freshly squeezed lemon juice	15 mL
1 tsp	Dijon mustard	5 mL
2 tbsp	olive oil	30 mL
¼ tsp	salt	1 mL
¼ tsp	freshly ground black pepper	1 mL

SALAD

6 cups	arugula or baby spinach	1.5 L
½ cup	toasted pine nuts (see tip, at left)	125 mL

1. *Mushrooms and Fennel:* In a small bowl, whisk together oil, garlic, tarragon, salt and pepper.

2. Arrange mushrooms, round side up, on a prepared baking sheet. Brush with half the oil mixture.

3. In a large bowl, toss fennel wedges with the remaining oil mixture. Place on the other baking sheet.

Nutrients per serving

Calories	267
Fat	25 g
Carbohydrate	10 g
Fiber	3 g
Protein	5 g
Vitamin A	535 IU
Iron	1.7 mg
Magnesium	46 mg
Zinc	1.4 mg
Selenium	16.3 mcg

MAKE AHEAD

Prepare dressing, cover and refrigerate for up to 2 days.

4. Convection roast mushrooms and fennel in preheated oven — mushrooms for 12 minutes, fennel for 18 to 20 minutes or until tender. Cool both slightly. Cut each mushroom diagonally into 4 slices.

5. *Vinaigrette:* In a small bowl or measuring cup, whisk together vinegar, lemon juice, mustard, oil, salt and pepper.

6. *Salad:* Toss arugula with vinaigrette and arrange on serving plates. Arrange mushrooms and fennel over greens. Sprinkle with pine nuts.

Health-Enhancing Tips

To increase the protein content of this recipe, top the salad with cooked chicken, tofu, shrimp or red meat.

To make this a more filling meal, toss 3 cups (750 mL) cooked quinoa with the arugula and vinegar in step 6.

Kasha and Beet Salad with Celery and Feta

Beets, parsley and feta are the perfect balance for assertive buckwheat in this hearty salad. It's a great combination and a wonderful buffet dish.

Makes 6 to 8 servings

TIP

Buckwheat, a gluten-free grain, contains beneficial antioxidants that help protect the body's cells. In addition, it may help you stay full longer than other grains.

2 cups	ready-to-use GF vegetable or chicken broth	500 mL
2	cloves garlic, minced	2
1 cup	kasha or buckwheat groats (see tip, opposite)	250 mL

DRESSING

¼ cup	red wine vinegar	60 mL
1 tsp	Dijon mustard	5 mL
½ tsp	salt	2 mL
½ tsp	freshly ground black pepper	2 mL
3 tbsp	extra virgin olive oil	45 mL
2 cups	diced peeled cooked beets	500 mL
4	stalks celery, diced	4
6	green onions, white part only, thinly sliced	6
½ cup	finely chopped parsley	125 mL
3 oz	crumbled feta cheese	90 g

1. In a saucepan over medium-high heat, bring broth and garlic to a boil. Gradually add kasha, stirring constantly to prevent clumping. Reduce heat to low. Cover and simmer until all the liquid is absorbed and kasha is tender, about 10 minutes. Remove from heat. Fluff up with a fork and transfer to a serving bowl and let cool slightly.

2. *Dressing:* In a small bowl, combine vinegar, mustard, salt and pepper, stirring until salt dissolves. Gradually whisk in olive oil until blended. Add to kasha and toss well.

3. Add beets, celery and green onions to kasha and toss again. Chill until ready to serve. Just before serving, garnish with parsley and sprinkle feta over top.

Nutrients per serving (1 of 8)

Calories	181
Fat	8 g
Carbohydrate	23 g
Fiber	4 g
Protein	6 g
Vitamin A	574 IU
Iron	1.4 mg
Magnesium	59 mg
Zinc	0.8 mg
Selenium	2.2 mcg

Buckwheat groats that are already toasted are known as kasha. If you prefer a milder buckwheat flavor, use groats rather than kasha in this dish. Just place them in a dry skillet over medium-high heat and cook, stirring constantly, until they are nicely fragrant, about 4 minutes. In the process they will darken from a light shade of sand to one with a hint of brown. Groats you toast yourself have a milder flavor than store-bought kasha.

Variation

Rice and Beet Salad with Celery and Feta: Substitute 3 cups (750 mL) cooked long-grain brown rice for the cooked kasha.

Health-Enhancing Tip

To increase the protein content of this recipe, top the salad with cooked chicken, fish, shrimp or tofu.

Cactus Salad

Nopales, the edible leaf pads of the prickly pear cactus (nopal), are very popular in Mexican cuisine. Many people believe nopal can prevent or manage diabetes by lowering blood sugar levels.

Makes 4 servings

TIPS

Panela cheese, also known as queso de canasta, has a mild "fresh milk" flavor. Only a small amount is used in this dish, as it is high in fat and saturated fat.

If you cannot find panela cheese, substitute farmer's cheese or feta.

SALAD

6	large cactus leaves (about 22 oz/660 g total)	6
$\frac{1}{8}$	red onion (left in one piece)	$\frac{1}{8}$
1 tsp	baking soda	5 mL
2 cups	water	500 mL
3	large plum (Roma) tomatoes, diced	3
1	serrano chile pepper, seeded and minced	1
$\frac{1}{2}$ cup	finely chopped red onion	125 mL
$\frac{1}{2}$ cup	finely chopped fresh cilantro	125 mL
$\frac{1}{4}$ cup	cubed panela cheese ($\frac{1}{8}$-inch/3 mm cubes)	60 mL

DRESSING

$\frac{1}{4}$ cup	freshly squeezed lime juice	60 mL
1 tbsp	olive oil	15 mL
$\frac{1}{2}$ tsp	salt	2 mL

1. *Salad:* Holding a knife parallel to the cutting board and aiming the blade away from you, use the tip of the knife to remove the cactus spines. Cut around the perimeter of the cactus leaves to remove the spines on the edges. Wash leaves and cut into 1-inch (2.5 cm) squares. You should have about $3\frac{1}{2}$ cups (875 mL).

2. In a large pot, combine cactus, $\frac{1}{8}$ onion, baking soda and water. Bring to a boil over high heat. Boil for 20 minutes or until cactus is tender. Discard onion. Drain and cool cactus under cold water.

3. In a medium bowl, combine cactus, tomatoes, chile, chopped onion, cilantro and cheese.

4. *Dressing:* In a small bowl, combine lime juice, oil and salt.

5. Add dressing to salad and toss to coat.

Nutrients per serving

Calories	126
Fat	6 g
Carbohydrate	15 g
Fiber	2 g
Protein	5 g
Vitamin A	1279 IU
Iron	0.6 mg
Magnesium	24 mg
Zinc	0.5 mg
Selenium	1.2 mcg

Quinoa Salad

This simple, delicious salad packs a nutritional punch. Thanks to the quinoa, it even provides a complete protein, so it's a great choice for vegetarians. Whether it serves 2 people or 4 depends on how much you're willing to share!

Makes 2 to 4 servings

TIP

If you have time to make Basic Vegetable Stock (page 194), use it in place of the ready-to-use broth.

1¼ cups	ready-to-use GF vegetable broth	300 mL
¾ cup	quinoa, rinsed	175 mL
½ cup	thawed frozen peas	125 mL
¼ cup	finely chopped orange bell pepper	60 mL
¼ cup	finely chopped yellow bell pepper	60 mL
1 tbsp	finely chopped red onion	15 mL
2 tbsp	extra virgin olive oil	30 mL
1 tbsp	chopped fresh parsley	15 mL
1 tsp	dried thyme	5 mL
1 tsp	freshly squeezed lemon juice	5 mL
	Salt and freshly ground black pepper	

1. In a saucepan, bring broth to a boil over high heat. Add quinoa, reduce heat to low, cover and simmer for 20 minutes or until quinoa is tender and liquid is almost absorbed. Remove from heat and let stand, covered, for 5 minutes or until liquid is absorbed.

2. In a large bowl, combine quinoa, peas, orange pepper, yellow pepper and red onion.

3. In a small bowl, whisk together oil, parsley, thyme and lemon juice. Drizzle over salad and toss to coat. Season to taste with salt and pepper. Serve warm or cover and refrigerate for 1 hour, until chilled, and serve cold.

Variation

If you're making this salad for non-vegetarians, you can substitute ready-to-use GF chicken or turkey broth, or Homemade Chicken Stock (page 195), for the vegetable broth.

Health-Enhancing Tip

To increase the protein content of this recipe, add half of a 6-oz (170 g) can of wild Alaskan salmon, drained and flaked, 5 to 7 cooked jumbo shrimp, 3 oz (90 g) baked chicken breast or 1 cup (250 mL) cooked diced tofu to each serving.

Nutrients per serving (1 of 4)

Calories	201
Fat	9 g
Carbohydrate	25 g
Fiber	4 g
Protein	6 g
Vitamin A	1178 IU
Iron	2.2 mg
Magnesium	71 mg
Zinc	1.2 mg
Selenium	3.1 mcg

Lentil Squash Salad

This is a good make-ahead dish for your next family get-together, and if you choose vegetable broth, it's vegetarian! It can be eaten cold or, if you prefer, heated in the microwave to serve hot.

Makes 12 servings

TIPS

A 3-lb (1.5 kg) butternut squash yields about 4 cups (1 L) diced.

Purchase unroasted, unsalted pumpkin seeds. To toast them, spread them in a single layer in a large skillet and toast over medium heat, shaking the pan frequently, for 5 to 8 minutes or until aromatic and lightly browned.

- **Large microwave-safe casserole dish**

DRESSING

1	clove garlic, minced	1
2 tbsp	cider vinegar	30 mL
2 tbsp	liquid honey	30 mL
2 tbsp	vegetable oil	30 mL
2 tsp	Dijon mustard	10 mL

SALAD

3 cups	ready-to-use GF vegetable or beef broth	750 mL
½ cup	dried red and/or green lentils	125 mL
½ cup	dried split peas	125 mL
1	butternut squash, diced	1
½ cup	dried cranberries	125 mL
½ cup	chopped green onions	125 mL
⅓ cup	green pumpkin seeds (pepitas), toasted (see tip, at left)	75 mL
3 tbsp	snipped fresh tarragon	45 mL
	Salt and freshly ground black pepper	

1. *Dressing:* In a small bowl, whisk together garlic, vinegar, honey, oil and mustard. Set aside.

2. *Salad:* In a large saucepan, bring broth to a boil over high heat. Add lentils and split peas; return to a boil. Reduce heat to medium-low and simmer for 25 to 30 minutes or until tender. Drain and let cool.

3. In casserole dish, combine squash and 2 tbsp (30 mL) water. Cover and microwave on High for 10 to 12 minutes or until squash is fork-tender. Drain and set aside.

4. In a large bowl, combine lentils, split peas, squash, cranberries, green onions, pumpkin seeds and tarragon. Pour in dressing and toss to coat.

5. Cover and refrigerate for at least 8 hours, until chilled, or for up to 3 days. Season to taste with salt and pepper.

Nutrients per serving

Calories	136
Fat	4 g
Carbohydrate	21 g
Fiber	4 g
Protein	5 g
Vitamin A	2053 IU
Iron	1.5 mg
Magnesium	41 mg
Zinc	0.9 mg
Selenium	1.3 mcg

You can use all lentils or all split peas.

Variations

A 14- to 19-oz (398 to 540 mL) can of beans, drained and rinsed, can be substituted for the lentils and broth.

Substitute Hubbard squash for the butternut, using about 4 cups (1 L) diced.

Substitute sunflower seeds for the pumpkin seeds.

Health-Enhancing Tips

To reduce the carbohydrate content and acidity in this recipe, omit the dried cranberries.

Add up to 1 cup (250 mL) roasted root vegetables to increase the alkalinity of this dish.

Grilled Salmon and Romaine Salad

Grilled salmon on a bed of freshly tossed greens makes for an easy and delicious dinner. The dressing, made in the food processor, does double duty as a marinade for the salmon and a dressing for the salad.

Makes 4 servings

TIP

Salmon is high in omega-3 fatty acids, which help reduce inflammation.

- **Preheat greased barbecue grill or stovetop grill pan to medium**
- **Food processor**
- **Four 8-inch (20 cm) bamboo skewers, soaked in water for 15 minutes**

1	clove garlic, coarsely chopped	1
2 cups	lightly packed fresh parsley leaves	500 mL
¼ tsp	salt	1 mL
¼ tsp	freshly ground black pepper	1 mL
1 tsp	grated orange zest	5 mL
¼ cup	freshly squeezed orange juice	60 mL
2 tbsp	extra virgin olive oil	30 mL
2 tbsp	red wine vinegar	30 mL
1 tbsp	Dijon mustard	15 mL
1 lb	skinless salmon fillet (in one piece)	500 g
8 cups	torn romaine lettuce	2 L
2 cups	halved cherry tomatoes	500 mL
½	English cucumber, halved lengthwise and sliced	½

1. In food processor, combine garlic, parsley, salt, pepper, orange juice, oil, vinegar and mustard; process, scraping down sides occasionally with a spatula, until parsley is very finely chopped. Transfer to a bowl and stir in orange zest.

2. Cut salmon lengthwise into 4 equal strips. Thread lengthwise onto skewers. Arrange skewers in a shallow dish and spread with ¼ cup (60 mL) of the dressing. Let marinate at room temperature for 10 minutes, turning occasionally.

3. Place salmon on preheated grill and cook, turning once, for 5 to 6 minutes per side or until fish is opaque and flakes easily when tested with a fork. Let stand for 5 minutes.

Nutrients per serving	
Calories	261
Fat	12 g
Carbohydrate	11 g
Fiber	4 g
Protein	26 g
Vitamin A	11,552 IU
Iron	3.6 mg
Magnesium	73 mg
Zinc	1.2 mg
Selenium	36.2 mcg

Before purchasing fish, always learn what you can about sustainability and fishing practices. Ask your fishmonger or check online resources. A great resource is the Monterey Bay Aquarium's Seafood Watch Guide, which can be found at www.seafoodwatch.org.

4. Meanwhile, in a bowl, combine romaine, tomatoes and cucumber. Pour the remaining dressing over salad and toss to lightly coat.

5. Divide salad among plates and top with salmon.

Health-Enhancing Tip

To reduce toxins (advanced glycation end products, or AGEs), instead of threading the salmon onto skewers to grill, place strips (or the whole fillet) in a shallow baking dish and bake at 350°F (180°C) for 15 to 25 minutes or until fish is opaque and flakes easily when tested with a fork.

Pork Quinoa Salad with Indian Dressing

You'll love this make-ahead salad when you're entertaining houseguests for the weekend — no need to worry about their arrival time!

Makes 4 servings

TIPS

If you have time to make Homemade Chicken Stock (page 195), use it in place of the ready-to-use broth.

Leave the peel on the cucumber for great color and added fiber.

The dressing can be stored in an airtight container in the refrigerator for up to 1 week.

VARIATION

Substitute raisins or peanuts for the currants.

CARDAMOM DRESSING

⅔ cup	plain yogurt	150 mL
1 tsp	ground coriander	5 mL
1 tsp	ground cardamom	5 mL
1 tsp	ground cumin	5 mL

SALAD

⅓ cup	quinoa, rinsed	75 mL
1 cup	ready-to-use GF chicken broth	250 mL
8 oz	cooked pork tenderloin, thinly sliced	250 g
16	strawberry or grape tomatoes	16
½	seedless cucumber, cubed	½
½ cup	dried currants	125 mL
2 tbsp	snipped fresh cilantro	30 mL

1. *Dressing:* In a small bowl, whisk together yogurt, coriander, cardamom and cumin. Set aside for at least 1 hour or cover and refrigerate overnight to let flavors develop and blend.

2. *Salad:* In a saucepan, bring quinoa and broth to a boil over high heat. Reduce heat to low, cover and simmer for 18 to 20 minutes or until quinoa is transparent and the tiny, spiral-like germ is separated. Remove from heat and let stand, covered, for 5 to 10 minutes or until broth is absorbed.

3. In a large bowl, combine quinoa, pork, tomatoes, cucumber, currants and cilantro. Pour in dressing and toss well to coat.

4. Cover and refrigerate for at least 4 hours or overnight to let flavors develop and blend.

Health-Enhancing Tips

To create a more alkaline meal, serve this dish with steamed vegetables or on top of a bed of greens.

To reduce the carbohydrate content of this recipe, substitute an equal amount of nuts or seeds for the dried currants.

Nutrients per serving

Calories	182
Fat	4 g
Carbohydrate	19 g
Fiber	3 g
Protein	19 g
Vitamin A	650 IU
Iron	2.3 mg
Magnesium	68 mg
Zinc	2.3 mg
Selenium	28.6 mcg

Green Goddess Salad Dressing

Attractive, colorful, contrasting flecks of green — this is the dressing everyone requests. Use as a dip on a tray with your favorite crudités. Serve as a dressing over potato, pasta or carrot coleslaw salads.

**Makes about
1 cup (250 mL)**

TIPS

This recipe can be halved or doubled, depending on the amount you require.

For the best color, be sure to use fresh parsley.

- **Food processor**

1	small clove garlic	1
1	green onion	1
¼ cup	fresh parsley	60 mL
1½ tsp	dried tarragon (or 1 to 2 tbsp/15 to 30 mL snipped fresh)	7 mL
½ cup	GF sour cream	125 mL
½ cup	plain yogurt	125 mL
1 tbsp	freshly squeezed lemon juice	15 mL

1. In food processor, combine garlic, green onion, parsley, tarragon, sour cream, yogurt and lemon juice. Process until smooth. Cover and refrigerate for a minimum of 2 hours to allow flavors to develop and blend. Refrigerate for up to 2 weeks.

Nutrients per
2 tbsp (30 mL)

Calories	33
Fat	2 g
Carbohydrate	2 g
Fiber	0 g
Protein	2 g
Vitamin A	95 IU
Iron	0.1 mg
Magnesium	3 mg
Zinc	0.1 mg
Selenium	0.5 mcg

Roasted Garlic and Sun-Dried Tomato Dressing

The colors of this dressing are reminiscent of the Mediterranean. Besides using it to dress a fresh green salad, enjoy it spread on a roast beef sandwich.

Makes about 1½ cups (375 mL)

1	head garlic	1
1 cup	plain yogurt	250 mL
½ cup	GF sour cream	125 mL
½ cup	snipped sun-dried tomatoes	125 mL
¼ cup	snipped fresh parsley	60 mL

1. *To roast garlic:* Cut off top of head to expose clove tips. Drizzle with ¼ tsp (1 mL) olive oil and microwave on High for 70 seconds or until fork-tender. Or bake in a pie plate or baking dish at 375°F (190°C) for 15 to 20 minutes.

2. In a small bowl, stir together yogurt, sour cream, garlic, sun-dried tomatoes and parsley. Cover and refrigerate for a minimum of 2 hours to allow flavors to develop and blend. Refrigerate for up to 2 weeks. The longer the dressing is refrigerated, the stronger the flavor and the deeper the color becomes.

Variations

Substitute mayonnaise for the sour cream to turn this dressing into a dip.

For a dill-flavored dressing, substitute ¼ cup (60 mL) snipped fresh dill for fresh parsley.

Nutrients per 2 tbsp (30 mL)

Calories	34
Fat	1 g
Carbohydrate	4 g
Fiber	0 g
Protein	2 g
Vitamin A	158 IU
Iron	0.3 mg
Magnesium	9 mg
Zinc	0.3 mg
Selenium	1.3 mcg

Dips and Sauces

Roasted Garlic Dip. 240

Chili Black Bean Dip. 241

Artichoke and White Bean Spread. 242

Anti-inflammatory Hummus 243

Lentil Tapenade. 244

Sardine Spread 245

Basic Pesto 246

Creamy Basil Pesto 247

Parsley Pesto Sauce. 248

Cucumber Mint Raita. 248

Tomato Avocado Salsa 249

Basic Tomato Sauce. 250

Roasted Garlic Dip

Roasting garlic takes the bitter bite out of it, so go ahead and enjoy.

**Makes about
2 cups (500 mL)**

TIPS

If you can only find smaller cans of black beans, use 2 cups (500 mL) drained rinsed beans.

Save money and cut back on sodium by soaking and cooking dried beans to use in place of canned.

To roast garlic, cut off top of head to expose clove tips. Drizzle with $\frac{1}{4}$ tsp (1 mL) olive oil, place in a pie plate or baking dish and roast in a 375°F (190°C) oven for 15 to 20 minutes or until fork-tender. Let cool slightly, then squeeze cloves from skins.

- **Food processor**

2 tsp	extra virgin olive oil	10 mL
1	onion, finely chopped	1
1	can (19 oz/540 mL) black beans, drained and rinsed	1
1	bulb garlic, roasted and cloves squeezed out (see tip, at left)	1
2 tbsp	snipped fresh sage	30 mL
1 tbsp	balsamic vinegar	15 mL
1 tsp	freshly squeezed lemon juice	5 mL
$\frac{1}{2}$ tsp	salt	2 mL
$\frac{1}{4}$ tsp	freshly ground black pepper	1 mL

1. In a skillet, heat oil over medium heat. Sauté onion for 2 to 3 minutes or until tender.

2. In food processor, combine onion, beans, roasted garlic cloves, sage, vinegar, lemon juice, salt and pepper; pulse, scraping down sides occasionally, until smooth.

3. Transfer to an airtight container and refrigerate for at least 2 hours to allow flavors to develop and blend. Store in the refrigerator for up to 2 weeks.

Variation

Choose any variety of canned beans, such as chickpeas (garbanzo beans), white beans or pinto beans.

Health-Enhancing Tips

Serve with cut-up raw vegetables, 2 to 3 GF crackers or 10 to 12 Beanitos (bean chips you can purchase at many health food and grocery stores).

To increase the alkalinity of this recipe, use canned lentils in place of black beans.

Nutrients per 2 tbsp (30 mL)

Calories	32
Fat	1 g
Carbohydrate	5 g
Fiber	1 g
Protein	2 g
Vitamin A	9 IU
Iron	0.4 mg
Magnesium	12 mg
Zinc	0.2 mg
Selenium	0.8 mcg

Chili Black Bean Dip

Making your own tasty bean dip couldn't be any easier. Just purée the ingredients in your food processor and it's ready — a bowl of wholesome goodness to serve with vegetables or use as a sandwich spread.

Makes about 2 cups (500 mL)

TIPS

Save money and cut back on sodium by soaking and cooking dried beans to use in place of canned.

The dip can be stored in an airtight container in the refrigerator for up to 5 days.

- **Food processor**

2 cups	well-rinsed drained canned black beans or red kidney beans	500 mL
1	clove garlic, chopped	1
1½ tsp	chili powder	7 mL
1 tsp	dried oregano	5 mL
Pinch	cayenne pepper (optional)	Pinch
⅔ cup	light (5%) sour cream	150 mL

1. In food processor, combine beans, garlic, chili powder, oregano and cayenne (if using); pulse until beans are partially mashed. Add sour cream and process until smooth. Transfer to a serving dish.

Variation

If you have a fresh jalapeño pepper on hand, mince it and add it to the dip, along with coarsely chopped fresh cilantro, if you have some handy.

> ### Health-Enhancing Tip
> Serve with cut-up raw vegetables, 2 to 3 GF crackers or 10 to 12 Beanitos (bean chips you can purchase at many health food and grocery stores).

Nutrients per ¼ cup (60 mL)

Calories	72
Fat	1 g
Carbohydrate	12 g
Fiber	3 g
Protein	4 g
Vitamin A	220 IU
Iron	0.9 mg
Magnesium	21 mg
Zinc	0.4 mg
Selenium	1.4 mcg

Artichoke and White Bean Spread

This exceptionally health-promoting spread is packed with flavor. Serve with cut-up raw vegetables to instantly turn a mundane carrot or bell pepper into an exciting snack.

Makes about 3 cups (750 mL)

TIPS

For this quantity of beans, soak, cook and drain 1 cup (250 mL) dried cannellini beans (see Basic Beans, page 255) or drain and rinse 1 can (14 to 19 oz/398 to 540 mL) no-salt added cannellini beans. Cannellini beans are also known as white kidney beans.

If you prefer, use frozen artichokes, thawed, to make this recipe. You will need 6 artichoke hearts.

- **Small (about 2-quart) slow cooker**
- **Food processor**

½	red onion, finely chopped	½
2	cloves garlic, minced	2
¼ cup	extra virgin olive oil, divided	60 mL
2 cups	drained cooked cannellini beans (see tip, at left)	500 mL
1	can (14 oz/398 mL) artichoke hearts, drained and coarsely chopped	1
½ cup	freshly grated Parmesan cheese or vegan alternative	125 mL
1 tsp	sweet paprika	5 mL
½ tsp	sea salt	2 mL
¼ tsp	freshly ground black pepper	1 mL
½ cup	finely chopped fresh parsley leaves	125 mL

1. In slow cooker stoneware, combine onion, garlic and 2 tbsp (30 mL) oil. Place a clean tea towel folded in half (so you will have two layers) over top of stoneware to absorb moisture. Cover and cook on High for 30 minutes, until onions are softened.

2. Meanwhile, in food processor, in batches if necessary, pulse beans and artichokes until desired consistency is achieved. After onions have softened, add bean mixture to stoneware along with Parmesan, paprika, salt, pepper and the remaining oil. Replace tea towel. Cover and cook on Low for 4 hours or on High for 2 hours, until hot and bubbly. Add parsley and stir well.

Nutrients per ¼ cup (60 mL)

Calories	98
Fat	5 g
Carbohydrate	11 g
Fiber	5 g
Protein	4 g
Vitamin A	313 IU
Iron	1.1 mg
Magnesium	28 mg
Zinc	0.5 mg
Selenium	0.6 mcg

Anti-inflammatory Hummus

This recipe turns ordinary hummus into a potent anti-inflammatory medicine. Not only will your body thank you, but your taste buds will be applauding.

Makes about 1²⁄₃ cups (400 mL)

TIPS

You can cook your own chickpeas (see Basic Beans, page 255) or use canned chickpeas, drained and rinsed.

The hummus can be stored in an airtight container in the refrigerator for up to 3 days.

- **Blender or food processor**

3	cloves garlic	3
1½ cups	cooked chickpeas (see tip, at left)	375 mL
½ tsp	ground turmeric	2 mL
¼ tsp	salt	1 mL
¼ cup	tahini	60 mL
3 tbsp	freshly squeezed lemon juice	45 mL
	Water, as necessary	

1. In blender, combine garlic, chickpeas, turmeric, salt, tahini and lemon juice; blend until smooth, adding water if needed to achieve the desired texture.

Health-Enhancing Tip

Serve with cut-up raw vegetables, 2 to 3 GF crackers or 10 to 12 Beanitos (bean chips you can purchase at many health food and grocery stores).

Nutrients per 5 tsp (25 mL)

Calories	49
Fat	2 g
Carbohydrate	6 g
Fiber	1 g
Protein	2 g
Vitamin A	7 IU
Iron	0.7 mg
Magnesium	11 mg
Zinc	0.4 mg
Selenium	1.9 mcg

Lentil Tapenade

Spread tapenade on your favorite whole-grain crackers or crisps for a wholesome snack. This robust spread also makes a superb sandwich filling on crusty bread with roasted vegetables and assertive greens such as arugula.

Makes about 1¼ cups (300 mL)

TIPS

Always rinse brined foods, such as olives and capers, to remove excess salt.

The spread can be stored in an airtight container in the refrigerator for up to 5 days.

- **Food processor**

3 cups	water	750 mL
½ cup	dried brown or green lentils, rinsed	125 mL
1	small bay leaf	1
1	clove garlic, coarsely chopped	1
⅓ cup	pitted kalamata olives, rinsed and coarsely chopped (about 12)	75 mL
1 tbsp	extra virgin olive oil	15 mL
¼ tsp	freshly ground black pepper	1 mL
¼ cup	chopped fresh parsley	60 mL
1 tsp	grated lemon zest	5 mL

1. In a medium saucepan, bring water to a boil over high heat. Add lentils and bay leaf. Reduce heat to medium-low, cover and simmer for 25 to 30 minutes or until lentils are tender. Drain and let cool to room temperature. Discard bay leaf.

2. In food processor, combine lentils, garlic, olives, olive oil and pepper; process until smooth. Add parsley and lemon zest; pulse until combined.

3. Transfer to a serving bowl, cover and refrigerate for 2 hours, until chilled, before serving.

Health-Enhancing Tip

Serve with cut-up raw vegetables, 2 to 3 GF crackers or 10 to 12 Beanitos (bean chips you can purchase at many health food and grocery stores).

Nutrients per ¼ cup (60 mL)

Calories	103
Fat	4 g
Carbohydrate	13 g
Fiber	3 g
Protein	5 g
Vitamin A	307 IU
Iron	2.0 mg
Magnesium	18 mg
Zinc	0.8 mg
Selenium	1.8 mcg

Sardine Spread

The next time you're wondering what to make for a simple appetizer or snack to serve with crostini, reach for a can of sardines — they are rich in omega-3 fats and good for your heart.

Makes about ¾ cup (175 mL)

TIPS

Canned sardines are great to have on hand, as they can be easily mashed for lunchtime sandwich fillings and to make this delicious spread.

To roast bell peppers, preheat the barbecue grill to high or preheat the broiler. Grill peppers on barbecue, or on a baking sheet under the broiler, turning often, until blackened and blistering on all sides. Transfer to a bowl and cover with plastic wrap (or transfer to a paper bag) and let cool. Peel off skins and remove core, ribs and seeds.

* **Food processor**

1	can (4 oz/125 g) boneless sardines, drained and patted dry	1
¼ cup	packed fresh parsley leaves	60 mL
¼ cup	roasted red bell pepper (see tip, at left), rinsed and patted dry	60 mL
2 tbsp	light mayonnaise	30 mL
½ tsp	grated lemon zest	2 mL
1 tsp	freshly squeezed lemon juice	5 mL
¼ tsp	hot pepper sauce	1 mL
	Freshly ground black pepper	

1. In food processor, combine sardines, parsley, red pepper, mayonnaise, lemon zest, lemon juice and hot pepper sauce; process until smooth. Season to taste with black pepper.

2. Transfer to a serving bowl, cover and refrigerate for 2 hours, until chilled, before serving. Store in the refrigerator for up to 3 days.

Health Enhancing Tips

Replace the mayonnaise with 2 tbsp (30 mL) mashed ripe avocado.

Serve with cut-up raw vegetables, 2 to 3 GF crackers or 10 to 12 Beanitos (bean chips you can purchase at many health food and grocery stores).

Nutrients per 2 tbsp (30 mL)

Calories	60
Fat	4 g
Carbohydrate	1 g
Fiber	0 g
Protein	5 g
Vitamin A	413 IU
Iron	0.5 mg
Magnesium	11 mg
Zinc	0.3 mg
Selenium	0.0 mcg

Basic Pesto

Pesto is the perfect condiment atop meat, pizza, vegetables, crackers and so much more! This one is bursting with flavor and packs a healing punch.

Makes about 2 cups (500 mL)

TIP

The pesto can be stored in an airtight container in the refrigerator for up to 3 days or frozen for up to 6 months.

- **Blender or food processor**

3	cloves garlic	3
4 cups	fresh basil leaves (about 3 large bunches)	1 L
1/3 cup	pine nuts	75 mL
1/4 cup	freshly grated Parmesan cheese	60 mL
1 tsp	coarse kosher salt	5 mL
1/2 cup	extra virgin olive oil	125 mL
1 tsp	freshly squeezed lemon juice	5 mL

1. In blender, combine garlic, basil, pine nuts, cheese, salt, oil and lemon juice; blend until smooth.

Nutrients per 1 tbsp (15 mL)

Calories	42
Fat	4 g
Carbohydrate	0 g
Fiber	0 g
Protein	1 g
Vitamin A	277 IU
Iron	0.3 mg
Magnesium	7 mg
Zinc	0.2 mg
Selenium	0.2 mcg

Creamy Basil Pesto

The classic Italian sauce gets a low-fat makeover, with creamy yogurt replacing most of the olive oil and feta cheese standing in for Parmesan and pine nuts.

Makes about ¾ cup (175 mL)

TIP

The pesto can be stored in an airtight container in the refrigerator for up to 2 days or in the freezer for up to 1 month.

- **Food processor**

2	cloves garlic, coarsely chopped	2
1½ cups	lightly packed fresh basil leaves	375 mL
⅓ cup	crumbled light feta cheese	75 mL
⅓ cup	nonfat plain yogurt	75 mL
4 tsp	extra virgin olive oil	20 mL
	Freshly ground black pepper	

1. In food processor, combine garlic, basil and feta; process until basil is finely chopped. Scrape down sides. Add yogurt and oil; process until smooth.

Variation

Mixed Herb Pesto: Instead of basil, use 1 cup (250 mL) lightly packed fresh parsley sprigs, ¼ cup (60 mL) lightly packed fresh oregano leaves and ¼ cup (60 mL) chopped fresh chives.

Nutrients per 2 tbsp (30 mL)

Calories	61
Fat	5 g
Carbohydrate	2 g
Fiber	0 g
Protein	2 g
Vitamin A	601 IU
Iron	0.4 mg
Magnesium	11 mg
Zinc	0.5 mg
Selenium	1.9 mcg

Parsley Pesto Sauce

**Makes about
2/3 cup (150 mL)**

Nutrients per 2 tbsp (30 mL)	
Calories	49
Fat	4 g
Carbohydrate	2 g
Fiber	1 g
Protein	2 g
Vitamin A	1233 IU
Iron	0.9 mg
Magnesium	10 mg
Zinc	0.3 mg
Selenium	0.9 mcg

- **Food processor**

2	large cloves garlic	2
1 cup	tightly packed fresh parsley leaves	250 mL
1/3 cup	tightly packed fresh basil leaves	75 mL
1 tbsp	extra virgin olive oil	15 mL
1/4 cup	freshly grated Parmesan cheese	60 mL
1/4 cup	ready-to-use GF vegetable broth	60 mL

1. In food processor, with motor running, drop garlic through the tube and process until chopped. Add parsley, basil, oil and Parmesan cheese. Process until well mixed. With a rubber spatula, scrape the sides once or twice. Add broth and process until well blended.

Variation

If you have time to make Basic Vegetable Stock (page 194), use it in place of the ready-to-use broth.

Cucumber Mint Raita

**Makes about
1 1/4 cups (300 mL)**

Nutrients per 2 tbsp (30 mL)	
Calories	17
Fat	0 g
Carbohydrate	2 g
Fiber	0 g
Protein	1 g
Vitamin A	35 IU
Iron	0.1 mg
Magnesium	5 mg
Zinc	0.2 mg
Selenium	0.8 mcg

3/4 cup	grated English cucumber (unpeeled)	175 mL
2 tbsp	chopped fresh mint or cilantro	30 mL
1/4 tsp	ground cumin	1 mL
1/8 tsp	salt	0.5 mL
Pinch	cayenne pepper	Pinch
1 cup	nonfat plain yogurt	250 mL

1. Place cucumber in a sieve and squeeze out excess water. Wrap in paper towels or a clean kitchen towel and squeeze out excess moisture.

2. In a bowl, combine cucumber, mint, cumin, salt, cayenne and yogurt.

Tomato Avocado Salsa

You'll love this quick, creative salsa. Spoon it over fish or chicken, or eat it as a snack, paired with gluten-free crackers.

Makes about 2 cups (500 mL)

TIPS

Avocados are often avoided as they contain a lot of fat and calories. But they are also packed with heart-friendly monounsaturated oil and other valuable nutrients, so enjoy them in moderation for their many health benefits.

Fresh cilantro lasts only a few days in the fridge before it deteriorates, so buy it shortly before you intend to use it. Wash it well in water to remove any dirt, spin dry and wrap in paper towels. Store in a plastic bag in the fridge.

2	tomatoes, seeded and diced	2
2	green onions, thinly sliced	2
1	Hass avocado, peeled and diced	1
1	jalapeño pepper, seeded and minced	1
⅓ cup	chopped fresh cilantro or parsley	75 mL
2 tsp	freshly squeezed lime juice	10 mL

1. In a bowl, combine tomatoes, green onions, avocado, jalapeño, cilantro and lime juice; toss well. Serve immediately or let stand for 1 hour before serving.

Health-Enhancing Tip

Enjoy with 10 to 12 Beanitos (bean chips you can purchase at many health food and grocery stores).

Nutrients per ¼ cup (60 mL)

Calories	47
Fat	4 g
Carbohydrate	4 g
Fiber	2 g
Protein	1 g
Vitamin A	329 IU
Iron	0.3 mg
Magnesium	11 mg
Zinc	0.2 mg
Selenium	0.1 mcg

Basic Tomato Sauce

Not only is this sauce tasty and easy to make, it is also much lower in sodium than prepared sauces. It keeps, covered, for up to 1 week in the refrigerator and can be frozen for up to 6 months.

Makes about 8 cups (2 L)

TIP

If you are in a hurry, you can soften the vegetables on the stovetop. Heat oil in a skillet for 30 seconds. Add onions and carrots and cook, stirring, until carrots are softened, about 7 minutes. Add garlic, thyme and peppercorns and cook, stirring, for 1 minute. Transfer to slow cooker stoneware. Add tomatoes and continue with step 2.

- **Medium to large (3½- to 6-quart) slow cooker**

1 tbsp	olive oil	15 mL
2	onions, finely chopped	2
2	carrots, diced	2
4	cloves garlic, minced	4
1 tsp	dried thyme, crumbled	5 mL
½ tsp	cracked black peppercorns	2 mL
2	cans (each 28 oz/796 mL) diced tomatoes, with juice	2

1. In slow cooker stoneware, combine olive oil, onions and carrots. Stir well to ensure vegetables are coated with oil. Cover and cook on High for 1 hour, until vegetables are softened. Add garlic, thyme and peppercorns. Stir well. Stir in tomatoes.

2. Place a tea towel folded in half (so you have two layers) over top of stoneware to absorb moisture. Cover and cook on Low for 6 to 8 hours or on High for 3 to 4 hours, until sauce is thickened and flavors are melded.

Nutrients per 1 cup (250 mL)

Calories	81
Fat	2 g
Carbohydrate	14 g
Fiber	4 g
Protein	2 g
Vitamin A	3209 IU
Iron	0.3 mg
Magnesium	4 mg
Zinc	0.1 mg
Selenium	0.3 mcg

Vegetarian Dishes

Spinach with Almonds. 252

Zucchini Patties 253

Wild Rice Cakes 254

Basic Beans. 255

Gingery Red Lentils with Spinach and Coconut 256

Indian Peas and Beans. 258

Butternut Chili 260

Celery Root and Mushroom Lasagna. 262

Thin Pizza Crust 264

Cauliflower Pizza Crust 266

Quinoa-Stuffed Tomatoes 267

Spinach and Tofu Curry. 268

Tofu Chop Suey 270

Tofu Vegetable Quiche 271

Vegetable Quiche with Oat Groat Crust 272

Crustless Dill Spinach Quiche with Mushrooms and Cheese. 274

Spinach with Almonds

Did you know that cooked spinach has more iron than raw spinach? And you can up the iron even more by topping it off with almonds.

Makes 1 serving

TIP

Almonds are a good source of protein and fiber, are loaded with vitamin E (an antioxidant) and magnesium, and are a good source of calcium and iron. They also contain the important flavonoids quercetin and kaempferol, which help to decrease inflammation and protect cells.

1	package (10 oz/300 g) fresh spinach, trimmed	1
2 tbsp	olive oil	30 mL
½ cup	slivered almonds	125 mL
	Salt and freshly ground black pepper	

1. Rinse spinach under cold running water. In a large saucepan, over medium-high heat, cook spinach in the water clinging to the leaves, stirring, for 3 to 5 minutes or until wilted. Drain and transfer to a serving platter.

2. Drizzle oil over spinach and sprinkle with almonds. Season to taste with salt and pepper.

Health-Enhancing Tip

If you don't follow a vegetarian diet, you can add protein to this meal while decreasing the fat content by reducing the amount of almonds and adding cooked chicken breast, shrimp, fish or lean red meat on top.

Nutrients per serving

Calories	614
Fat	55 g
Carbohydrate	22 g
Fiber	13 g
Protein	20 g
Vitamin A	26,584 IU
Iron	9.8 mg
Magnesium	369 mg
Zinc	3.2 mg
Selenium	4.2 mcg

Zucchini Patties

These patties are fantastic as either a main dish or a side dish, and either hot or cold.

Makes 4 servings

TIP

If you are using pre-shredded cheese, check the label to make sure the manufacturer has not added a product containing gluten to prevent sticking.

- **Spray bottle of grapeseed oil**

4	large eggs, beaten	4
4	cloves garlic, minced	4
2 cups	shredded zucchini	500 mL
½ cup	shredded mozzarella cheese or mozzarella-style rice cheese	125 mL
½ cup	shredded reduced-fat Cheddar cheese or Cheddar-style rice cheese	125 mL
½ cup	sorghum flour or white rice flour	125 mL
	Salt and freshly ground black pepper	

1. In a large bowl, combine eggs, garlic, zucchini, mozzarella, Cheddar and flour.

2. Spray a large skillet with oil and heat over medium-high heat. For each patty, pour in ¼ cup (60 mL) batter. Cook for 1 to 2 minutes or until edges are firm. Flip over and cook for 1 to 2 minutes or until golden and hot in the center. Transfer to a plate and keep warm. Repeat with the remaining batter, spraying skillet with oil and adjusting heat between batches as needed.

Nutrients per serving

Calories	214
Fat	9 g
Carbohydrate	17 g
Fiber	2 g
Protein	16 g
Vitamin A	509 IU
Iron	2.0 mg
Magnesium	24 mg
Zinc	1.6 mg
Selenium	20.3 mcg

Wild Rice Cakes

These make a nice light dinner accompanied by a salad, or you can serve them as a substantial side dish. Top them with pesto (page 246 or 247) or Tomato Avocado Salsa (page 249) for a colorful, tasty treat!

Makes 4 main servings or 8 side servings

TIPS

Adding the coulis to this dish will increase the carbohydrate to 43 g and the protein to 26 g.

The basil adds a nice note to the coulis, but if you can't get fresh leaves, omit it — the coulis will be quite tasty anyway.

Be careful when turning the cakes, as they have a tendency to fall apart until they are thoroughly cooked.

Nutrients per main serving (without coulis)

Calories	343
Fat	13 g
Carbohydrate	38 g
Fiber	2 g
Protein	19 g
Vitamin A	676 IU
Iron	1.2 mg
Magnesium	96 mg
Zinc	3.8 mg
Selenium	12.3 mcg

- **Preheat oven to 400°F (200°C)**
- **Large rimmed baking sheet, lightly greased**
- **Food processor**

2½ cups	water	625 mL
1 cup	wild and brown rice mixture, rinsed	250 mL
½ tsp	salt	2 mL
1½ cups	shredded reduced-fat Swiss cheese	375 mL
½ cup	plain yogurt (preferably full-fat)	125 mL
¼ cup	chopped red or green onion	60 mL
¼ cup	finely chopped parsley	60 mL
2	large eggs, beaten	2
	Freshly ground black pepper	

RED PEPPER COULIS (OPTIONAL)

2	roasted red bell peppers (see tip, page 245)	2
3	drained oil-packed sun-dried tomatoes, chopped	3
2 tbsp	extra virgin olive oil	30 mL
1 tbsp	balsamic vinegar	15 mL
10	fresh basil leaves (optional)	10

1. In a large saucepan, bring water to a rolling boil. Add rice and salt. Return to a boil. Reduce heat, cover and simmer until rice is tender and about half of the wild rice grains have split, about 1 hour. Set aside until cool enough to handle, about 20 minutes.

2. In a bowl, combine rice, Swiss cheese, yogurt, red onion, parsley, eggs and pepper to taste. Mix well. Using a large spoon, drop mixture in 8 batches onto prepared baking sheet. Flatten lightly with a spatula or large spoon.

3. Bake in preheated oven for 15 minutes, then flip and cook until lightly browned and heated through, for 5 minutes. Let cool on pan for 5 minutes before serving. Top with Red Pepper Coulis, if using.

4. *Red Pepper Coulis:* In food processor, combine roasted peppers, sun-dried tomatoes, oil, balsamic vinegar and basil, if using, and process until smooth.

Basic Beans

Loaded with nutrition and high in fiber, dried beans are one of our most healthful edibles. And using a slow cooker to cook them is extraordinarily convenient. Put presoaked beans into the slow cooker before you go to bed, and in the morning they are ready for whatever recipe you intend to make.

Makes about 2 cups (500 mL) cooked beans

TIPS

If you have difficulty digesting legumes, add 2 tsp (10 mL) cider vinegar or lemon juice to the water when soaking dried beans.

Once cooked, legumes should be covered and stored in the refrigerator, where they will keep for 4 to 5 days. Cooked legumes can also be frozen in an airtight container. They will keep, frozen, for up to 6 months.

Nutrients per ½ cup (125 mL)

Calories	139
Fat	1 g
Carbohydrate	25 g
Fiber	7 g
Protein	10 g
Vitamin A	0 IU
Iron	2.4 mg
Magnesium	48 mg
Zinc	1.1 mg
Selenium	1.2 mcg

- **Medium to large (3½- to 5-quart) slow cooker**

1 cup	dried white beans (see tip, at left)	250 mL
3 cups	water	750 mL
	Garlic (optional)	
	Bay leaves (optional)	
	Bouquet garni (optional)	

1. *Long soak:* In a bowl, combine beans and water. Soak for at least 6 hours or overnight. Drain and rinse thoroughly with cold water. Beans are now ready for cooking.

2. *Quick soak:* In a pot, combine beans and water. Cover and bring to a boil. Boil for 3 minutes. Turn off heat and soak for 1 hour. Drain and rinse thoroughly under cold water. Beans are now ready to cook.

3. *Cooking:* In slow cooker stoneware, combine 1 cup (250 mL) presoaked beans and 3 cups (750 mL) fresh cold water. If desired, season with garlic, bay leaves or a bouquet garni made from your favorite herbs tied together in a cheesecloth. Cover and cook on Low for 10 to 12 hours or overnight or on High for 5 to 6 hours, until beans are tender. Drain and rinse. If not using immediately, cover and refrigerate. The beans are now ready for use in your favorite recipe.

Variations

Substitute any dried bean (for instance, red kidney beans, pinto beans, white navy beans), chickpeas or split yellow peas for the white beans. Soybeans and chickpeas take longer than other legumes to cook. They will likely take the full 12 hours on Low (about 6 hours on High).

These instructions also work for brown or green lentils or large yellow lentils, with the following changes: Unless you have problems digesting legumes, they do not need to be presoaked. If you have problems digesting legumes, presoak or use sprouted lentils, which are available in natural food stores. Reduce the cooking time to about 6 hours on Low.

Gingery Red Lentils with Spinach and Coconut

As this dish cooks, the red lentils and shredded potato melt into the sauce, creating a luscious texture, and the flavors are so appealing, even non-vegetarians will lap it up. It makes a generous serving, so you won't need to add much if you are serving it as a main course.

Makes 6 servings

TIPS

You can halve this recipe, but be sure to use a small (1½- to 3-quart) slow cooker.

If you have time to make Basic Vegetable Stock (page 194), use it in place of the ready-to-use broth.

- **Medium to large (3½- to 5-quart) slow cooker**

1 tbsp	olive or coconut oil	15 mL
2	onions, finely chopped	2
2	stalks celery, diced	2
2	carrots, diced	2
4	cloves garlic, minced	4
2 tbsp	minced gingerroot	30 mL
2 tsp	ground cumin	10 mL
2 tsp	ground turmeric	10 mL
½ tsp	salt	2 mL
½ tsp	cracked black peppercorns	2 mL
1 cup	dried red lentils, rinsed	250 mL
3 cups	ready-to-use GF vegetable broth	750 mL
1	potato, peeled and shredded	1
1 cup	coconut milk	250 mL
¼ tsp	cayenne pepper	1 mL
1 lb	fresh spinach leaves, or 1 package (10 oz/300 g) fresh or frozen spinach, thawed and drained if frozen, stems removed and coarsely chopped	500 g

1. In a skillet, heat oil over medium heat. Add onions, celery and carrots and cook, stirring, until carrots are softened, about 7 minutes. Add garlic, ginger, cumin, turmeric, salt and peppercorns and cook, stirring, for 1 minute. Add lentils and toss to coat. Add broth and bring to a boil.

2. Transfer to slow cooker stoneware. Stir in potato. Cover and cook on Low for 8 hours or on High for 4 hours, until lentils are very tender and slightly puréed.

Nutrients per serving	
Calories	294
Fat	13 g
Carbohydrate	36 g
Fiber	8 g
Protein	12 g
Vitamin A	8201 IU
Iron	5.5 mg
Magnesium	95 mg
Zinc	2.1 mg
Selenium	6.3 mcg

MAKE AHEAD

Complete step 1. When you're ready to cook, complete the recipe.

3. In a small bowl, combine 1 tbsp (15 mL) coconut milk and cayenne. Stir until blended. Add to stoneware along with the remaining coconut milk and spinach. Cover and cook on High for 20 minutes, until spinach is wilted and flavors meld. Serve immediately.

> ### Health-Enhancing Tip
>
> To increase the protein content of this meal, serve it with cooked tofu, chicken or shrimp.

Indian Peas and Beans

Simple, yet delicious, this Indian-inspired dish makes a great weeknight dinner, served with a cucumber salad. It also makes a nice addition to a multi-dish Indian meal.

Makes 6 servings

TIPS

Can sizes vary. If your supermarket carries 19-oz (540 mL) cans of diced tomatoes with no salt added, by all means substitute for the 14-oz (398 mL) can called for in the recipe.

Keep a bag of frozen green beans in the freezer. They contain valuable nutrients: vitamins K and C, a selection of the B vitamins, including folate, and the minerals manganese, iron and magnesium. They also contain fiber.

• Medium to large (3½- to 5-quart) slow cooker

1 cup	yellow split peas, rinsed	250 mL
1 tbsp	cumin seeds	15 mL
2 tsp	coriander seeds	10 mL
1 tbsp	olive oil or virgin coconut oil	15 mL
2	onions, finely chopped	2
4	cloves garlic, minced	4
1 tbsp	minced gingerroot	15 mL
1 tsp	ground turmeric	5 mL
1 tsp	cracked black peppercorns	5 mL
2	bay leaves	2
1	can (14 oz/398 mL) no-salt-added diced tomatoes, with juice (see tip, at left)	1
2 cups	ready-to-use GF vegetable broth	500 mL
2 cups	frozen sliced green beans	500 mL
¼ tsp	cayenne, dissolved in 1 tbsp (15 mL) freshly squeezed lemon juice	1 mL
1 cup	coconut milk (optional)	250 mL
½ cup	finely chopped fresh cilantro leaves	125 mL

1. In a large saucepan, combine peas with 6 cups (1.5 L) cold water. Bring to a boil and boil rapidly for 3 minutes. Remove from heat and set aside for 1 hour. Rinse thoroughly under cold water, drain and set aside.

2. In a large dry skillet over medium heat, toast cumin and coriander seeds, stirring, until fragrant and cumin seeds just begin to brown, about 3 minutes. Immediately transfer to a mortar or a spice grinder and grind. Set aside.

3. In same skillet, heat oil over medium heat. Add onions and cook, stirring, until softened, about 3 minutes. Add garlic, ginger, turmeric, peppercorns, bay leaves and reserved cumin and coriander and cook, stirring, for 1 minute. Add tomatoes and reserved split peas and bring to a boil. Transfer to slow cooker stoneware.

Nutrients per serving

Calories	185
Fat	3 g
Carbohydrate	31 g
Fiber	11 g
Protein	10 g
Vitamin A	575 IU
Iron	3.6 mg
Magnesium	65 mg
Zinc	1.4 mg
Selenium	1.5 mcg

MAKE AHEAD

This dish can be partially prepared before it is cooked. Complete steps 1 through 3. Cover and refrigerate overnight or for up to 2 days. When you're ready to cook, continue with step 4.

4. Add broth and green beans and stir well. Cover and cook on Low for 8 hours or on High for 4 hours, until peas are tender. Stir in cayenne solution and coconut milk (if using). Add cilantro and stir well. Cover and cook on High for 20 minutes, until heated through. Discard bay leaves.

Health-Enhancing Tip

To increase the protein content of this meal, serve it with cooked chicken or tofu.

Butternut Chili

The combination of beef, butternut squash, ancho chiles and cilantro is a real winner. Don't be afraid to make extra, because it's great reheated.

Makes 8 servings

TIPS

To toast and grind cumin seeds, place them in a dry skillet over medium heat and cook, stirring, until fragrant, about 3 minutes. Immediately transfer to a spice grinder or mortar and grind finely.

If you prefer, you can soak and purée the chiles while preparing the chili and refrigerate until you're ready to add them to the recipe.

- **Large (minimum 5-quart) slow cooker**
- **Blender**

1 tbsp	olive oil	15 mL
1 lb	lean ground beef	500 g
2	onions, finely chopped	2
4	cloves garlic, minced	4
1 tbsp	cumin seeds, toasted and ground (see tip, at left)	15 mL
2 tsp	dried oregano	10 mL
1 tsp	salt	5 mL
½ tsp	cracked black peppercorns	2 mL
1	2-inch (5 cm) cinnamon stick	1
1	can (28 oz/796 mL) diced tomatoes, with juice	1
3 cups	cubed peeled butternut squash (1-inch/2.5 cm cubes)	750 mL
2 cups	cooked dried or canned kidney beans, drained and rinsed	500 mL
2	dried New Mexico, ancho or guajillo chile peppers	2
2 cups	boiling water	500 mL
½ cup	coarsely chopped fresh cilantro	125 mL

1. In a skillet, heat oil over medium-high heat for 30 seconds. Add beef and onions and cook, stirring, until beef is no longer pink, about 5 minutes. Add garlic, toasted cumin, oregano, salt, peppercorns and cinnamon stick and cook, stirring, for 1 minute. Add diced tomatoes and bring to a boil.

2. Place squash and beans in slow cooker stoneware and cover with sauce. Cover and cook on Low for 6 to 8 hours or on High for 3 to 4 hours, until squash is tender.

Nutrients per serving

Calories	213
Fat	6 g
Carbohydrate	25 g
Fiber	7 g
Protein	18 g
Vitamin A	6589 IU
Iron	4.6 mg
Magnesium	70 mg
Zinc	3.6 mg
Selenium	11.3 mcg

MAKE AHEAD

This dish can be partially prepared before it is cooked. Complete steps 1 and 3. Cover and refrigerate tomato and chile mixtures separately overnight. The next morning, continue with the recipe.

3. An hour before recipe is finished cooking, in a heatproof bowl, soak dried chile peppers in boiling water for 30 minutes, weighing down with a cup to ensure they are submerged. Drain, reserving $\frac{1}{2}$ cup (125 mL) of the soaking liquid. Discard stems and chop coarsely. In blender, combine rehydrated chiles, cilantro and reserved soaking liquid. Purée. Add to stoneware and stir well. Cover and cook on High for 30 minutes, until hot and bubbly and flavors meld.

Health-Enhancing Tips

To increase the alkalinity of this recipe, substitute cooked dried brown or green lentils or canned lentils for the kidney beans.

Lean ground organic turkey, chicken or buffalo can be used in place of the ground beef.

Celery Root and Mushroom Lasagna

If you're tired of the same old thing, try this delightfully different lasagna, which combines celery root and mushrooms with more traditional tomatoes and cheese.

Makes 10 servings

TIP

If you are using pre-shredded cheese, check the label to make sure the manufacturer has not added a product containing gluten to prevent sticking.

- **Large (minimum 5-quart) oval slow cooker, stoneware greased**

9	brown rice lasagna noodles	9
2 tbsp	extra virgin olive oil, divided	30 mL
4 cups	shredded peeled celery root (about 1 medium)	1 L
2 tbsp	freshly squeezed lemon juice	30 mL
1	large sweet onion, such as Spanish or Vidalia, finely chopped	1
1 lb	cremini mushrooms, stems removed and caps sliced	500 g
4	cloves garlic, minced	4
1 tbsp	fresh thyme leaves (or 1 tsp/5 mL dried thyme, crumbled)	15 mL
1 tbsp	fresh rosemary leaves, finely chopped (or 1 tsp/5 mL dried rosemary, crumbled)	15 mL
4 cups	Basic Tomato Sauce (page 250), divided	1 L
1	container (16 oz/475 g) light (5%) ricotta cheese	1
2 cups	shredded part-skim mozzarella cheese	500 mL

1. Cook lasagna noodles in a pot of boiling salted water until slightly undercooked, or according to package instructions, undercooking by 2 minutes. Drain, toss with 1 tbsp (15 mL) oil and set aside.

2. In a bowl, toss celery root with lemon juice. Set aside.

3. In a skillet, heat the remaining oil over medium heat for 30 seconds. Add onion and mushrooms and cook, stirring, for 2 minutes. Add garlic, thyme and rosemary and cook, stirring, for 1 minute. Add celery root and 2 cups (500 mL) of the tomato sauce and bring to a boil. Remove from heat.

Nutrients per serving

Calories	263
Fat	12 g
Carbohydrate	25 g
Fiber	3 g
Protein	16 g
Vitamin A	771 IU
Iron	2.3 mg
Magnesium	48 mg
Zinc	2.1 mg
Selenium	17.1 mcg

MAKE AHEAD

This dish can be partially prepared before it is cooked. Complete steps 1 through 4. Cover and refrigerate overnight. In the morning, continue with step 5.

4. Spread 1 cup (250 mL) tomato sauce over bottom of prepared stoneware. Cover with 3 noodles. Spread with half of the ricotta, half of the mushroom mixture and one-third of the mozzarella. Repeat. Cover with final layer of noodles. Pour the remaining tomato sauce over top. Sprinkle with the remaining mozzarella.

5. Cover and cook on Low for 6 hours or on High for 3 hours, until mushrooms are tender and mixture is hot and bubbly.

Thin Pizza Crust

Try this tasty thin crust for a lower-carbohydrate pizza. The dough is so flavorful you won't miss the deep-dish crust. Be creative with your toppings!

Makes 2 crusts, 6 slices per crust

TIPS

This dough is thin enough to pour onto the pizza pans. It can be quickly spread to the edges with a moist rubber spatula.

Don't worry about the cracks on the surface of this crust after 10 minutes of baking. Expect slight shrinkage from the edges.

- **Two 12-inch (30 cm) pizza pans, lightly greased**

1 cup	whole bean flour	250 mL
1 cup	sorghum flour	250 mL
1/3 cup	tapioca starch	75 mL
1 tsp	granulated sugar	5 mL
1/2 tsp	xanthan gum	2 mL
1 1/2 tsp	bread machine or instant yeast	7 mL
1 tsp	salt	5 mL
1 tsp	dried oregano	5 mL
1 3/4 cups	water	425 mL
1 tsp	cider vinegar	5 mL
2 tbsp	vegetable oil	30 mL
	Pizza toppings of choice	

BREAD MACHINE METHOD

1. In a large bowl or plastic bag, combine whole bean flour, sorghum flour, tapioca starch, sugar, xanthan gum, yeast, salt and oregano. Mix well and set aside.

2. Pour water, vinegar and oil into the bread machine baking pan. Select the Dough Cycle.

3. Gradually add the dry ingredients as the bread machine is mixing, scraping with a rubber spatula while adding. Try to incorporate all the dry ingredients within 1 to 2 minutes. Allow the bread machine to complete the cycle.

MIXER METHOD

1. In a large bowl or plastic bag, combine whole bean flour, sorghum flour, tapioca starch, sugar, xanthan gum, yeast, salt and oregano. Mix well and set aside.

2. In a separate bowl, using a heavy-duty electric mixer with paddle attachment, combine water, vinegar and oil until well blended.

3. With the mixer on the lowest speed, slowly add the dry ingredients until combined. With a rubber spatula, scrape the bottom and sides of the bowl. With the mixer on medium speed, beat for 4 minutes.

Nutrients per 2 slices

Calories	249
Fat	7 g
Carbohydrate	39 g
Fiber	5 g
Protein	9 g
Vitamin A	3 IU
Iron	2.5 mg
Magnesium	1 mg
Zinc	0.0 mg
Selenium	0.0 mcg

Substitute 1 tbsp (15 mL) chopped fresh oregano for the dried herb.

FOR BOTH METHODS

4. Immediately pour onto prepared pans. Spread evenly with a water-moistened rubber spatula. Allow to rise in a warm, draft-free place for 15 minutes. Bake in 400°F (200°C) preheated oven for 12 to 15 minutes or until firm. Spread with your choice of toppings. Return to oven and bake until toppings are heated through and any cheese is melted and lightly browned.

Health-Enhancing Tip

For the toppings, spread with Basic Pesto (page 246), cover with your favorite chopped vegetables and sprinkle with a light dusting of cheese.

This dough can be divided into equal portions to make eight 6-inch (15 cm) individual pizzas. Bake on greased baking sheets for 10 to 12 minutes.

Cauliflower Pizza Crust

If you're looking for a lower-carbohydrate, more alkaline pizza crust you can enjoy anytime, this is the recipe for you.

Makes 6 slices

TIPS

Use a box grater or the shredding blade of a food processor to grate the cauliflower. You'll need about $\frac{1}{2}$ head for 3 cups (750 mL) grated cauliflower.

Ghee is a type of clarified butter highly valued in Indian cooking as it can be heated to a very high temperature. It is available in grocery stores specializing in Indian ingredients and will keep, refrigerated, for as long as a year.

- **Preheat oven to 400°F (200°C)**
- **Baking sheet, lightly oiled with ghee**

3 cups	grated cauliflower (see tip, at left)	750 mL
Pinch	dried rosemary	Pinch
$\frac{1}{8}$ tsp	fine sea salt	0.5 mL
3	large eggs	3
2 tbsp	ghee (see tip, at left), softened	30 mL
	Pizza toppings of choice	

1. In a bowl, using an electric mixer, mix cauliflower, rosemary, salt, eggs and ghee until a dough-like texture is achieved. Using your hands, spread dough on prepared baking sheet, making a circle or rectangle about $\frac{1}{2}$ inch (1 cm) thick.

2. Bake in preheated oven for 10 to 20 minutes or until edges are golden brown. Add toppings and bake for 10 to 15 minutes or until toppings are heated through and any cheese is melted and lightly browned.

Nutrients per slice

Calories	93
Fat	7 g
Carbohydrate	3 g
Fiber	1 g
Protein	4 g
Vitamin A	302 IU
Iron	0.7 mg
Magnesium	11 mg
Zinc	0.5 mg
Selenium	8.0 mcg

Quinoa-Stuffed Tomatoes

Here's a delightfully different main course. Make this in late summer or early fall when field tomatoes are in season and use the largest, reddest tomatoes you can find for a spectacular presentation.

Makes 6 servings

TIPS

A grapefruit spoon makes easy work of scooping out the tomato pulp.

If you are using pre-shredded cheese, check the label to make sure the manufacturer has not added a product containing gluten to prevent sticking.

If you're shredding your own cheese, you'll need about a 6-oz (175 g) block.

Chipotle peppers are dried smoked jalapeño peppers. Not all brands of chipotle peppers in adobo sauce are gluten-free, so be sure to check the label.

Nutrients per serving

Calories	179
Fat	4 g
Carbohydrate	22 g
Fiber	4 g
Protein	14 g
Vitamin A	1858 IU
Iron	1.7 mg
Magnesium	69 mg
Zinc	1.7 mg
Selenium	7.3 mcg

- **Preheat oven to 350°F (180°C)**

6	large firm tomatoes	6
FILLING		
2 cups	cooked quinoa	500 mL
2 cups	shredded Cheddar cheese, divided	500 mL
¼ cup	finely chopped red onion	60 mL
1	finely chopped chipotle pepper in adobo sauce (see tip, at left)	1
1 tsp	sweet paprika	5 mL
½ tsp	salt	2 mL
	Freshly ground black pepper	

1. Cut $\frac{1}{2}$ inch (1 cm) off tops of tomatoes. Remove the core and discard. Carefully scoop out the remaining pulp, leaving a thin wall and being careful not to puncture the shell. Place tomatoes in a baking dish. Finely chop pulp and set aside.

2. *Filling:* In a bowl, combine quinoa, $1\frac{1}{2}$ cups (375 mL) cheese, onion, chipotle pepper with sauce, paprika, salt, pepper to taste and reserved tomato pulp. Mix well. Spoon into tomato shells. Sprinkle the remaining cheese over top. Bake in preheated oven until cheese is melted and browned and tomatoes are tender, about 30 minutes. Serve hot.

Variation

Millet-Stuffed Tomatoes: Substitute an equal quantity of toasted cooked millet for the quinoa.

Health-Enhancing Tips

Enjoy with a side salad or steamed vegetables.

To increase the protein content of your meal, top your side salad with cooked chicken, tofu, shrimp, hard-cooked eggs or beef.

Spinach and Tofu Curry

This recipe is one of the most popular and delicious vegetarian dishes in India, and it will make you love eating green leafy vegetables! Traditionally, it is made with paneer, a fresh cheese common in Indian cuisine, and is called palak paneer. However, to reduce the saturated fat while keeping the same texture, the paneer has been replaced with light tofu.

Makes 6 servings

TIP

For the spinach, you can use 3 lbs (1.5 kg) baby spinach or 4 large bunches of regular spinach. To blanch it, place it in a large pot, add a pinch of salt and cover with cold water. Bring to a boil, then quickly transfer spinach to a strainer.

- **Food processor**

3	tomatoes	3
4 cups	blanched finely chopped spinach leaves (see tip, at left)	1 L
1 tbsp	vegetable oil	15 mL
2 cups	finely chopped onion	500 mL
¼ cup	minced garlic	60 mL
2 tbsp	minced gingerroot	30 mL
2 tbsp	ground coriander	30 mL
2 tsp	ground cumin	10 mL
2 tsp	dried fenugreek leaves (kasuri methi)	10 mL
1 tsp	garam masala	5 mL
4	small green chile peppers, chopped (with seeds)	4
½ tsp	salt	2 mL
12 oz	firm light tofu, cut into ¼-inch (1 cm) cubes	375 g

1. In food processor, purée tomatoes; set aside. Purée spinach until smooth. Set aside separately.

2. In a large skillet, heat oil over medium heat. Add onion, reduce heat to medium-low and cook, stirring, for about 10 minutes or until golden.

3. Add garlic and ginger; cook, stirring, for 1 minute. Add coriander, cumin, fenugreek and garam masala; cook, stirring, for 1 minute.

4. Add chiles, increase heat to medium and cook, stirring, for 1 minute. Add tomato purée and cook, stirring, for 2 minutes or until liquid has evaporated.

Nutrients per serving

Calories	159
Fat	5 g
Carbohydrate	22 g
Fiber	8 g
Protein	12 g
Vitamin A	15,933 IU
Iron	6.1 mg
Magnesium	137 mg
Zinc	1.1 mg
Selenium	3.0 mcg

When cooking with a small amount of oil, be sure to heat it well before adding the other ingredients; otherwise, they may simply absorb the oil, which can cause sticking and burning.

5. Add puréed spinach and salt; cook, stirring, for 5 minutes. Add tofu and cook, stirring, for 1 minute.

Health-Enhancing Tip

For a healthier, less inflammatory fat, use melted virgin coconut oil or ghee (see tip, page 266) in place of the vegetable oil.

Tofu Chop Suey

Tofu supplies the protein, and tastes similar to chicken breasts, in this quick-to-prepare, colorful vegetarian main dish.

Makes 2 servings

TIPS

If you have time to make Basic Vegetable Stock (page 194), use it in place of the ready-to-use broth.

All produce should be rinsed well under running water before it is prepared. After rinsing the bean sprouts, drain them well and pat them dry so they don't water down the flavor.

8 oz	firm or extra-firm tofu	250 g
¼ cup	ready-to-use GF vegetable or chicken broth, divided	60 mL
2 tsp	vegetable oil	10 mL
¼ tsp	ground ginger	1 mL
1	small onion, coarsely chopped	1
¼	red bell pepper, cut into thin slices	¼
1 cup	sliced celery	250 mL
1½ cups	bean sprouts	375 mL
1 tbsp	reduced-sodium GF soy sauce	15 mL
⅛ tsp	salt (or less)	0.5 mL
	Freshly ground black pepper	

1. Drain tofu and cut into ¾-inch (2 cm) pieces. Place between layers of paper towels and weigh down with a dinner plate. Let stand for 10 minutes to compress and remove excess water.

2. In a skillet, heat 2 tbsp (30 mL) broth, oil and ginger over medium heat. Sauté onion, red pepper and celery for 3 minutes. Add bean sprouts and sauté for 1 minute.

3. Stir in the remaining broth, soy sauce and tofu; cook, stirring gently, for about 5 minutes or until vegetables are tender-crisp and liquid has evaporated. Taste and add up to ⅛ tsp (0.5 mL) salt. Season to taste with pepper.

Nutrients per serving

Calories	200
Fat	10 g
Carbohydrate	13 g
Fiber	3 g
Protein	18 g
Vitamin A	2918 IU
Iron	3.4 mg
Magnesium	52 mg
Zinc	0.8 mg
Selenium	0.9 mcg

Health-Enhancing Tips

To increase the bulk and alkalinity of this recipe, add 1 cup (250 mL) sliced broccoli, cauliflower and/or baby kale with the bean sprouts. For a post-workout meal, serve it with ½ cup (125 mL) cooked wild rice or quinoa.

Replace the soy sauce with tamari or liquid coconut amino acids.

For a healthier, less inflammatory fat, use sesame oil or ghee (see tip, page 266) in place of the vegetable oil.

Tofu Vegetable Quiche

Quiche is a great meal for breakfast, lunch or dinner. It takes only minutes to make and is sure to be a go-to favorite on your menu.

Makes 4 servings

- **Preheat oven to 350°F (180°C)**
- **10-inch (25 cm) quiche pan or deep plate, lightly greased**
- **Food processor or blender**

2 cups	coarsely chopped vegetables, such as bell peppers or zucchini	500 mL
1/2 cup	finely chopped onion	125 mL
2	large eggs	2
1	package (19 oz/550 g) silken tofu, drained	1
	Salt and freshly ground black pepper	

1. In a large nonstick skillet, over medium-high heat, cook vegetables and onion for 10 minutes or until tender (add water if sticking occurs). Place in prepared pan.

2. In food processor, purée eggs and tofu until smooth and creamy. Season with salt and pepper. Pour tofu mixture over reserved vegetables.

3. Bake in preheated oven for 50 minutes or until knife inserted in the center comes out clean. Cut into 4 wedges and serve.

Nutrients per serving

Calories	150
Fat	6 g
Carbohydrate	10 g
Fiber	2 g
Protein	13 g
Vitamin A	2468 IU
Iron	2.2 mg
Magnesium	50 mg
Zinc	1.4 mg
Selenium	7.9 mcg

Vegetable Quiche with Oat Groat Crust

Beth Armour of Cream Hill Estates developed this recipe and has given us permission to include it for you. It's a good way to use up leftover vegetables from dinner, or you can plan to cook extras just to make this quiche.

Makes 6 servings

TIPS

If you are using pre-shredded cheese, check the label to make sure the manufacturer has not added a product containing gluten to prevent sticking.

For the vegetables, you can use any combination you like; just keep the total to 1 cup (250 mL) cooked vegetables. Try a mixture of bite-size pieces of broccoli, spinach, tomatoes and red, yellow or orange bell peppers. For a more intense flavor, try using roasted vegetables.

Nutrients per serving

Calories	243
Fat	8 g
Carbohydrate	22 g
Fiber	3 g
Protein	20 g
Vitamin A	740 IU
Iron	2.3 mg
Magnesium	66 mg
Zinc	2.9 mg
Selenium	19.3 mcg

• **Preheat oven to 350°F (180°C)**

1	Oat Groat Crust (see recipe, opposite)	1
5	large eggs	5
2 tbsp	milk	30 mL
½ tsp	salt	2 mL
1⅔ cups	shredded Swiss cheese (about 7 oz/210 g)	400 mL
1 cup	cooked vegetables (see tip, at left)	250 mL
¼ cup	chopped fresh rosemary	60 mL

1. Bake crust in preheated oven for 5 minutes.

2. Meanwhile, in a large bowl, using an electric mixer, beat eggs, milk and salt until combined. Stir in cheese, vegetables and rosemary. Spoon into partially baked crust.

3. Bake for 25 to 30 minutes or until center bubbles up. Let cool for 10 minutes before serving.

Health-Enhancing Tips

To increase the alkalinity of this meal, serve steamed greens or a green salad on the side.

If you juice vegetables for drinking, this is a great way to use up the solid portion of the vegetables (wash and peel the vegetables before juicing). Just add them raw in step 2.

Oat Groat Crust

This is a great alternative to a regular pie or quiche crust. In addition to being gluten-free, it is higher in fiber and has a ton of flavor.

Makes 1 crust

TIPS

Be sure to press the oat groat mixture evenly into the bottom and up the sides of the quiche dish. Don't let it get too thick where the sides meet the bottom. Use the back of a dessert spoon for easier spreading.

Crust can be covered and refrigerated for up to 2 days or frozen for up to 3 weeks.

Use this crust as the base of a meat pie.

- **9-inch (23 cm) quiche dish or deep-dish pie plate, lightly greased**

2 cups	water	500 mL
1 cup	whole oat groats	250 mL
1	large egg, lightly beaten	1

1. In a saucepan, bring water to a boil over high heat. Add oat groats and return to a boil. Remove from heat, cover and let stand for 30 minutes.

2. Bring groats mixture to a simmer over medium-low heat. Simmer for 20 to 25 minutes or until softened but still firm. Remove from heat, drain and let stand for 10 minutes.

3. Add egg and stir until well coated. Press mixture into bottom and up sides of prepared dish.

4. Bake according to recipe directions.

Nutrients per $\frac{1}{6}$ crust

Calories	85
Fat	3 g
Carbohydrate	18 g
Fiber	3 g
Protein	6 g
Vitamin A	45 IU
Iron	1.4 mg
Magnesium	48 mg
Zinc	1.2 mg
Selenium	2.6 mcg

Crustless Dill Spinach Quiche with Mushrooms and Cheese

There is no need for a crust to distract from the rich flavor of this quiche. The cheeses, vegetables and dill combine to create an unforgettably mouth-watering meal.

Makes 6 servings

TIPS

Use a 10-oz (300 g) package of frozen spinach instead of fresh spinach.

All ricotta or all cottage cheese can be used, but ricotta gives a creamy texture.

If you are using pre-shredded cheese, check the label to make sure the manufacturer has not added a product containing gluten to prevent sticking.

- **Preheat oven to 350°F (180°C)**
- **8-inch (20 cm) springform pan sprayed with vegetable spray**

10 oz	fresh spinach	300 g
2 tsp	vegetable oil	10 mL
1 tsp	minced garlic	5 mL
¾ cup	chopped onions	175 mL
¾ cup	chopped mushrooms	175 mL
⅔ cup	5% ricotta cheese	150 mL
⅔ cup	2% cottage cheese	150 mL
⅓ cup	shredded Cheddar cheese	75 mL
2 tbsp	freshly grated Parmesan cheese	30 mL
1	large egg	1
1	large egg white	1
3 tbsp	chopped fresh dill (or 2 tsp/10 mL dried)	45 mL
¼ tsp	freshly ground black pepper	1 mL

1. Wash spinach and shake off excess water. In the water clinging to the leaves, cook the spinach over high heat just until it wilts. Squeeze out excess moisture, chop and set aside.

2. In a large nonstick skillet, heat oil over medium heat. Add garlic, onions and mushrooms and cook for 5 minutes or until softened. Remove from heat and add chopped spinach, ricotta, cottage, Cheddar and Parmesan cheeses, egg, egg white, dill and pepper; mix well. Pour into prepared pan.

3. Bake in preheated oven for 35 to 40 minutes or until a knife inserted in the center comes out clean.

Health-Enhancing Tip

For a healthier, less inflammatory fat, use ghee (see tip, page 266) or olive oil in place of the vegetable oil.

Nutrients per serving

Calories	144
Fat	8 g
Carbohydrate	7 g
Fiber	2 g
Protein	12 g
Vitamin A	4700 IU
Iron	1.8 mg
Magnesium	50 mg
Zinc	1.2 mg
Selenium	13.3 mcg

Fish and Seafood

Poached Fish 276

Fish Fillets with Corn and Red Pepper Salsa 277

Peruvian Ceviche 278

Bengali Fish Curry 279

Mediterranean-Style Mahi-Mahi 280

Salmon and Wild Rice Cakes with Avocado-Chili Topping 281

Baked Salmon Patties 282

Baked Salmon with Ginger and Lemon 283

Grilled Salmon with Lemon Oregano Pesto 284

Fish for the Sole 285

Pan-Roasted Trout with Fresh Tomato Basil Sauce 286

Sweet Potato Coconut Curry with Shrimp 287

Shrimp and Vegetable Spring Rolls 288

Mexican-Style Seafood Stew with Hominy 290

Valencia Seafood Paella 292

Onion-Braised Shrimp. 294

Poached Fish

Onion, lemon and bay leaf flavor white fish for an appealing entrée that's easy on the cook and great for your health.

Makes 4 servings

TIPS

Before purchasing fish, always learn what you can about sustainability and fishing practices. Ask your fishmonger or check online resources. A great resource is the Monterey Bay Aquarium's Seafood Watch Guide, which can be found at www.seafoodwatch.org.

This cooking time is for fillets that are about 1 inch (2.5 cm) thick; if you have thinner fillets, check earlier for doneness.

1	onion, chopped	1
6	whole black peppercorns	6
4	slices lemon	4
3	sprigs parsley	3
1	bay leaf	1
1 tsp	salt	5 mL
1 lb	skinless white fish fillets, such as haddock or halibut	500 g

1. In a large skillet, combine onion, peppercorns, lemon, parsley, bay leaf, salt and $1\frac{1}{2}$ cups (375 mL) water. Bring to a boil over high heat. Arrange fish in a single layer in pan; reduce heat to low, cover and simmer for 10 to 12 minutes or until fish is opaque and flakes easily when tested with a fork.

2. Using a slotted spoon, transfer fish to a serving platter, along with onions and lemon slices, if desired.

Nutrients per serving

Calories	93
Fat	1 g
Carbohydrate	2 g
Fiber	1 g
Protein	19 g
Vitamin A	133 IU
Iron	0.4 mg
Magnesium	27 mg
Zinc	0.4 mg
Selenium	29.5 mcg

Fish Fillets with Corn and Red Pepper Salsa

Everyone loves an easy-to-prepare, delicious fish recipe. This one is also loaded with healing nutrients to help you on your journey to regaining your health.

Makes 4 servings

TIPS

The fresh pepper can be replaced with 4 oz (125 g) bell pepper packed in water in a jar.

Before purchasing fish, always learn what you can about sustainability and fishing practices. Ask your fishmonger or check online resources. A great resource is the Monterey Bay Aquarium's Seafood Watch Guide, which can be found at www.seafoodwatch.org.

MAKE AHEAD

Prepare salsa earlier in the day and refrigerate.

Nutrients per serving

Calories	207
Fat	6 g
Carbohydrate	15 g
Fiber	2 g
Protein	23 g
Vitamin A	1472 IU
Iron	0.7 mg
Magnesium	53 mg
Zinc	0.8 mg
Selenium	52.2 mcg

- **Preheat broiler**
- **Baking dish sprayed with vegetable spray**

1	large red bell pepper	1
1½ cups	corn kernels	375 mL
⅓ cup	chopped red onion	75 mL
¼ cup	chopped fresh cilantro	60 mL
2 tbsp	freshly squeezed lime or lemon juice	30 mL
3 tsp	olive oil, divided	15 mL
2 tsp	minced garlic, divided	7 mL
1 lb	fish fillets	500 g

1. Broil red pepper for 15 to 20 minutes, turning occasionally, until charred on all sides. Remove pepper and set oven at 425°F (220°C). Place pepper in a small bowl and cover tightly with plastic wrap. When pepper is cool, remove skin, seeds and stem. Chop and put in small bowl along with corn, onion, cilantro, lime juice, 2 tsp (10 mL oil and 1 tsp (5 mL) garlic; mix well.

2. Put fish in single layer in prepared baking dish and brush with the remaining garlic and oil. Bake uncovered for 10 minutes per inch (2.5 cm) thickness of fish or until fish flakes easily when pierced with a fork. Serve with salsa.

Health-Enhancing Tip

Purchase non-GMO or organic corn.

Peruvian Ceviche

Ceviche is a cooking method in which acid is used instead of heat to cook fish or seafood. The traditional acid choice is the juice of the bitter orange, but today, lemon, lime or orange juice is more commonly used.

Makes 6 servings

TIPS

Very fresh fish is the key to this dish. The thickness of the fish will dictate how long it needs to "cook."

Any white fish can be used in place of the tilapia.

The ginger and milk are added to counteract the sourness of the lime juice. Traditionally, condensed milk is used, but this adds a lot of fat and sugar; skim milk is a better choice.

2	cloves garlic, minced	2
¾ tsp	salt	3 mL
½ tsp	freshly ground black pepper	2 mL
1 cup	freshly squeezed lime juice	250 mL
2 lbs	skinless tilapia fillets, rinsed and cut into ½-inch (1 cm) cubes	1 kg
¼ cup	very finely diced celery leaves and stalk (from the thin top part of the stalk only)	60 mL
½	red onion, thinly sliced	½
3 tbsp	finely chopped fresh cilantro	45 mL
1½ tsp	finely minced gingerroot (approx.)	7 mL
3 tbsp	skim milk (approx.)	45 mL

1. In a large bowl, combine garlic, salt, pepper and lime juice. Add fish and toss to coat. Cover and let "cook" in the refrigerator for 15 to 30 minutes or until fish has turned white.

2. In another bowl, combine celery, onion and cilantro. Remove fish from marinade, discarding marinade, and add fish to celery mixture. Stir in ginger and milk. Taste and, if too sour, add more ginger or milk.

Nutrients per serving

Calories	163
Fat	3 g
Carbohydrate	5 g
Fiber	0 g
Protein	31 g
Vitamin A	59 IU
Iron	0.9 mg
Magnesium	47 mg
Zinc	0.6 mg
Selenium	63.7 mcg

Bengali Fish Curry

Doi maach, which translates literally as "yogurt fish," is a very popular spicy fish dish in Bangladesh. It is traditionally eaten with a side of hot white rice on festive occasions, but can instead be served with brown rice, quinoa or roasted vegetables. The serving of fish in this dish is small, so be sure to balance your meal with enough additional protein.

Makes 3 servings

TIPS

If sole is not available, any other carp species, haddock or salmon will also work in this recipe.

Rinse fish thoroughly under cold water before cooking it, to remove as much salt as possible, especially if it is frozen.

Before purchasing fish, always learn what you can about sustainability and fishing practices. Ask your fishmonger or check online resources. A great resource is the Monterey Bay Aquarium's Seafood Watch Guide, which can be found at www.seafoodwatch.org.

Nutrients per serving

Calories	201
Fat	8 g
Carbohydrate	17 g
Fiber	3 g
Protein	15 g
Vitamin A	702 IU
Iron	2.2 mg
Magnesium	52 mg
Zinc	1.1 mg
Selenium	26.7 mcg

1/3 cup	nonfat plain yogurt	75 mL
2 tbsp	water	30 mL
3/4 tsp	salt	3 mL
3/4 tsp	ground turmeric	3 mL
10 oz	skinless sole fillets (see tips, at left), rinsed and patted dry	300 g
1 tbsp	mustard oil	15 mL
1	large yellow onion, finely chopped	1
1 tbsp	minced gingerroot	15 mL
1 tbsp	minced garlic	15 mL
1	large bay leaf	1
1	1½-inch (4 cm) cinnamon stick	1
4 tsp	ground green cardamom seeds	20 mL
1 tsp	ground cumin	5 mL
2	dried red chile peppers, broken in half	2
2	small green chile peppers, finely chopped	2

1. In a bowl, combine yogurt and water until smooth. Set aside.

2. Combine salt and turmeric and rub over fish. Set aside.

3. In a skillet, heat oil over medium-high heat. Add onion, ginger and garlic; cook, stirring, for about 3 minutes or until onions are starting to turn golden. Add bay leaf, cinnamon, cardamom, cumin and dried red chiles; cook, stirring, for 30 seconds.

4. Stir in yogurt mixture and green chiles. Place fish on top, reduce heat and simmer, gently moving the fish in the sauce occasionally, for about 5 minutes or until fish is firm and flakes easily when tested with a fork. Discard bay leaf and cinnamon.

Mediterranean-Style Mahi-Mahi

This recipe is great for entertaining because you can assemble it just before your guests arrive and turn the slow cooker on when they come through the door. By the time everyone is enjoying drinks and nibbles, the conversation is flowing and you're thinking about moving to the table, the fish will be cooked. Serve this with a big platter of sautéed spinach or Swiss chard.

Makes 4 servings

TIPS

You can halve this recipe, but be sure to use a small (1½- to 3-quart) slow cooker.

It is difficult to be specific about the timing because of the configuration of the fish, but you should begin checking for doneness after 1 hour. Be aware it may take up to 1½ hours.

Before purchasing fish, always learn what you can about sustainability and fishing practices. Ask your fishmonger or check online resources.

- **Medium to large (3½- to 5-quart) oval slow cooker**

2 lbs	mahi-mahi steaks	1 kg
1 tsp	dried oregano	5 mL
1	lemon, thinly sliced	1
1	can (28 oz/796 mL) no-salt added tomatoes, with juice, coarsely chopped	1
½ cup	dry white wine	125 mL
¼ cup	extra virgin olive oil, divided	60 mL
½ tsp	sea salt	2 mL
	Freshly ground black pepper	

GREMOLATA

½ cup	finely chopped fresh parsley leaves	125 mL
3 tbsp	drained capers, minced	45 mL
2	whole anchovies, rinsed and finely chopped	2
	Freshly ground black pepper	
	Chopped black olives	

1. Place fish in slow cooker stoneware. Sprinkle with oregano and lay lemon slices evenly over top. In a bowl, combine tomatoes, wine, 2 tbsp (30 mL) oil, salt and pepper to taste. Pour over fish. Cover and cook on High for about 1 hour (see tip, at left) or until fish flakes easily when pierced with a knife.

2. *Gremolata:* Meanwhile, in a bowl, combine parsley, capers, anchovies, the remaining oil and pepper to taste. Mix well and set aside in refrigerator until fish is cooked.

3. To serve, transfer fish and tomato sauce to a warm platter. Spoon gremolata evenly over top and garnish with olives.

Nutrients per serving

Calories	377
Fat	15 g
Carbohydrate	11 g
Fiber	3 g
Protein	44 g
Vitamin A	649 IU
Iron	4.8 mg
Magnesium	92 mg
Zinc	1.3 mg
Selenium	83.1 mcg

Salmon and Wild Rice Cakes with Avocado-Chili Topping

These tasty burgers make a light weeknight meal. For convenience, cook the rice ahead.

Makes 4 servings

TIPS

With additions such as salad, one burger makes a light meal for most people. However, hungry people might want an extra half or whole one.

Salmon bones add calcium, but if you prefer you can remove them.

Tamari is a type of soy sauce that shouldn't contain wheat.

When mixed, the cakes are very wet and not easily shaped into patties. However, they dry out and solidify quickly on cooking.

Nutrients per serving

Calories	293
Fat	16 g
Carbohydrate	20 g
Fiber	5 g
Protein	18 g
Vitamin A	265 IU
Iron	1.4 mg
Magnesium	61 mg
Zinc	1.7 mg
Selenium	26.2 mcg

- **Food processor**

1½ cups	cooked brown and wild rice mixture, cooled	375 mL
1	can (7.5 oz/213 g) salmon, drained	1
1	large egg	1
4	green onions, white part only, with a bit of green, chopped	4
1 tbsp	GF soy sauce or tamari	15 mL
	Freshly ground black pepper	
1 tbsp	olive oil	15 mL

AVOCADO-CHILI TOPPING

1	avocado, mashed	1
1 tbsp	freshly squeezed lemon juice	15 mL
¼ tsp	salt	1 mL
	Freshly ground black pepper	
½ tsp	Asian chili sauce, such as sambal oelek	2 mL

1. In food processor, combine salmon, egg, green onions, soy sauce and pepper to taste. Process until smooth. Add rice and pulse to blend.

2. In a skillet, heat oil over medium heat for 30 seconds. Using a large spoon, drop salmon mixture into the pan in 4 blobs (see tip, at left). Cook until crispy outside and hot in the center, about 5 minutes per side.

3. *Topping:* Meanwhile, in a bowl, combine avocado, lemon juice, salt, pepper to taste and Asian chili sauce. Mix well.

4. Serve burgers warm with a large dollop of topping.

Health-Enhancing Tip

To create a more alkaline meal, add a side of steamed non-starchy vegetables or a side salad. You could also wrap each cooked salmon cake in a steamed collard green leaf. Steam whole large collard leaves in ½ inch (1 cm) of water for about 5 minutes or until tender. Wrap the salmon cake like a burrito. Note that the collard greens will be slightly chewy.

Baked Salmon Patties

This great twist on the usual burger has added anti-inflammatory properties. But you'll forget how good for you it is when you take your first mouth-watering bite!

Makes 4 servings

TIPS

If you prefer, you can remove the bones from the salmon, but they contribute a significant amount of calcium.

If you are using pre-shredded cheese, check the label to make sure the manufacturer has not added a product containing gluten to prevent sticking.

In addition to making cleanup easier, parchment paper is biodegradable.

- **Preheat oven to 350°F (180°C)**
- **Rimmed baking sheet, lined with parchment paper**

2	cans (each 6 oz/170 g) salmon, drained	2
1	large egg, beaten	1
1 cup	shredded reduced-fat Cheddar cheese	250 mL
1 cup	finely chopped celery	250 mL
¼ cup	finely chopped onion	60 mL
2 tsp	chopped fresh parsley	10 mL
	Juice of ½ lemon	

1. In a large bowl, mash salmon with a fork, crushing the bones. Stir in egg, cheese, celery, onion, parsley and lemon juice until well combined. Using your hands, form mixture into eight ½-inch (1 cm) thick patties.

2. Place on prepared baking sheet and bake in preheated oven for 20 minutes. Flip patties over and bake for 10 minutes or until golden brown and hot in the center.

Health-Enhancing Tips

To create a more alkaline meal, wrap each salmon patty in a steamed collard green leaf (see the Health-Enhancing Tip on page 281). You can also add sprouts to your wrap. Another option for increasing both alkalinity and fiber is to lay the salmon patties on a bed of greens or enjoy them with steamed vegetables.

If you need additional carbohydrates in this meal, add ½ cup (125 mL) cooked lentils, ⅓ cup (75 mL) cooked quinoa or ½ cup (125 mL) cooked chopped starchy vegetables (such as yam, pumpkin, winter squash or sweet potato).

Nutrients per serving

Calories	191
Fat	7 g
Carbohydrate	2 g
Fiber	1 g
Protein	28 g
Vitamin A	357 IU
Iron	1.2 mg
Magnesium	39 mg
Zinc	1.7 mg
Selenium	41.7 mcg

Baked Salmon with Ginger and Lemon

Fresh ginger gives such a sparkling flavor to salmon — or any fish, for that matter. Dried ground ginger just doesn't impart the same crisp taste.

Makes 4 servings

TIPS

Salmon is high in omega-3 fatty acids, which help reduce inflammation.

Buy gingerroot that is firm and unwrinkled, with a gingery aroma. Mature, thick-skinned ginger has a more intense flavor than tender, thin-skinned roots. Store gingerroot in a sealable plastic bag in the refrigerator. It will keep for several weeks. Or peel the ginger and freeze it in a freezer bag. Grate what you need for a recipe while it's still frozen and return the rest to the freezer.

Nutrients per serving

Calories	166
Fat	6 g
Carbohydrate	3 g
Fiber	0 g
Protein	24 g
Vitamin A	158 IU
Iron	0.7 mg
Magnesium	35 mg
Zinc	0.5 mg
Selenium	35.8 mcg

- **Preheat oven to 375°F (190°C)**
- **Shallow baking dish**

4	skinless salmon fillets (each 4 oz/125 g)	4
2	green onions	2
1	clove garlic, minced	1
1½ tsp	minced gingerroot	7 mL
1 tsp	granulated sugar	5 mL
2 tbsp	reduced-sodium GF soy sauce	30 mL
1 tsp	grated lemon zest	5 mL
1 tbsp	freshly squeezed lemon juice	15 mL
1 tsp	sesame oil	5 mL

1. Arrange salmon in a single layer in baking dish.

2. Thinly slice green onions and set aside green parts for garnish. In a bowl, combine white part of green onions, garlic, ginger, sugar, soy sauce, lemon zest, lemon juice and oil. Pour marinade over salmon. Let stand at room temperature for 15 minutes, or cover and refrigerate for up to 1 hour.

3. Bake, uncovered, in preheated oven for 17 to 20 minutes or until fish is opaque and flakes easily when tested with a fork.

4. Arrange salmon on serving plates and spoon sauce from dish over top. Sprinkle with reserved green onions.

Health-Enhancing Tips

Use wild Alaskan salmon for increased omega-3 fatty acids and to reduce your total toxic load (PCBs, dioxins, toxaphene, etc.) from consuming farm-raised fish.

Replace the soy sauce with tamari or liquid coconut amino acids.

Grilled Salmon with Lemon Oregano Pesto

This simple pesto sauce keeps the salmon extra-moist and adds a burst of fresh flavor and health-enhancing nutrition.

Makes 4 servings

TIPS

Double the quantity of the pesto ingredients. Use half to marinate the fish and refrigerate the other half to use as a quick baste when grilling chicken, pork or lamb. Pesto can be stored in an airtight container in the refrigerator for up to 2 days.

Broiler Method: Preheat broiler, with rack set 4 inches (10 cm) from heat. In step 3, arrange salmon on a broiler pan and broil for 5 minutes per side or until fish is opaque and flakes easily when tested with a fork.

Nutrients per serving	
Calories	209
Fat	12 g
Carbohydrate	2 g
Fiber	0 g
Protein	23 g
Vitamin A	728 IU
Iron	1.4 mg
Magnesium	39 mg
Zinc	0.9 mg
Selenium	41.5 mcg

- **Preheat greased barbecue grill to medium**
- **Food processor or mini chopper**
- **Shallow glass baking dish**

1	clove garlic, chopped	1
½ cup	lightly packed fresh parsley sprigs	125 mL
2 tbsp	lightly packed fresh oregano (or 2 tsp/10 mL dried)	30 mL
2 tsp	grated lemon zest	10 mL
2 tbsp	freshly squeezed lemon juice	30 mL
4 tsp	olive oil	20 mL
¼ tsp	freshly ground black pepper	1 mL
4	skinless salmon fillets (each 4 oz/125 g)	4

1. In food processor, combine garlic, parsley, oregano, lemon zest, lemon juice, oil and pepper; purée until very smooth.

2. Pat salmon dry with paper towels. Arrange in baking dish and coat both sides with pesto. Marinate at room temperature for 15 minutes, or cover and refrigerate for up to 1 hour.

3. Place salmon on preheated grill and cook for 5 to 7 minutes per side (depending on thickness) or until fish is opaque and flakes easily when tested with a fork.

Health-Enhancing Tip

Grill on a lower heat, making sure the flame doesn't touch the fish.

Fish for the Sole

Forgive the pun, but this cracker-crusted fish really is comfort food for the soul — and it does your body good, too!

Makes 2 servings

TIP

To crush the crackers, place them in a sealable plastic bag. Seal and use a rolling pin to crush them to the consistency of dry bread crumbs. Alternatively, you can crush them in a blender.

- **Preheat oven to 350°F (180°C)**
- **13- by 9-inch (33 by 23 cm) glass baking dish, greased**

2	cloves garlic, minced	2
¼ cup	GF cracker crumbs	60 mL
2 tbsp	chopped fresh parsley	30 mL
2 tbsp	olive oil (approx.)	30 mL
	Juice of ½ lemon	
3	pieces skinless sole fillet (each about 3½ oz/100 g)	3

1. In a small bowl, combine garlic, cracker crumbs, parsley, oil and lemon juice; stir until a paste forms, adding more oil if mixture is too dry.

2. Arrange sole in prepared baking dish. Spread paste over fish.

3. Cover dish with foil and bake in preheated oven for 20 to 30 minutes or until fish flakes easily when tested with a fork. Uncover and bake for 5 minutes or until crust is crispy.

Nutrients per serving

Calories	274
Fat	17 g
Carbohydrate	9 g
Fiber	1 g
Protein	20 g
Vitamin A	370 IU
Iron	1.0 mg
Magnesium	33 mg
Zinc	0.6 mg
Selenium	41.1 mcg

Pan-Roasted Trout with Fresh Tomato Basil Sauce

Here's a simplified cooking method for trout. It's served with a vibrant fresh tomato topping that is more popularly associated with bruschetta.

Makes 4 servings

TIP

Learn more about how to choose sustainable seafood by checking out these websites: Marine Stewardship Council (www.msc.org), Monterey Bay Aquarium Seafood Watch (www.seafoodwatch.org) or SeaChoice (www.seachoice.org).

FRESH TOMATO BASIL SAUCE

2	large ripe red tomatoes, seeded and diced	2
½	clove garlic, minced	½
2 tbsp	minced green onion	30 mL
2 tbsp	chopped fresh basil	30 mL
⅛ tsp	salt	0.5 mL
	Freshly ground black pepper	
1 tbsp	balsamic vinegar	15 mL
1 tbsp	extra virgin olive oil	15 mL

FISH

1 tsp	extra virgin olive oil	5 mL
1 lb	trout fillets with skins	500 g

1. *Sauce:* Shortly before serving, in a bowl, combine tomatoes, garlic, green onion, basil, salt, pepper to taste, vinegar and oil.

2. *Fish:* Pat trout dry with paper towels. Brush a large nonstick skillet with oil and heat over medium-high heat. Place trout, skin side down, in skillet. Cook for 2 minutes, without turning. Reduce heat to medium-low, cover and cook for 3 to 5 minutes or until fish is opaque and flakes easily when tested with a fork (time depends on thickness of fish; increase time as needed).

3. Arrange fish on plates and top with sauce.

Variation

Substitute Mexico's famous pico de gallo (also called salsa fresca) for the fresh tomato basil sauce. The preparation is very similar; just use cilantro instead of basil, replace the vinegar with freshly squeezed lime juice, and add 1 minced jalapeño pepper.

Nutrients per serving

Calories	197
Fat	9 g
Carbohydrate	5 g
Fiber	1 g
Protein	24 g
Vitamin A	929 IU
Iron	1.2 mg
Magnesium	47 mg
Zinc	1.4 mg
Selenium	14.4 mcg

Sweet Potato Coconut Curry with Shrimp

The combination of sweet and spicy flavors in this luscious dish is wonderful over brown basmati rice. For a lower-carbohydrate option, skip the rice and serve the curry with a platter of steamed spinach sprinkled with toasted sesame seeds.

Makes 2 servings

TIPS

Check the label to make sure your curry paste does not contain gluten.

If you are adding the almond garnish, try to find slivered almonds with the skin on. They add color and nutrients to the dish.

MAKE AHEAD

Complete step 1. Cover and refrigerate overnight or for up to 2 days. When you're ready, complete the recipe.

Nutrients per serving

Calories	274
Fat	17 g
Carbohydrate	9 g
Fiber	1 g
Protein	20 g
Vitamin A	370 IU
Iron	1.0 mg
Magnesium	33 mg
Zinc	0.6 mg
Selenium	41.1 mcg

• **Medium to large (3½- to 5-quart) slow cooker**

1 tbsp	olive or virgin coconut oil	15 mL
2	onions, finely chopped	2
4	cloves garlic, minced	4
1 tbsp	minced gingerroot	15 mL
1 cup	ready-to-use GF vegetable broth	250 mL
2	sweet potatoes, peeled and cut into 1-inch (2.5 cm) cubes	2
2 tsp	Thai green curry paste (see tip, at left)	10 mL
1 tbsp	freshly squeezed lime juice	15 mL
½ cup	coconut milk	125 mL
1 lb	cooked peeled shrimp, thawed if frozen	500 g
¼ cup	toasted slivered almonds (optional)	60 mL
¼ cup	finely chopped fresh cilantro leaves	60 mL

1. In a skillet, heat oil over medium heat. Add onions and cook, stirring, until softened, about 3 minutes. Add garlic and ginger and cook, stirring, for 1 minute. Add broth. Transfer to slow cooker stoneware.

2. Add sweet potatoes and stir well. Cover and cook on Low for 6 hours or on High for 3 hours, until sweet potatoes are tender.

3. In a small bowl, combine curry paste and lime juice. Add to slow cooker stoneware and stir well. Stir in coconut milk and shrimp. Cover and cook on High for 20 minutes, until shrimp are hot. Transfer to a serving dish. Garnish with almonds (if using), and cilantro and serve.

Shrimp and Vegetable Spring Rolls

Rice paper wrappers make great covers for a variety of fillings, like this colorful salad combo with shrimp and peanut dressing. If you haven't worked with rice paper wrappers, it may initially require a bit of practice to assemble them — it's similar to rolling a wrap sandwich. Once the rice paper roll is softened in water, assemble and roll the wrapper before going on to the next one.

Makes 2 servings

TIPS

Rice paper wrappers are sold in the specialty food section of most supermarkets or at Asian food shops.

To prevent the rolls from getting soggy, prepare them no more than 4 hours ahead of serving.

Nutrients per 2 rolls

Calories	242
Fat	8 g
Carbohydrate	29 g
Fiber	3 g
Protein	18 g
Vitamin A	6783 IU
Iron	1.8 mg
Magnesium	69 mg
Zinc	1.5 mg
Selenium	20.6 mcg

PEANUT DRESSING

1 tsp	packed brown sugar	5 mL
1 tbsp	unsalted smooth peanut butter	15 mL
1 tbsp	freshly squeezed lime juice	15 mL
2 tsp	reduced-sodium GF soy sauce	10 mL
¼ tsp	Asian chili sauce	1 mL

SPRING ROLLS

1	small red bell pepper, cut into thin strips	1
1 cup	shredded napa cabbage or romaine lettuce	250 mL
1 cup	bean sprouts	250 mL
½ cup	shredded carrots	125 mL
2	green onions, sliced	2
4	8½-inch (22 cm) round rice paper wrappers	4
4 oz	small cooked peeled shrimp	125 g
8	fresh cilantro stems with leaves	8

1. *Dressing:* In a small bowl, whisk together brown sugar, peanut butter, lime juice, soy sauce and chili sauce. Set aside.

2. *Spring Rolls:* In a bowl, combine red pepper, cabbage, bean sprouts, carrots and green onions; toss lightly.

3. Working with one rice paper wrapper at a time, dip the wrapper in a large, shallow bowl of cold water for about 10 seconds or until pliable. Place on a clean wooden board or dry work surface. Mound one-quarter of the salad mixture on the lower half of the wrapper, leaving a 1-inch (2.5 cm) edge all around. Top with shrimp and 2 cilantro stems with leaves. Pat down lightly. Drizzle with 2 tsp (10 mL) peanut dressing. Carefully fold in sides of wrapper, then, starting at the bottom, tightly roll up to enclose filling. Place on a plate.

TIPS

Prepare extra peanut dressing and keep it handy in the fridge for when you make these rolls another time. The sauce keeps well for several weeks in an airtight container in the refrigerator.

Soy sauce is a popular condiment and ingredient, but it is also high in sodium. Choose reduced-sodium soy sauce. Brands vary, but there is typically about 1000 mg of sodium in 1 tbsp (15 mL) of regular soy sauce and 500 mg in the same amount of reduced-sodium soy sauce.

4. Repeat with the remaining rice papers and filling to make 3 more rolls. Serve immediately or cover rolls with plastic wrap and refrigerate for up to 4 hours. To serve, cut each roll on the diagonal into halves.

Health-Enhancing Tips

Replace the soy sauce with tamari or liquid coconut amino acids.

Serve with a side salad or steamed vegetables.

Mexican-Style Seafood Stew with Hominy

This rustic dish has an abundance of flavors that combine in intriguing ways. The chiles add depth with a hint of heat, and the hominy and clams add robustness. Try finishing it with a garnish of avocado cubes drizzled with lime juice, which inserts creaminess and a hit of acidity into the mix.

Makes 6 servings

TIPS

Fish stock provides the best flavor base, but you can substitute an equal quantity of ready-to-use GF vegetable stock or equal parts bottled clam juice and water.

If purchasing fish stock rather than making your own, check the label to make sure it is gluten-free.

Nutrients per serving

Calories	239
Fat	6 g
Carbohydrate	21 g
Fiber	4 g
Protein	26 g
Vitamin A	1467 IU
Iron	3.1 mg
Magnesium	61 mg
Zinc	1.8 mg
Selenium	42.8 mcg

• **Blender**

2	dried ancho, guajillo or mild New Mexico chile peppers	2
1 cup	packed fresh cilantro leaves	250 mL
4 cups	fish stock, divided (see tips, at left)	1 L
1 tbsp	olive oil	15 mL
2	onions, finely chopped	2
3	cloves garlic, minced	3
1 tsp	ground cumin	5 mL
1 tsp	dried oregano (preferably Mexican)	5 mL
1	can (14 oz/398 mL) diced tomatoes with juice	1
1	can (15 oz/412 mL) hominy, drained and rinsed	1
	Salt and freshly ground black pepper	
12	clams, thoroughly scrubbed and rinsed	12
12 oz	skinless snapper fillets or other firm white fish, cut into bite-size pieces	375 g
6 oz	medium shrimp, peeled and deveined	175 g
	Finely chopped fresh cilantro	
	Avocado cubes (optional)	
	Lime wedges	

1. In a heatproof bowl, soak chiles in boiling water for 30 minutes, weighing down with a cup to ensure they remain submerged. Drain, discarding soaking liquid and stems, and chop coarsely. Transfer to blender. Add cilantro and 1 cup (250 mL) stock. Purée and set aside.

2. In a large saucepan or stockpot, heat oil over medium heat for 30 seconds. Add onions and cook, stirring, until softened, about 3 minutes. Add garlic, cumin and oregano and cook, stirring, for 1 minute. Add tomatoes, reserved chile mixture, the remaining stock and hominy. Season to taste with salt and pepper and bring to a boil. Reduce heat to low. Cover and simmer until flavors meld, about 30 minutes.

If using the avocado, cut it a few minutes ahead and toss with about 1 tbsp (15 mL) lime juice, which will prevent browning.

3. Increase heat to medium-high. Return mixture to a full boil. Add clams. Cover and cook, shaking the pot, until all the clams open, about 5 minutes. Discard any that do not open. Add snapper and shrimp and cook, stirring, until fish is tender and shrimp turn pink and are cooked through, 3 to 5 minutes.

4. Ladle stew into soup plates. Garnish with cilantro and avocado (if using). Pass lime wedges at the table.

Health-Enhancing Tip

Serve with a side salad or add up to 1 cup (250 mL) chopped non-starchy vegetables (broccoli, cauliflower, spinach, zucchini, baby kale, sea vegetables, tomato) with the clams in step 3.

Valencia Seafood Paella

Versions of paella can be found all over Spain and Portugal, but the best-known recipe is from Valencia, Spain. Most restaurants in Spain serve paella at lunch, when the heavier meal is traditionally eaten. The key to this dish is the Spanish saffron, which gives paella its characteristic color and flavor.

Makes 5 servings

TIPS

Paella is often made with a short-grain white rice called bomba, which is similar to risotto but not as starchy. It can be difficult to find, however, and long-grain white rice is just as authentic and works just as well.

When purchasing ready-to-use chicken broth, check the label to make sure it is gluten-free. Or prepare Homemade Chicken Stock (page 195) to use in this recipe.

Nutrients per serving

Calories	327
Fat	13 g
Carbohydrate	35 g
Fiber	1 g
Protein	16 g
Vitamin A	927 IU
Iron	3.6 mg
Magnesium	41 mg
Zinc	1.8 mg
Selenium	42.1 mcg

- **12- to 13-inch (30 to 33 cm) skillet or paella pan**

1 tsp	minced garlic	5 mL
4 tbsp	extra virgin olive oil, divided	60 mL
3½ oz	calamari, cut lengthwise into strips	100 g
½ cup	Basic Tomato Sauce (page 250)	125 mL
1 cup	long-grain white rice	250 mL
3 cups	ready-to-use no-salt-added chicken broth	750 mL
½ tsp	Spanish saffron threads	2 mL
½ tsp	salt	2 mL
6½ oz	large tiger shrimp (unpeeled), rinsed	200 g
6½ oz	small mussels, scrubbed and debearded (see tips, opposite)	200 g
¼ cup	fresh or frozen green peas	60 mL
¼	roasted red bell pepper (see tip, page 245), cut into ⅛-inch (3 mm) thick slices	¼
¼	roasted green bell pepper, cut into ⅛-inch (3 mm) thick slices	¼
2 tsp	freshly squeezed lemon juice (or 4 lemon wedges)	10 mL
2 tbsp	finely chopped fresh parsley	30 mL

1. In a shallow bowl, combine garlic and 3 tbsp (45 mL) oil. Add calamari and toss to coat. Cover and refrigerate for at least 30 minutes or overnight.

2. Remove calamari from marinade, discarding marinade. Heat the skillet over medium-low heat. Add calamari and cook for 2 minutes. Add tomato sauce and the remaining oil; increase heat to medium and cook, stirring, for 3 to 4 minutes to combine the flavors.

3. Stir in rice and cook, stirring occasionally, for about 3 minutes. Stir in broth and bring to a boil. Stir in saffron and salt.

TIPS

When purchasing
mussels, tap each one to
make sure it snaps shut.
Tap again just before
cooking. Discard any
mussels that don't close,
as they are no longer alive.
After cooking, discard
any mussels that have
not opened.

Store mussels in the
coolest part of the
refrigerator, wrapped
loosely in a damp
cloth (allowing them
to breathe), but not in
water. Clean them just
before use so as to not
disturb them. To do so,
hold them under cool
running water and scrub
them with a firm brush to
ensure that all the sand
is removed. Remove the
"beards" by firmly tugging
them toward the hinge
of the shell.

4. Gently stir in shrimp, one at a time. Reduce heat to low and
simmer for 2 minutes.

5. Add mussels, one at a time. Gently stir in peas. Place roasted
red and green pepper on top, and drizzle with lemon juice.
Cover with foil and simmer for 20 minutes or until rice is
tender and liquid is absorbed. Remove from heat, remove foil
and let stand for 10 minutes. Discard any mussels that have
not opened.

6. Serve garnished with parsley.

Onion-Braised Shrimp

This is a great dish for a buffet, an Indian-style meal with numerous small plates, or a light dinner. The substantial quantity of onions, which are cooked until they begin to caramelize and release their sugars, produces a dish that is pleasantly sweet. Serve it with a side salad or steamed vegetables.

Makes 4 servings

TIP

The quantity of chile pepper in the recipe produces a mildly spicy result. Heat seekers can add an extra half of a fresh chile, finely chopped, or more cayenne pepper. You can add up to $\frac{1}{2}$ tsp (2 mL) cayenne pepper in addition to the fresh red chile or, if you don't have a fresh chile, substitute that amount of cayenne instead. Just be sure to dissolve the powdered pepper in the lemon juice before adding to the slow cooker.

Nutrients per serving

Calories	242
Fat	6 g
Carbohydrate	17 g
Fiber	3 g
Protein	29 g
Vitamin A	553 IU
Iron	2.0 mg
Magnesium	72 mg
Zinc	2.5 mg
Selenium	58.0 mcg

• **Medium to large (3$\frac{1}{2}$- to 5-quart) slow cooker**

1 tsp	coriander seeds	5 mL
1 tbsp	olive oil	15 mL
4	onions, finely chopped	4
2	cloves garlic, minced	2
1 tbsp	minced gingerroot	15 mL
1 tsp	ground turmeric	5 mL
$\frac{1}{2}$ tsp	sea salt (or to taste)	2 mL
$\frac{1}{2}$ tsp	cracked black peppercorns	2 mL
1	can (14 oz/398 mL) no-salt-added diced tomatoes, with juice	1
1	long red chile pepper, seeded and finely chopped (see tip, at left)	1
1 tbsp	freshly squeezed lemon juice	15 mL
1 lb	peeled cooked shrimp, thawed if frozen	500 g
$\frac{1}{2}$ cup	plain yogurt	125 mL
2 tbsp	finely chopped fresh cilantro leaves	30 mL

1. In a dry skillet over medium heat, toast coriander seeds, stirring, until fragrant, about 3 minutes. Immediately transfer to a mortar or a spice grinder and grind. Set aside.

2. In same skillet, heat oil over medium heat. Add onions and cook, stirring, until they turn golden and just begin to brown, about 7 minutes. Add garlic, ginger, turmeric, salt, peppercorns and reserved coriander and cook, stirring, for 1 minute. Add tomatoes and stir well.

3. Transfer to slow cooker stoneware. Cover and cook on Low for 6 hours or on High for 3 hours, until mixture is hot and bubbly. Stir in chile pepper and lemon juice. Add shrimp and stir well. Cover and cook on High for 20 minutes, until shrimp are heated through. Stir in yogurt. Garnish with cilantro and serve.

Meaty Mains

Crunchy Almond Chicken 296

French Basil Chicken 297

Italian-Style Chicken in White Wine with Olives and Polenta 298

Lemon Garlic Chicken 300

Jerk Chicken. 301

Indian-Style Grilled Chicken Breasts 302

Tandoori Chicken with Cucumber Mint Raita 304

Miso Mushroom Chicken with Chinese Cabbage. 305

Indian-Style Chicken with Puréed Spinach 306

Spicy Peanut Chicken 308

Turkey Ratatouille Chili 309

Turkey Mole 310

Pork Vindaloo. 312

Catalan Beef Stew 313

Zesty Braised Beef with New Potatoes. 314

Meatballs for Everyday 316

Country Supper Cabbage Rolls 317

Grilled Lamb Chops with Rosemary Mustard Baste 318

Segovia-Style Lamb. 319

Spicy Lamb with Chickpeas 320

Lamb with Lentils and Chard. 322

Crunchy Almond Chicken

Need a quick main dish for dinner? Sprinkle extra almonds on the pan to toast as the chicken bakes.

Makes 6 servings

TIP

For best results when making fresh GF bread crumbs, the bread should be at least 1 day old. Using a food processor or blender, pulse until crumbs are of the desired consistency. Store bread crumbs in an airtight container in the freezer for up to 3 months.

- **Preheat oven to 350°F (180°C)**
- **15- by 10-inch (40 by 25 cm) jelly roll pan, lightly greased**

⅓ cup	plain yogurt	75 mL
¼ cup	Dijon mustard	60 mL
½ cup	fresh GF bread crumbs (see tip, at left)	125 mL
⅓ cup	sliced almonds	75 mL
1 tsp	dried rosemary	5 mL
½ tsp	salt	2 mL
¼ tsp	freshly ground black pepper	1 mL
6	boneless skinless chicken breasts	6

1. On a pie plate, combine yogurt and Dijon mustard. Set aside. On a second pie plate, combine bread crumbs, almonds, rosemary, salt and pepper.

2. Roll chicken first in yogurt-mustard mixture and then in the seasoned bread crumbs.

3. Place in a single layer on prepared pan. Bake in a preheated oven for 30 to 35 minutes or until chicken is no longer pink inside.

Variations

Use commercial GF rice crackers to make crumbs as a substitute for the bread crumbs.

Substitute dried basil, marjoram or thyme for the rosemary.

Substitute boneless fish fillets for the chicken and bake until fish is firm and opaque and flakes easily when tested with a fork.

Nutrients per serving

Calories	193
Fat	6 g
Carbohydrate	6 g
Fiber	1 g
Protein	27 g
Vitamin A	49 IU
Iron	0.9 mg
Magnesium	48 mg
Zinc	1.0 mg
Selenium	39.0 mcg

French Basil Chicken

Chicken never tasted so good. Serve with a side of sautéed spinach or Swiss chard, or a tossed salad.

Makes 6 to 8 servings

TIPS

If you prefer, substitute an equal amount of ready-to-use GF chicken broth for the wine.

If you have time to make Homemade Chicken Stock (page 195), use it in place of the ready-to-use broth.

MAKE AHEAD

Complete step 1. Cover and refrigerate for up to 2 days. When you're ready to cook, complete the recipe.

Nutrients per serving (1 of 8)

Calories	291
Fat	9 g
Carbohydrate	13 g
Fiber	6 g
Protein	37 g
Vitamin A	1483 IU
Iron	3.0 mg
Magnesium	76 mg
Zinc	3.7 mg
Selenium	23.5 mcg

- **Medium to large (3½- to 5-quart) slow cooker**

1 tbsp	extra virgin olive oil	15 mL
2	onions, finely chopped	2
4	cloves garlic, minced	4
1 tsp	dried herbes de Provence	5 mL
½ tsp	sea salt (or to taste)	2 mL
½ tsp	cracked black peppercorns	2 mL
½ cup	dry white wine (see tip, at left)	125 mL
1 cup	ready-to-use GF chicken broth	250 mL
1	can (14 oz/398 mL) diced no-salt-added tomatoes, with juice	1
1	can (14 oz/398 mL) artichoke hearts, drained, rinsed and quartered	1
3 lbs	skinless bone-in chicken thighs (about 12 thighs)	1.5 kg
2 cups	finely chopped red bell pepper	500 mL
½ cup	finely chopped fresh basil leaves	125 mL

1. In a skillet, heat oil over medium heat. Add onions and cook, stirring, until softened, about 3 minutes. Add garlic, herbes de Provence, salt and peppercorns and cook, stirring, for 1 minute. Add wine and cook, stirring, for 1 minute. Add broth and tomatoes and bring to a boil. Stir in artichoke hearts and remove from heat.

2. Arrange chicken pieces evenly over the bottom of slow cooker stoneware and cover with tomato mixture. Cover and cook on Low for 6 hours or on High for 3 hours, until juices run clear when chicken is pierced with a fork. Stir in red pepper and basil. Cover and cook on High for 30 minutes or until pepper is tender.

Italian-Style Chicken in White Wine with Olives and Polenta

This is a fairly straightforward recipe for chicken cooked in white wine, distinguished by the addition of fresh sage and sliced green olives, which add pleasant acidity to the sauce. Served over polenta, it makes a delicious one-dish meal.

Makes 8 servings

TIP

Have your butcher cut chicken breasts into quarters.

• **Preheat oven to 350°F (180°C)**

1	batch Creamy Polenta (page 346)	1
1 tbsp	olive oil	15 mL
3 lbs	skin-on bone-in chicken breasts, cut into serving-size pieces, rinsed and patted dry	1.5 kg
2	onions, finely chopped	2
2	carrots, diced	2
2	stalks celery, diced	2
2	cloves garlic, minced	2
2 tsp	dried Italian seasoning	10 mL
6	fresh sage leaves, chopped (or ½ tsp/2 mL dried sage)	6
½ tsp	freshly ground black pepper	2 mL
¼ tsp	cayenne pepper	1 mL
	Salt	
2 tbsp	corn flour (see tip, opposite)	30 mL
1 cup	dry white wine	250 mL
1 cup	ready-to-use GF chicken broth	250 mL
1 cup	sliced pitted green olives	250 mL
1 tbsp	freshly squeezed lemon juice	15 mL

1. In a Dutch oven, heat oil over medium heat for 30 seconds. Add chicken, in batches, and brown, turning once, about 6 minutes per batch. Transfer to a plate as completed and set aside.

Nutrients per serving

Calories	427
Fat	18 g
Carbohydrate	26 g
Fiber	2 g
Protein	34 g
Vitamin A	2984 IU
Iron	2.3 mg
Magnesium	58 mg
Zinc	1.7 mg
Selenium	27.8 mcg

Corn flour is dried corn that has been ground into flour. It is available in natural foods stores. Check to make sure it has been produced in a gluten-free facility. Do not confuse it with cornstarch. In some parts of the world (not North America) cornstarch is called corn flour.

2. Add onions, carrots and celery to pan and cook, stirring, until vegetables are softened, about 7 minutes. Add garlic, Italian seasoning, sage, black pepper, cayenne and salt to taste and cook, stirring, for 1 minute. Add corn flour and cook, stirring, until mixture congeals, for 1 minute. Add wine and broth and bring to a boil. Cook, stirring, until mixture thickens, about 3 minutes. Return chicken to pot. Cover and bake in preheated oven until chicken is no longer pink inside, about 45 minutes. Stir in olives and lemon juice.

3. Spread polenta over a deep platter and top with chicken and sauce.

Health-Enhancing Tip

Look for non-GMO or organic corn flour.

Lemon Garlic Chicken

This is not your usual lemon garlic chicken. The nutmeg and paprika give it a distinct flavor that will awaken and delight your taste buds.

Makes 4 servings

TIPS

Chicken can be marinated at room temperature for up to 30 minutes if you are short of time. Any longer, make sure it is refrigerated. Throw out the plastic bag used for marinating.

Can't find the cover that fits your casserole? Cover it with foil, dull side out. Trace around the rim with your fingers to be sure foil forms a tight seal.

• **8-cup (2 L) covered casserole dish**

1	clove garlic, minced	1
2 tbsp	freshly squeezed lemon juice	30 mL
1 tbsp	extra virgin olive oil	15 mL
1 tsp	dried thyme	5 mL
1/4 tsp	salt	1 mL
Pinch	ground nutmeg	Pinch
Pinch	paprika	Pinch
Pinch	freshly ground white pepper	Pinch
4	boneless skinless chicken breasts	4

1. In a sealable plastic freezer bag set in a bowl, combine garlic, lemon juice, olive oil, thyme, salt, nutmeg, paprika and white pepper. Add chicken breasts to marinade, seal bag and refrigerate for 1 hour.

2. Preheat oven to 375°F (190°C). Place chicken breasts with marinade in the casserole dish, and cover tightly. Bake for 45 minutes or until chicken is no longer pink inside.

Variation

Substitute an equal amount of oregano for the thyme. Or use 1 tbsp (15 mL) snipped fresh thyme or oregano.

Nutrients per serving

Calories	170
Fat	7 g
Carbohydrate	1 g
Fiber	0 g
Protein	25 g
Vitamin A	81 IU
Iron	0.8 mg
Magnesium	32 mg
Zinc	0.7 mg
Selenium	37.9 mcg

Jerk Chicken

Traditionally, jerk chicken is made with the skin on, which keeps it tender and gives it a dark color, but skin also contributes a lot of fat. If you would like to reduce the saturated fat in this recipe, use skinless chicken and remove any excess fat before preparing the dish.

Makes 4 servings

TIPS

It is best to make your own jerk marinade, as store-bought versions can have more than 900 mg of sodium per 2 tbsp (30 mL).

You can increase the amount of Scotch bonnet pepper in the marinade or leave the seeds in if you like your jerk chicken spicier.

- **Small food processor or mini chopper**
- **8-inch (20 cm) square shallow glass baking dish**

3	green onions, chopped	3
½	Scotch bonnet chile pepper, seeded	½
3	cloves garlic	3
1½ tsp	minced gingerroot	7 mL
1½ tsp	ground allspice	7 mL
1 tsp	chopped fresh thyme	5 mL
½ tsp	salt	2 mL
½ tsp	freshly ground black pepper	2 mL
½ tsp	ground cinnamon	2 mL
¼ tsp	ground nutmeg	1 mL
1½ tbsp	water	22 mL
1 tbsp	freshly squeezed lime juice	15 mL
1 lb	boneless skinless chicken thighs (about 6)	500 g

1. In food processor, combine green onions, Scotch bonnet, garlic, ginger, allspice, thyme, salt, pepper, cinnamon, nutmeg, water and lime juice; process until a thick paste forms.

2. Score meaty side of chicken thighs with 1-inch (2.5 cm) slits and place in baking dish. Rub paste over chicken and into slits. Cover and refrigerate for at least 1 hour or preferably overnight.

3. Preheat oven to 375°F (190°C).

4. Uncover dish. Bake chicken for 30 minutes or until golden. Increase oven temperature to 400°F (200°C) and bake for 15 minutes or until juices run clear when chicken is pierced and a meat thermometer inserted in the thickest part of a thigh registers 165°F (74°C).

Nutrients per serving

Calories	148
Fat	5 g
Carbohydrate	3 g
Fiber	1 g
Protein	23 g
Vitamin A	196 IU
Iron	1.5 mg
Magnesium	33 mg
Zinc	2.3 mg
Selenium	15.7 mcg

Indian-Style Grilled Chicken Breasts

Indian spices have long been recognized for their healing properties, including anti-inflammatory, anti-cancer and antioxidant effects, increasing bile flow and reducing plaque buildup in the arteries. The chicken in this recipe is truly bathed in medicinal spices to help heal your body. Serve with a side salad.

Makes 4 servings

TIP

If you have time, let the chicken marinate for several hours or overnight in the refrigerator to intensify the flavors. To avoid bacterial contamination, baste the chicken only once, halfway through cooking, then discard any leftover marinade.

- **Food processor**
- **Preheat barbecue grill or oven to 350°F (180°C)**

½ cup	plain low-fat yogurt	125 mL
1 tbsp	tomato paste	15 mL
2	green onions, coarsely chopped	2
2	cloves garlic, quartered	2
1	1-inch (2.5 cm) piece gingerroot, coarsely chopped (or 1 tsp/5 mL ground ginger)	1
½ tsp	ground cumin	2 mL
½ tsp	ground coriander	2 mL
½ tsp	salt	2 mL
¼ tsp	cayenne pepper	1 mL
4	chicken breasts (bone-in)	4
2 tbsp	chopped fresh cilantro or parsley	30 mL

1. In food processor, combine yogurt, tomato paste, green onions, garlic, ginger, cumin, coriander, salt and cayenne; purée until smooth.

2. Arrange chicken in a shallow dish; coat with yogurt mixture. Cover and refrigerate for 1 hour or up to 1 day ahead. Remove from refrigerator 30 minutes before cooking.

3. Place chicken skin-side down on greased grill over medium-high heat; cook for 15 minutes. Brush with marinade; turn and cook for 10 to 15 minutes or until golden and juices run clear. (Or place chicken on rack set on baking sheet; roast, basting after 30 minutes with marinade, for 50 to 55 minutes or until juices run clear.) Serve garnished with cilantro.

Nutrients per serving

Calories	162
Fat	4 g
Carbohydrate	4 g
Fiber	0 g
Protein	27 g
Vitamin A	190 IU
Iron	0.8 mg
Magnesium	39 mg
Zinc	1.0 mg
Selenium	39.2 mcg

Buy gingerroot that is firm and unwrinkled, with a gingery aroma. Mature, thick-skinned ginger has a more intense flavor than tender, thin-skinned roots. Store gingerroot in a sealable plastic bag in the refrigerator. It will keep for several weeks. Or peel the ginger and freeze it in a freezer bag. Grate what you need for a recipe while it's still frozen and return the rest to the freezer.

Health-Enhancing Tip

If you grill the chicken, do so on a lower heat, making sure the flame doesn't touch the meat. To further reduce the formation of advanced glycation end products (AGEs), follow the baking option instead. AGEs cause increased inflammation in the body, which will negatively impact thyroid function.

Tandoori Chicken with Cucumber Mint Raita

Ginger, cumin, coriander and cayenne pepper are signature ingredients in Indian cooking. Not only do they make chicken taste wonderful, but the spicy yogurt marinade keeps it moist and tender.

Makes 4 servings

TIPS

If you have time, let the chicken marinate for several hours or overnight to intensify the flavors.

For food safety reasons, discard any leftover marinade.

Double the recipe and place half the uncooked chicken with marinade in a storage container. Freeze for up to 1 month. Let thaw in the refrigerator overnight before cooking as directed.

Nutrients per serving

Calories	168
Fat	4 g
Carbohydrate	5 g
Fiber	1 g
Protein	27 g
Vitamin A	207 IU
Iron	0.9 mg
Magnesium	42 mg
Zinc	1.2 mg
Selenium	38.2 mcg

- **Food processor**
- **13- by 9-inch (33 by 23 cm) glass baking dish with a metal rack, rack sprayed with vegetable oil cooking spray**

1	large green onion, coarsely chopped	1
1	clove garlic, quartered	1
1	1-inch (2.5 cm) piece gingerroot, coarsely chopped	1
½ tsp	ground cumin	2 mL
½ tsp	ground coriander	2 mL
¼ tsp	ground turmeric	1 mL
¼ tsp	salt	1 mL
⅛ tsp	cayenne pepper (optional)	0.5 mL
⅓ cup	nonfat plain yogurt	75 mL
1 tbsp	no-salt-added tomato paste	15 mL
1 lb	boneless skinless chicken breasts (2 large)	500 g
½ cup	Cucumber Mint Raita (page 248)	125 mL

1. In food processor, combine green onion, garlic, ginger, cumin, coriander, turmeric, salt, cayenne (if using), yogurt and tomato paste; process until smooth.

2. On a cutting board, cut each chicken breast lengthwise to make two thinner halves. Arrange in a shallow glass dish and coat both sides with yogurt mixture. (Can be covered and refrigerated for up to 1 day.)

3. Preheat oven to 375°F (190°C).

4. Remove chicken from marinade, discarding marinade. Place chicken on rack in baking dish. Bake for 20 to 25 minutes or until chicken is no longer pink inside. Serve with Cucumber Mint Raita.

Miso Mushroom Chicken with Chinese Cabbage

Serve this luscious, nutritious stew over hot brown rice or quinoa for a delicious, hearty meal.

Makes 8 servings

TIPS

You can halve this recipe, but be sure to use a small (2- to 3-quart) slow cooker.

Brown rice miso, unlike other kinds of miso, is gluten-free.

MAKE AHEAD

Complete step 2. Cover and refrigerate mixture for up to 2 days. When you're ready to cook, complete the recipe.

Nutrients per serving

Calories	241
Fat	7 g
Carbohydrate	18 g
Fiber	4 g
Protein	26 g
Vitamin A	710 IU
Iron	2.0 mg
Magnesium	48 mg
Zinc	2.8 mg
Selenium	18.7 mcg

- **Large (about 5-quart) slow cooker**

1	package (½ oz/14 g) dried wood ear mushrooms	1
1 cup	hot water	250 mL
1 tbsp	vegetable oil	15 mL
2	onions, finely chopped	2
4	stalks celery, diced	4
6	cloves garlic, minced	6
1 tbsp	minced gingerroot	15 mL
1 tsp	cracked black peppercorns	5 mL
½ tsp	sea salt	2 mL
8 oz	shiitake mushrooms, stems discarded, sliced	250 g
½ cup	mirin	125 mL
¼ cup	reduced-sodium GF soy sauce or liquid coconut amino acids	60 mL
2 cups	ready-to-use GF chicken broth	500 mL
2 lbs	skinless bone-in chicken thighs (about 8)	1 kg
2 tbsp	brown rice miso	30 mL
6 cups	packed shredded napa cabbage	1.5 L

1. In a bowl, combine dried mushrooms and hot water. Let stand for 30 minutes. Drain through a fine sieve, discarding soaking liquid. Pat mushrooms dry with paper towel, chop finely and set aside.

2. In a skillet, heat oil over medium heat. Add onions and celery and cook, stirring, until softened, about 5 minutes. Add garlic, ginger, peppercorns, salt and reserved dried mushrooms and cook, stirring, for 1 minute. Add shiitake mushrooms and toss until coated. Add mirin and bring to a boil. Boil for 1 minute. Stir in soy sauce and broth.

3. Arrange chicken evenly over bottom of stoneware and pour mushroom mixture over top. Cover and cook on Low for 6 hours or on High for 3 hours, until chicken is falling off the bone. Stir in miso. Add cabbage, in batches, stirring until each batch is submerged. Cover and cook on High for 15 minutes, until cabbage is wilted and flavors meld.

Indian-Style Chicken with Puréed Spinach

This is a great dish to make on a rainy afternoon. While your chicken cooks, snuggle up and watch a movie. At dinnertime, you'll enjoy a mouth-watering, healing dish that tastes like you spent hours slaving in the kitchen.

Makes 8 servings

TIPS

If using fresh spinach, be sure to remove the stems, and if it has not been prewashed, rinse it thoroughly in a basin of lukewarm water.

One chile produces a medium-hot result. Add a second chile only if you're a true heat seeker.

- **Large (about 5-quart) oval slow cooker**
- **Food processor or blender**

4 lbs	skinless bone-in chicken thighs (about 16 thighs)	2 kg
¼ cup	freshly squeezed lemon juice	60 mL
2 tbsp	olive oil	30 mL
2	onions, thinly sliced on the vertical	2
1 tbsp	minced gingerroot	15 mL
1 tbsp	minced garlic	15 mL
1 tbsp	ground cumin (see tip, page 320)	15 mL
2 tsp	ground coriander	10 mL
1 tsp	cracked black peppercorns	5 mL
1 tsp	sea salt (or to taste)	5 mL
1	can (14 oz/398 mL) diced tomatoes, with juice	1
1 tsp	ground turmeric	5 mL
	Juice of 1 lime or lemon	
2	packages (each 10 oz/300 g) fresh or frozen spinach (see tip, at left)	2
1 to 2	long red or green chile peppers, chopped (see tip, at left)	1 to 2
1 cup	ready-to-use GF chicken broth	250 mL

Nutrients per serving

Calories	247
Fat	10 g
Carbohydrate	9 g
Fiber	3 g
Protein	31 g
Vitamin A	6853 IU
Iron	4.5 mg
Magnesium	101 mg
Zinc	3.2 mg
Selenium	19.7 mcg

1. Rinse chicken under cold running water and pat dry. In a bowl, combine chicken and lemon juice. Toss well and set aside for 20 to 30 minutes.

2. In a skillet, heat oil over medium-high heat. Add onions and cook, stirring, until they begin to color, about 5 minutes. Reduce heat to medium and cook, stirring, until golden, about 12 minutes. Add ginger, garlic, cumin, coriander, peppercorns and salt and cook, stirring, for 1 minute. Stir in tomatoes and bring to a boil. Remove from heat.

MAKE AHEAD

This dish can be partially prepared before it is cooked. Complete step 1. Cover and refrigerate chicken. Complete step 2. Cover and refrigerate separately from chicken. The next day, continue with steps 3, 4 and 5.

3. Arrange marinated chicken evenly over the bottom of slow cooker stoneware. Pour tomato mixture over top. Cover and cook on Low for 6 hours or on High for 3 hours, until juices run clear when chicken is pierced with a fork.

4. In a small bowl, combine turmeric and lime juice. Set aside.

5. In food processor, combine spinach, chile(s) and broth. Pulse until spinach is puréed. Add to chicken along with turmeric mixture and stir well. Cover and cook on High for 20 minutes, until mixture is bubbly.

Spicy Peanut Chicken

This is a lively dish, chock-full of many flavors, all of which work together to create the "yum" factor. Serve it over brown basmati rice to add fiber and complete the meal. To create a more alkaline meal, serve this dish with a side salad or steamed vegetables.

Makes 6 to 8 servings

TIPS

You can halve this recipe, but be sure to use a small (1½- to 3½- quart) slow cooker.

Using virgin coconut oil to soften the onions adds a depth of coconut flavor to the sauce.

Always check the labels of prepared products, such as curry paste, to ensure they don't contain gluten.

MAKE AHEAD

Complete step 1. Cover and refrigerate for up to 2 days. When you're ready to cook, complete the recipe.

Nutrients per serving (1 of 8)	
Calories	370
Fat	17 g
Carbohydrate	14 g
Fiber	4 g
Protein	40 g
Vitamin A	3916 IU
Iron	3.3 mg
Magnesium	85 mg
Zinc	4.3 mg
Selenium	27.8 mcg

- **Medium to large (3½- to 5-quart) slow cooker**

1 tbsp	olive oil or virgin coconut oil	15 mL
2	onions, finely chopped	2
2	carrots, diced	2
4	stalks celery, diced	4
4	cloves garlic, minced	4
1 tbsp	minced gingerroot	15 mL
½ tsp	cracked black peppercorns	2 mL
1 cup	ready-to-use GF chicken broth	250 mL
3 lbs	skinless bone-in chicken thighs (about 12 thighs)	1.5 kg
3 tbsp	smooth natural peanut butter	45 mL
2 tbsp	freshly squeezed lemon juice	30 mL
2 tbsp	reduced-sodium GF soy sauce	30 mL
2 tsp	Thai red curry paste (see tip, at left)	10 mL
½ cup	coconut milk	125 mL
2 cups	sweet green peas, thawed if frozen	500 mL
1	red bell pepper, diced	1
¼ cup	chopped roasted peanuts	60 mL
½ cup	finely chopped fresh cilantro leaves	125 mL

1. In a skillet, heat oil over medium heat. Add onions, carrots and celery and cook, stirring, until carrots are softened, about 7 minutes. Add garlic, ginger and peppercorns and cook, stirring, for 1 minute. Add broth and bring to a boil.

2. Arrange chicken over bottom of slow cooker stoneware and add vegetable mixture. Cover and cook on Low for 5 hours or on High for 2½ hours, until juices run clear when chicken is pierced with a fork.

3. In a bowl, combine peanut butter, lemon juice, soy sauce and red curry paste. Mix well. Add to slow cooker stoneware and stir well. Add coconut milk, peas and red pepper and stir well. Cover and cook on High for 20 minutes, until pepper is tender and mixture is hot. Garnish with peanuts and cilantro and serve.

Turkey Ratatouille Chili

Here's a great combination of ratatouille and chili in one dish, perfect for a family meal!

Makes 4 to 6 servings

MAKE AHEAD

Prepare up to a day ahead and reheat gently, adding extra GF chicken broth if too thick.

2 tsp	vegetable oil	10 mL
2 tsp	minced garlic	10 mL
1 cup	chopped onions	250 mL
1⅔ cups	chopped zucchini	400 mL
1⅔ cups	chopped peeled eggplant	400 mL
1½ cups	chopped mushrooms	375 mL
12 oz	lean ground turkey	375 g
2 tbsp	tomato paste	30 mL
1	can (19 oz/540 mL) tomatoes, puréed	1
2 cups	ready-to-use GF chicken broth	500 mL
1⅓ cups	peeled chopped potatoes	325 mL
1 cup	canned red kidney beans, drained	250 mL
1 tbsp	chili powder	15 mL
1½ tsp	dried basil	7 mL
1	bay leaf	1

1. In a large nonstick saucepan sprayed with vegetable spray, heat oil over medium heat. Add garlic, onions, zucchini and eggplant; cook for 5 minutes or until softened. Add mushrooms and cook for 2 minutes. Remove vegetables from skillet and set aside. Add turkey to skillet and cook, stirring to break it up, for 3 minutes or until no longer pink. Drain fat and add cooked vegetables to skillet.

2. Add tomato paste, tomatoes, broth, potatoes, beans, chili powder, basil and bay leaf; bring to a boil. Cover, reduce heat to low and simmer for 40 minutes, stirring occasionally.

Variation

Lean ground pork, veal or chicken can replace the turkey.

Health-Enhancing Tips

Look for BPA-free cans of beans and tomatoes.

For a healthier fat, substitute olive oil for the vegetable oil.

Nutrients per serving (1 of 6)

Calories	238
Fat	8 g
Carbohydrate	27 g
Fiber	7 g
Protein	19 g
Vitamin A	1230 IU
Iron	3.5 mg
Magnesium	70 mg
Zinc	2.3 mg
Selenium	15.9 mcg

Turkey Mole

In many parts of Mexico, no special occasion is complete without turkey cooked in mole poblano. The authentic version is quite a production, but this simplified slow cooker version is delicious nonetheless. Serve with steamed vegetables, a side salad or a low-carb vegetable side dish.

Makes 8 servings

TIP

Turkey is an excellent source of complete protein and a good source of important B vitamins — niacin, B_6 and B_{12} — as well as zinc, which helps to keep your immune system strong. Turkley is also a good source of selenium, which acts as an antioxidant.

- **Large (minimum 5-quart) slow cooker**
- **Blender**

1 tbsp	olive oil	15 mL
1	skin-on turkey breast (about 2 lbs/1 kg)	1
2	onions, sliced	2
4	cloves garlic, sliced	4
4	whole cloves	4
1	2-inch (5 cm) cinnamon stick	1
1 tsp	salt	5 mL
1 tsp	cracked black peppercorns	5 mL
1	can (28 oz/796 mL) tomatillos, drained	1
½ oz	unsweetened chocolate, broken into pieces	15 g
1 cup	ready-to-use GF chicken broth, divided	250 mL
2	dried ancho, New Mexico or guajillo chile peppers	2
2 cups	boiling water	500 mL
½ cup	coarsely chopped fresh cilantro stems and leaves	125 mL
1 tbsp	chili powder	15 mL
1 to 2	jalapeño peppers, chopped	1 to 2
3 tbsp	diced mild green chile peppers (optional)	45 mL

1. In a skillet, heat oil over medium-high heat for 30 seconds. Add turkey and brown on all sides. Transfer to slow cooker stoneware.

2. Reduce heat to medium. Add onions to pan and cook, stirring, until softened, about 3 minutes. Add garlic, cloves, cinnamon stick, salt and peppercorns and cook, stirring, for 1 minute. Transfer mixture to blender. Add tomatillos, chocolate and ½ cup (125 mL) broth and process until smooth.

Nutrients per serving

Calories	284
Fat	12 g
Carbohydrate	16 g
Fiber	3 g
Protein	29 g
Vitamin A	1199 IU
Iron	2.5 mg
Magnesium	44 mg
Zinc	2.2 mg
Selenium	26.2 mcg

MAKE AHEAD

This dish can be partially prepared before it is cooked. Complete steps 2 and 4, heating 1 tbsp (15 mL) oil in pan before softening onions. Cover and refrigerate puréed sauces separately for up to 2 days, being aware that the chile mixture will lose some of its vibrancy if held for this long. (For best results, complete step 4 while the turkey is cooking or no sooner than the night before you plan to cook.) When you're ready to cook, brown turkey (step 1), or remove skin from turkey, omit browning and place directly in stoneware. Continue with the recipe.

3. Pour sauce over turkey, cover and cook on Low for 8 hours or on High for 4 hours, until juices run clear when turkey is pierced with a fork or meat thermometer reads 170°F (77°C).

4. An hour before recipe has finished cooking, in a heatproof bowl, soak dried chiles in boiling water for 30 minutes, weighing down with a cup to ensure they remain submerged. Drain, discarding soaking liquid and stems, and chop coarsely. Transfer to blender. Add cilantro, the remaining broth, chili powder and jalapeño pepper and purée. Add to stoneware along with mild green chiles (if using), and stir gently to combine. Cover and cook on High for 30 minutes, until flavors meld.

Pork Vindaloo

Vindaloo is a popular curry dish served in many parts of India. Like many Indian recipes, it includes several health-promoting ingredients to help heal your body.

Makes 8 servings

TIP

Ghee is a type of clarified butter highly valued in Indian cooking as it can be heated to a very high temperature. It is available in grocery stores specializing in Indian ingredients and will keep, refrigerated, for as long as a year.

MAKE AHEAD

This dish must be assembled the night before it is cooked as it needs to be marinated overnight. Follow preparation directions and refrigerate overnight. The next day, transfer to stoneware and cook as directed.

Nutrients per serving

Calories	173
Fat	6 g
Carbohydrate	3 g
Fiber	1 g
Protein	24 g
Vitamin A	107 IU
Iron	2.0 mg
Magnesium	40 mg
Zinc	2.3 mg
Selenium	36.1 mcg

• **Large (minimum 5-quart) slow cooker**

1 tbsp	cumin seeds	15 mL
2 tsp	coriander seeds	10 mL
1 tbsp	clarified butter or ghee (see tip, at left)	15 mL
1	onion, finely chopped	1
8	cloves garlic, minced	8
1 tbsp	minced gingerroot	15 mL
1	2-inch (5 cm) cinnamon stick	1
6	whole cloves	6
1/2 tsp	salt	2 mL
2 tsp	mustard seeds	10 mL
1/4 tsp	cayenne pepper	1 mL
2 lbs	stewing pork, cut into 1-inch (2.5 cm) cubes	1 kg
4	bay leaves	4
1/2 cup	red wine vinegar	125 mL

1. In a skillet, over medium heat, cook cumin and coriander seeds, stirring constantly, until they release their aroma and just begin to turn golden. Remove pan from heat and transfer seeds to a mortar or a cutting board. Using a pestle or a rolling pin, crush seeds coarsely. Set aside.

2. In a skillet, heat butter or ghee over medium heat. Add onion, garlic and ginger and cook for 1 minute. Add cumin and coriander seeds, cinnamon, cloves, salt, mustard seeds and cayenne and cook for 1 more minute. Remove from heat. Let cool.

3. Place pork in a mixing bowl. Add bay leaves and contents of pan. Add vinegar and stir to combine. Cover and marinate overnight in refrigerator. The next day, transfer to slow cooker stoneware, cover and cook on Low for 8 to 10 hours or on High for 4 to 5 hours, until pork is tender. Discard bay leaves, cinnamon stick and whole cloves.

Catalan Beef Stew

The region of Catalonia, best known for its capital, Barcelona, has some great cuisine! This version of the famous dish uses fresh tomatoes instead of tomato sauce, and leeks and long beans in place of mushrooms.

Makes 5 servings

TIPS

Although this recipe is delicious just as it is, for true authenticity it requires an additional ingredient: chocolate. If you're feeling bold, add 1 oz (30 g) unsweetened chocolate with the chicken broth. This will increase the carbohydrate content by 1 g per serving.

When purchasing ready-to-use chicken broth, check the label to make sure it is gluten-free. Or prepare Homemade Chicken Stock (page 195) to use in this recipe.

1½ tsp	extra virgin olive oil	7 mL
½ cup	chopped onion	125 mL
2	cloves garlic, minced	2
½	stalk celery, chopped	½
1 lb	boneless beef bottom round, visible fat removed, cut into 1-inch (2.5 cm) cubes	500 g
½ tsp	salt	2 mL
¼ tsp	freshly ground black pepper	1 mL
2	plum (Roma) tomatoes, chopped	2
1	leek (white and light green parts only), chopped	1
1 tbsp	finely chopped fresh oregano	15 mL
¼ tsp	ground cinnamon	1 mL
1	carrot, thinly sliced	1
1 cup	halved Chinese long beans	250 mL
2 cups	water	500 mL
1½ cups	ready-to-use reduced-sodium chicken broth	375 mL
½ cup	dry red wine	125 mL

1. In a large, deep pot, heat oil over medium heat. Add onion and cook, stirring, for about 2 minutes or until translucent. Add garlic and celery; cook, stirring, for 1 minute.

2. Stir in beef, salt and pepper; cook, stirring, for 10 minutes.

3. Stir in tomatoes, leek, oregano and cinnamon; cook, stirring, for 8 minutes.

4. Stir in carrot and cook, stirring, for 5 minutes.

5. Stir in green beans, water, broth and wine; reduce heat to medium-low, cover and simmer, stirring occasionally, for 1 hour and 20 minutes or until beef is tender.

Nutrients per serving

Calories	209
Fat	7 g
Carbohydrate	10 g
Fiber	2 g
Protein	22 g
Vitamin A	2716 IU
Iron	3.3 mg
Magnesium	44 mg
Zinc	3.9 mg
Selenium	29.9 mcg

Zesty Braised Beef with New Potatoes

It's hard to believe that a simple combination of ingredients can taste so luscious. Serve this with a big platter of roasted carrots. Save leftovers and enjoy them in a bowl like a hearty soup.

Makes 8 servings

TIPS

You can halve this recipe, but be sure to use a small (2- to 3½-quart) slow cooker.

If you have time to make Homemade Chicken Stock (page 195), use it in place of the ready-to-use broth.

Nutrients per serving

Calories	341
Fat	13 g
Carbohydrate	24 g
Fiber	3 g
Protein	30 g
Vitamin A	192 IU
Iron	3.2 mg
Magnesium	55 mg
Zinc	4.7 mg
Selenium	27.8 mcg

- **Medium to large (3½- to 5-quart) slow cooker**

2 tbsp	olive oil, divided	30 mL
2 oz	chunk pancetta (preferably hot pancetta), diced	60 g
2 lbs	trimmed stewing beef, cut into 1-inch (2.5 cm) cubes and patted dry	1 kg
2	onions, finely chopped	2
4	cloves garlic, minced	4
1 tsp	dried thyme	5 mL
½ tsp	sea salt	2 mL
½ tsp	cracked black peppercorns	2 mL
½ cup	dry white wine	125 mL
2 cups	ready-to-use GF chicken broth	500 mL
2 lbs	small new potatoes (about 30 tiny ones), thinly sliced	1 kg
¼ tsp	cayenne pepper, dissolved in 1 tbsp (15 mL) freshly squeezed lemon juice	1 mL
¼ cup	finely chopped fresh parsley leaves	60 mL

1. In a skillet, heat 1 tbsp (15 mL) oil over medium-high heat. Add pancetta and cook, stirring, until nicely browned, about 3 minutes. Transfer to slow cooker stoneware.

2. Add beef to skillet, in batches, and cook, stirring, until browned, about 4 minutes per batch. Transfer to stoneware as completed.

3. Reduce heat to medium. Add the remaining oil to pan. Add onions and cook, stirring, until softened, about 3 minutes. Add garlic, thyme, salt and peppercorns and cook, stirring, for 1 minute. Add wine, bring to a boil and boil, stirring and scraping up brown bits from bottom of pan, for 2 minutes. Add broth and potatoes and bring to a boil. Simmer for 2 minutes.

TIP

Because it's important to bring the potatoes to a boil in order to ensure that they cook in the slow cooker, making part of this dish ahead of time is not recommended.

4. Transfer to stoneware. Cover and cook on Low for 8 hours or on High for 4 hours, until potatoes are tender. Stir in cayenne solution. Cover and cook on High for 10 minutes. Transfer to a serving dish and garnish with parsley.

> ## Health-Enhancing Tip
>
> To create a more alkaline meal, serve this dish with a side salad or steamed vegetables.

Meatballs for Everyday

Whether you serve these meatballs with spaghetti or sweet-and-sour sauce, or as hot hors d'oeuvres, they are sure to be a hit.

| **Makes 42 meatballs** | | |

TIP

To freeze: Let cool slightly, then freeze baked meatballs on the jelly roll pan. Once frozen, remove meatballs from pan and place in a heavy-duty freezer bag. Remove only the number you need — they won't stick together. Reheat meatballs from frozen directly in sauce or microwave just until thawed and then add to the sauce.

- **Preheat oven to 400°F (200°C)**
- **15- by 10-inch (40 by 25 cm) jelly roll pan, lightly greased**

1 lb	extra lean ground beef	500 g
8 oz	ground pork	250 g
½ cup	finely chopped onion	125 mL
1	large egg, lightly beaten	1
1 cup	soft GF bread crumbs (see tip, page 296)	250 mL
2 tbsp	snipped fresh parsley	30 mL
2 tbsp	snipped fresh basil leaves	30 mL
2 tbsp	snipped fresh oregano	30 mL
¼ tsp	freshly ground black pepper	1 mL

1. In a large bowl, gently mix together beef, pork, onion, egg, bread crumbs, parsley, basil, oregano and pepper. Shape into 1-inch (2.5 cm) balls. Place in a single layer on prepared pan.

2. Bake in a preheated oven for 20 minutes or until no longer pink in the center.

Variations

Use commercial GF rice crackers to make crumbs and substitute for GF bread crumbs. If using flavored crackers, such as barbecue or teriyaki, omit the basil and oregano.

Substitute ground turkey or chicken for all or part of the ground beef and pork.

Nutrients per 6 meatballs

Calories	242
Fat	13 g
Carbohydrate	10 g
Fiber	1 g
Protein	21 g
Vitamin A	198 IU
Iron	2.2 mg
Magnesium	24 mg
Zinc	4.2 mg
Selenium	21.5 mcg

Health-Enhancing Tips

For a low-carb option, serve these meatballs over spaghetti squash. To prepare it, cut spaghetti squash in half and remove seeds. Place squash halves in a casserole dish with ½ inch (1 cm) of water and cover with foil. Bake at 350°F (180°C) for 30 minutes or until squash is fork-tender. Scoop pulp into a bowl and, using a fork, rake into strands.

Serve the meatballs with Basic Tomato Sauce (page 250) or Basic Pesto (page 246).

Country Supper Cabbage Rolls

Freezing the cabbage is an easy way to wilt the leaves, which makes them easier to remove from the core.

Makes 24 cabbage rolls

TIPS

Holding the frozen cabbage under warm water as you work may make it easier to remove the leaves.

Save any remaining cabbage to serve as a vegetable at another meal.

Portion extra baked cabbage rolls into airtight containers, let cool, cover and freeze for up to 3 months. Let thaw overnight in the refrigerator or defrost in the microwave before reheating.

Nutrients per 3 cabbage rolls

Calories	186
Fat	4 g
Carbohydrate	18 g
Fiber	3 g
Protein	20 g
Vitamin A	615 IU
Iron	2.5 mg
Magnesium	41 mg
Zinc	2.9 mg
Selenium	27.6 mcg

• **8-cup (2 L) casserole dish**

1	head green cabbage	1
1 lb	lean ground pork	500 g
8 oz	lean ground beef	250 g
½ cup	long-grain white rice	125 mL
⅓ cup	chopped onion	75 mL
1	clove garlic, finely chopped (optional)	1
1 tsp	salt	5 mL
¼ tsp	freshly ground black pepper	1 mL
1 cup	reduced-sodium tomato juice	250 mL

1. Place cabbage in freezer overnight to wilt leaves.

2. Preheat oven to 300°F (150°C).

3. Carefully remove 24 cabbage leaves from the frozen head, one at a time, cutting each from the core with a sharp knife. Trim the center rib on individual leaves to make the leaf the same thickness throughout, but do not remove the rib.

4. In a large bowl, combine pork, beef, rice, onion, garlic (if using), salt, pepper and ½ cup (125 mL) water; mix thoroughly.

5. Place about 5 tsp (30 mL) meat mixture on the rib end of each cabbage leaf. Roll up and tuck in sides. Pack cabbage rolls tightly into casserole dish, a single layer at a time, layering them with tomato juice. Pour ½ cup (125 mL) water over rolls.

6. Cover and bake in preheated oven for 2 hours. Reduce oven temperature to 250°F (120°C) and bake for 1 hour or until meat is no longer pink and rice is tender.

Grilled Lamb Chops with Rosemary Mustard Baste

Lamb chops are wonderful au naturel, but even more delicious with a mustard glaze flavored with rosemary. Here's a quick and tasty way to dress up lamb chops for the barbecue.

Makes 4 servings

TIPS

The marinade is also fantastic with lamb kabobs, as well as with chicken and pork.

It may be helpful to use a food scale to weigh portions of meat, poultry, seafood and cheese to ensure accuracy, especially if you are concerned about weight loss or are strictly monitoring your diet to manage your blood glucose levels.

- **Preheat barbecue grill or stovetop grill pan to medium**

2	cloves garlic, minced	2
1 tbsp	chopped fresh rosemary	15 mL
1/4 tsp	freshly ground black pepper	1 mL
2 tbsp	honey-Dijon mustard	30 mL
2 tbsp	balsamic vinegar	30 mL
8	lamb loin chops (1 inch/2.5 cm thick), trimmed (1 1/2 lbs/750 g total)	8

1. In a shallow glass dish, combine garlic, rosemary, pepper, mustard and vinegar. Add lamb and turn to coat. Marinate at room temperature for 15 minutes, or cover and refrigerate, turning occasionally, for up to 8 hours.

2. Remove lamb from marinade, discarding marinade, and place on preheated grill. Cook for 6 to 7 minutes per side for medium-rare, or to desired doneness.

Health-Enhancing Tip

Grill on a lower heat, making sure the flame doesn't touch the meat. Or, to further reduce the formation of advanced glycation end products (AGEs), bake the lamb chops at 375°F (190°C) for 30 to 40 minutes, turning them halfway through. AGEs cause increased inflammation in the body, which will negatively impact thyroid function.

Nutrients per serving

Calories	283
Fat	13 g
Carbohydrate	3 g
Fiber	0 g
Protein	36 g
Vitamin A	16 IU
Iron	3.4 mg
Magnesium	48 mg
Zinc	5.5 mg
Selenium	40.4 mcg

Segovia-Style Lamb

The rocky, arid land around Segovia, Spain, is ideal for raising sheep and lamb, and their meats are traditionally roasted in Roman-style ovens, so it's no surprise that Segovia is known for its lamb dishes. This one is simple but full of flavor.

Makes 5 servings

TIPS

In this recipe, lamb shoulder and beef bottom round were used, as they are lower-fat cuts. When using lower-fat meats, it's important to watch the cooking time, as they can easily overcook and become tough.

In Spanish cuisine, sherry vinegar is often used to cook beef, duck or game. Look for it in specialty or gourmet food stores or well-stocked supermarkets. If you can't find it, substitute $1\frac{1}{2}$ tsp (7 mL) white wine vinegar.

1 tsp	extra virgin olive oil	5 mL
1	large onion, finely chopped	1
1	clove garlic, minced	1
$\frac{1}{4}$ cup	chopped fresh parsley	60 mL
8 oz	boneless lamb shoulder, visible fat removed, cut into 2-inch (5 cm) cubes	250 g
8 oz	boneless beef bottom round, visible fat removed, cut into 2-inch (5 cm) cubes	250 g
4	large portobello mushrooms, stems removed, caps cut into 1-inch (2.5 cm) slices	4
2	bay leaves	2
$\frac{1}{2}$ tsp	salt	2 mL
$\frac{1}{2}$ tsp	freshly ground black pepper	2 mL
1 tbsp	sherry vinegar	15 mL
1 cup	dry white wine	250 mL

1. In a small, deep pot, heat oil over medium heat. Add onion, garlic and parsley; cook, stirring, for 4 minutes or until onion is translucent.

2. Stir in lamb and beef; cook, stirring, for 15 minutes.

3. Stir in mushrooms, bay leaves, salt, pepper and vinegar; cook, stirring, for 5 minutes.

4. Stir in wine, reduce heat to low, cover and simmer, stirring occasionally, for $1\frac{1}{2}$ hours or until lamb and beef are tender. Discard bay leaves.

Nutrients per serving

Calories	204
Fat	6 g
Carbohydrate	7 g
Fiber	2 g
Protein	21 g
Vitamin A	263 IU
Iron	2.4 mg
Magnesium	26 mg
Zinc	4.1 mg
Selenium	30.9 mcg

Spicy Lamb with Chickpeas

Here's a dish with robust flavor that will delight even your most discriminating guests. Serve over hot quinoa, with a side of vegetables or a salad.

Makes 8 servings

TIPS

You can halve this recipe, but be sure to use a small (2- to 3½-quart) slow cooker.

For the best flavor, toast and grind the cumin and coriander yourself, rather than buying the ground versions. Place seeds in a dry skillet over medium heat, stirring until fragrant, about 3 minutes. Using a mortar and pestle or a spice grinder, pound or grind as finely as you can.

- **Medium to large (3½- to 5-quart) slow cooker**

1 tbsp	ground cumin (see tip, at left)	15 mL
2 tsp	ground coriander	10 mL
1 tsp	ground turmeric	5 mL
1½ tsp	cracked black peppercorns, divided	7 mL
¾ tsp	salt, divided	3 mL
1 tsp	finely grated lime zest	5 mL
2 tbsp	freshly squeezed lime juice	30 mL
2 lbs	trimmed stewing lamb, cut into 1-inch (2.5 cm) cubes	1 kg
2 tbsp	olive oil, divided	30 mL
2	onions, finely chopped	2
2	carrots, diced	2
2	parsnips, diced	2
4	cloves garlic, minced	4
2 tbsp	minced gingerroot	30 mL
4	black cardamom pods, crushed	4
1	2-inch (5 cm) cinnamon stick	1
6	whole cloves	6
1	can (28 oz/796 mL) no-salt added tomatoes, with juice, coarsely chopped	1
1 cup	ready-to-use GF chicken or vegetable broth	250 mL
3 cups	cooked chickpeas, mashed (see tip, opposite)	750 mL
1 tsp	Aleppo pepper (see tip, opposite)	5 mL
¼ tsp	cayenne pepper	1 mL

1. In a bowl, combine cumin, coriander, turmeric, 1 tsp (5 mL) peppercorns, ¼ tsp (1 mL) salt, lime zest and lime juice. Stir well. Add lamb and toss to coat. Cover and set aside in refrigerator for 4 hours or overnight.

Nutrients per serving

Calories	361
Fat	12 g
Carbohydrate	34 g
Fiber	9 g
Protein	31 g
Vitamin A	2737 IU
Iron	5.7 mg
Magnesium	90 mg
Zinc	6.1 mg
Selenium	29.6 mcg

You can cook your own chickpeas (see Basic Beans, page 255) or use canned chickpeas, with no salt added, drained and rinsed.

Aleppo pepper is a mild Syrian chile pepper. It is increasingly available in specialty shops or well-stocked supermarkets. If you don't have it, substitute another mild chile powder such as ancho or New Mexico, or add another $\frac{1}{4}$ tsp (1 mL) cayenne.

MAKE AHEAD

Complete steps 1 and 3. Cover and refrigerate overnight. When you're ready to cook, complete the recipe.

2. Pat lamb dry. In a skillet, heat 1 tbsp (15 mL) oil over medium heat. Add lamb, in batches, and cook, stirring, until lightly browned, about 4 minutes per batch. Transfer to slow cooker as completed.

3. Add the remaining oil to pan. Add onions, carrots and parsnips and cook, stirring and scraping up brown bits, until carrots are softened, about 7 minutes. Add garlic, ginger, cardamom, cinnamon stick, cloves, the remaining salt and the remaining peppercorns and cook, stirring, for 1 minute. Add tomatoes and broth and bring to a boil, scraping up brown bits from bottom of pan. Transfer to stoneware. Stir in chickpeas.

4. Cover and cook on Low for 8 hours or on High for 4 to 5 hours, until meat is very tender. Stir in Aleppo and cayenne. Cover and cook on High for 10 minutes.

Lamb with Lentils and Chard

Rich with the flavors of the French countryside, this hearty stew is perfect for guests or a family meal. All it needs is a simple green salad, finished with a scattering of shredded carrots.

Makes 10 servings

TIPS

If you can't find Swiss chard, use 2 packages (each 10 oz/300 g) fresh or frozen spinach. If using fresh spinach, remove the stems and chop before using. If it has not been prewashed, rinse it thoroughly in a basin of lukewarm water. If using frozen spinach, thaw it first.

Although this makes a large quantity, don't worry about leftovers. It reheats very well and may even be better the day after it is made.

Nutrients per serving

Calories	336
Fat	9 g
Carbohydrate	34 g
Fiber	7 g
Protein	31 g
Vitamin A	9998 IU
Iron	6.8 mg
Magnesium	90 mg
Zinc	5.5 mg
Selenium	33.1 mcg

- **Large (minimum 5-quart) slow cooker**

2 tbsp	olive oil, divided (approx.)	30 mL
2 lbs	trimmed stewing lamb, cut into 1-inch (2.5 cm) cubes	1 kg
2	onions, finely chopped	2
8	carrots, sliced	8
4	stalks celery, sliced	4
4	cloves garlic, minced	4
2 tsp	dried herbes de Provence	10 mL
1 tsp	salt	5 mL
½ tsp	cracked black peppercorns	2 mL
2	bay leaves	2
1 cup	ready-to-use GF vegetable or chicken broth	250 mL
1	can (28 oz/796 mL) tomatoes, with juice, coarsely chopped	1
2 cups	dried green or brown lentils, rinsed	500 mL
8 cups	chopped stemmed Swiss chard (about 2 bunches)	2 L

1. In a skillet, heat 1 tbsp (15 mL) of the oil over medium-high heat for 30 seconds. Add lamb, in batches, and cook, stirring, adding more oil as necessary, until browned, about 4 minutes per batch. Transfer to slow cooker stoneware.

2. Reduce heat to medium. Drain all but 1 tbsp (15 mL) of the fat from pan. Add onions, carrots and celery to pan and cook, stirring, until carrots are softened, about 7 minutes. Add garlic, herbes de Provence, salt and peppercorns and cook, stirring, for 1 minute. Add bay leaves, broth and tomatoes and bring to a boil, Transfer to slow cooker stoneware. Stir in lentils.

3. Cover and cook on Low for 8 hours or on High for 4 hours, until mixture is bubbly and lamb and lentils are tender. Add chard, in batches, stirring each batch into the stew until wilted. Cover and cook on High for 20 to 30 minutes, until chard is tender. Discard bay leaves.

Side Dishes

Stuffed Artichokes 324

Roasted Asparagus 325

Asparagus with Lemon and Garlic 326

Cumin Beets 327

Sautéed Broccoli and Red Peppers 328

Broccoli Cilantro Pesto with Pasta 329

Braised Brussels Sprouts 330

Herb-Glazed Brussels Sprouts 331

Thyme-Scented Carrots 332

Lemon Almond Sautéed Greens 333

New Orleans Braised Onions 334

Lentil-Stuffed Tomatoes 335

Cherry Tomato and Zucchini Sauté 336

Mix 'n' Mash Vegetables 337

Steamed Vegetables with Toasted Almonds 338

Roasted Butternut Squash with Onion and Sage 340

Baked Sweet Potato Fries 341

Creamy Mashed Potatoes with Cauliflower 342

Savoury Vegetarian Quinoa Pilaf 343

Red Beans and Greens 344

Creamy Polenta 346

Stuffed Artichokes

Not only are artichokes a great source of iron and soluble fiber, but they're also a great deal of fun to eat. Peel off one petal, place it between your teeth and pull, leaving the tender part in your mouth and discarding the unwanted leaf. When you reach the center, discard the choke and enjoy the tender base.

Makes 4 servings

TIP

The cooking time depends on the size of the artichoke. When choosing your artichokes, make sure they are all the same size, so they'll all be done at the same time.

8	small artichokes (about 1 lb/500 g)	8
	Lemon wedges	
½ cup	GF cracker crumbs	125 mL
2 to 3	cloves garlic, minced	2 to 3
2 tsp	dried parsley	10 mL
	Salt and freshly ground black pepper	
2 tbsp	olive oil	30 mL

1. Cut the stems off the artichokes, creating a flat base. Trim off the tough outer leaves. Cut about ½ inch (1 cm) off the tops, then use scissors to snip off the sharp leaf tips. Push open the leaves and rinse. Rub all cut surfaces with lemon.

2. In a small bowl, combine cracker crumbs, garlic to taste and parsley. Season to taste with salt and pepper. Stir in oil to make a paste.

3. Stuff artichokes with cracker mixture and place upright in a large pot. Add enough water to come halfway up artichokes. Cover and bring to a boil over high heat. Reduce heat to low and simmer for 45 minutes or until tender.

Nutrients per serving

Calories	194
Fat	8 g
Carbohydrate	30 g
Fiber	3 g
Protein	3 g
Vitamin A	31 IU
Iron	4.5 mg
Magnesium	25 mg
Zinc	0.3 mg
Selenium	2.2 mcg

Roasted Asparagus

Roasting brings out the best in many vegetables, including asparagus.

Makes 4 servings

TIP

The roasting time will depend on the thickness of the asparagus stalks.

- **Preheat oven to 400°F (200°C)**
- **Rimmed baking sheet or shallow roasting pan**

1 lb	asparagus	500 g
1 tbsp	extra virgin olive oil	15 mL
1 tbsp	balsamic or red wine vinegar	15 mL
	Freshly ground black pepper	

1. Snap off tough asparagus ends and peel any large stalks. Arrange in a single layer on baking sheet. Drizzle with oil and vinegar. Season with pepper.

2. Roast in preheated oven, stirring occasionally, for 14 to 18 minutes or until asparagus is glazed and tender-crisp. Serve immediately.

Nutrients per serving

Calories	56
Fat	4 g
Carbohydrate	5 g
Fiber	2 g
Protein	3 g
Vitamin A	857 IU
Iron	2.5 mg
Magnesium	16 mg
Zinc	0.6 mg
Selenium	2.6 mcg

Asparagus with Lemon and Garlic

This health-enhancing side dish is loaded with nutrients to heal your body, and it's delicious, too!

Makes 4 servings

TIPS

If asparagus is not available, try broccoli.

Adjust the lemon juice to taste.

If you have time to make Homemade Chicken Stock (page 195), use it in place of the ready-to-use broth.

MAKE AHEAD

Make this early in the day if it is to be served cold, to allow the asparagus a chance to marinate.

8 oz	asparagus, trimmed	250 g
2 tsp	vegetable oil	10 mL
1 tsp	crushed garlic	5 mL
¼ cup	finely chopped red bell pepper	60 mL
1	green onion, sliced	1
2 tbsp	white wine	30 mL
4 tsp	freshly squeezed lemon juice	20 mL
2 tbsp	ready-to-use GF chicken broth	30 mL
	Freshly ground black pepper	

1. Steam or boil asparagus just until tender-crisp. Do not overcook. Drain and set aside.

2. In large nonstick skillet, heat oil; sauté garlic and red pepper until softened.

3. Reduce heat and add green onion, wine, lemon juice, broth, pepper to taste and asparagus. Cook for 1 minute. Place asparagus mixture in serving dish.

Health-Enhancing Tip

For a healthier, less inflammatory fat, use sesame oil or ghee (see tip, page 312) in place of the vegetable oil.

Nutrients per serving

Calories	47
Fat	3 g
Carbohydrate	4 g
Fiber	1 g
Protein	2 g
Vitamin A	733 IU
Iron	1.3 mg
Magnesium	10 mg
Zinc	0.3 mg
Selenium	1.3 mcg

Cumin Beets

The flavors of garlic, cumin and tomatoes complement the earthy beets in this recipe, a perfect side dish to quinoa and chickpeas.

Makes 6 servings

TIP

Peeling the beets before they are cooked ensures that all the delicious cooking juices end up on your plate.

MAKE AHEAD

This dish can be assembled the night before it is cooked. Complete step 1, add beets to mixture and refrigerate overnight. The next day, continue cooking as directed in step 2.

- **Medium to large (3½- to 5-quart) slow cooker**

1 tbsp	vegetable oil	15 mL
1	onion, finely chopped	1
3	cloves garlic, minced	3
1 tsp	cumin seeds	5 mL
1 tsp	salt	5 mL
½ tsp	freshly ground black pepper	2 mL
2	tomatoes, peeled and coarsely chopped	2
1 cup	water	250 mL
1 lb	beets, peeled and used whole, if small, or sliced thinly (see tip, at left)	500 g

1. In a skillet, heat oil over medium-high heat. Add onion and cook, stirring, until softened. Stir in garlic, cumin, salt and pepper and cook for 1 minute. Add tomatoes and water and bring to a boil.

2. Place beets in slow cooker stoneware and pour tomato mixture over them. Cover and cook on Low for 8 to 10 hours or on High for 4 to 5 hours, until beets are tender.

Nutrients per serving

Calories	66
Fat	3 g
Carbohydrate	10 g
Fiber	3 g
Protein	2 g
Vitamin A	78 IU
Iron	0.9 mg
Magnesium	22 mg
Zinc	0.4 mg
Selenium	0.9 mcg

Sautéed Broccoli and Red Peppers

Jam-packed with nutrients, this yummy vegetable side dish is perfect with chicken, pork chops or broiled salmon. For a vegetarian main dish, prepare the variation with chickpeas (below).

Makes 4 servings

TIP

Do not discard the broccoli stalks — they have plenty of flavor and crunch. Peel away the thick outer layer and shred the stalks with a food processor or on the coarse side of a box grater. Add to a cabbage slaw or vegetable soup, or sprinkle into a mixed salad.

1 tbsp	olive oil	15 mL
1	red onion, chopped	1
1	clove garlic, minced	1
1/4 tsp	salt	1 mL
	Freshly ground black pepper	
3 cups	small broccoli florets	750 mL
1	red bell pepper, chopped	1
1/2 tsp	dried oregano	2 mL
2 tbsp	red wine vinegar	30 mL

1. In a large nonstick skillet, heat oil over medium-high heat. Sauté onion, garlic, salt, and pepper to taste for about 4 minutes or until onion is softened.

2. Stir in broccoli and red pepper; sauté for 4 to 5 minutes or until tender-crisp. Stir in oregano and vinegar; sauté for 1 minute.

Variation

Add 1 cup (250 mL) drained rinsed cooked or canned chickpeas and sauté for 1 minute before adding the oregano and vinegar.

Health-Enhancing Tip

Sauté the vegetables over medium heat, adjusting the cooking time as necessary.

Nutrients per serving

Calories	64
Fat	4 g
Carbohydrate	7 g
Fiber	3 g
Protein	2 g
Vitamin A	2532 IU
Iron	0.8 mg
Magnesium	20 mg
Zinc	0.3 mg
Selenium	1.8 mcg

Broccoli Cilantro Pesto with Pasta

Make good use of homegrown produce when it's at its best. Turn it into a meal by topping it with cooked tofu and fresh grape tomatoes.

Makes 4 servings

TIPS

Four cups (1 L) of broccoli florets weigh 1 pound (500 g).

Add more GF chicken broth if the pesto seems too thick.

Make lots of pesto during the summer, when herbs are plentiful, and freeze in small quantities.

Vary the herbs and the amounts used.

Nutrients per serving (with 1 cup/250 mL GF pasta)

Calories	224
Fat	17 g
Carbohydrate	14 g
Fiber	4 g
Protein	7 g
Vitamin A	2303 IU
Iron	0.9 mg
Magnesium	32 mg
Zinc	0.6 mg
Selenium	3.2 mcg

- **Food processor**

4 cups	broccoli florets	1 L
1	clove garlic, minced	1
½ cup	snipped fresh cilantro	125 mL
¼ cup	snipped fresh basil	60 mL
¼ cup	freshly grated Parmesan cheese	60 mL
¼ cup	extra virgin olive oil	60 mL
¼ cup	ready-to-use GF chicken broth	60 mL
¼ tsp	salt	1 mL
	Cooked GF pasta	

1. In a glass bowl, microwave broccoli florets, covered, on High (100%) for 3 to 5 minutes or until tender-crisp, or steam in a vegetable steamer until tender-crisp.

2. In food processor, combine broccoli, garlic, cilantro, basil, Parmesan, olive oil, broth and salt. Process until coarsely chopped.

3. Toss pesto with hot cooked GF pasta.

Health-Enhancing Tips

If you're not following a vegetarian diet, increase the protein content of this recipe by topping with cooked chicken, shrimp, steak or lamb.

To add both protein and fiber, substitute 4 cups (1 L) cooked quinoa for the GF pasta.

To increase the alkalinity of this recipe, add more raw or steamed vegetables and toss them with the pesto and pasta.

Braised Brussels Sprouts

Brussels sprouts, with their delicate, nutty flavor, take on a pleasant sweetness in this easy-to-prepare recipe that can be doubled to serve a crowd.

Makes 4 servings

TIPS

The sprouts can be blanched up to 1 day ahead. Chill in ice water, then drain well and wrap in a clean, dry kitchen towel to absorb moisture. Refrigerate in an airtight container.

Like other vegetables in the cabbage family, the key is not to overcook Brussels sprouts. Serve them when they are tender-crisp and bright green.

1 lb	Brussels sprouts, trimmed and halved	500 g
2 tbsp	ready-to-use GF chicken broth	30 mL
1 tsp	granulated sugar	5 mL
4 tsp	red wine vinegar	20 mL
2 tsp	extra virgin olive oil	10 mL
1	clove garlic, minced	1
	Freshly ground black pepper	

1. In a saucepan of boiling water, blanch Brussels sprouts for 2 minutes or until bright green and crisp. Drain well.

2. In a bowl, stir together broth, sugar and vinegar. Set aside.

3. In a large nonstick skillet, heat oil over medium-high heat. Stir-fry garlic for 20 seconds or until fragrant. Add Brussels sprouts and stir-fry for 2 minutes or until lightly browned.

4. Stir in broth mixture, reduce heat to medium and cook, stirring often, for 1 to 2 minutes or until sprouts are barely tender and are still bright green. Season to taste with pepper. Serve immediately.

Health-Enhancing Tips

To reduce the carbohydrate content of this recipe, omit the sugar.

In step 2, stir-fry the vegetables over medium heat, adjusting the cooking time as necessary.

Nutrients per serving

Calories	76
Fat	3 g
Carbohydrate	12 g
Fiber	4 g
Protein	4 g
Vitamin A	855 IU
Iron	1.7 mg
Magnesium	27 mg
Zinc	0.5 mg
Selenium	1.9 mcg

Herb-Glazed Brussels Sprouts

These nutrient-packed vegetables are delicious smothered in this mouth-watering herbal sauce.

Makes 6 servings

TIP

Basil has strong antioxidant properties and provides important phytochemicals that help lower inflammation and protect cells from damage.

¼ cup	coarsely chopped fresh mint	60 mL
¼ cup	coarsely chopped fresh basil	60 mL
¼ cup	olive oil	60 mL
2 tbsp	freshly squeezed lemon juice	30 mL
1 tbsp	Dijon mustard	15 mL
¼ tsp	salt	1 mL
¼ tsp	freshly ground black pepper	1 mL
2 lbs	small Brussels sprouts, stems and outer leaves trimmed (if necessary) and a slit cut in stem end of each	1 kg
	Fresh mint or basil leaves and/or grated lemon zest	

1. In a mini chopper or in a bowl and using a whisk, combine mint, basil, olive oil, lemon juice, mustard, salt and pepper; process or whisk until well combined.

2. In a saucepan of boiling salted water, cook Brussels sprouts for 3 to 5 minutes or until just tender but still a little crisp. (Check by cutting one in half.) Drain well; return to saucepan.

3. Spoon dressing over Brussels sprouts; stir gently to combine. Spoon into a warm serving dish; sprinkle with mint or basil leaves and/or lemon zest. Serve at once.

Nutrients per serving

Calories	150
Fat	10 g
Carbohydrate	15 g
Fiber	6 g
Protein	5 g
Vitamin A	1279 IU
Iron	2.3 mg
Magnesium	37 mg
Zinc	0.7 mg
Selenium	2.4 mcg

Thyme-Scented Carrots

These carrots are simple enough to prepare for everyday meals, yet they are sure to impress dinner guests, too.

Makes 4 servings

TIPS

Leave packaged carrots in their bags and refrigerate them in the vegetable crisper. To avoid bitter carrots, keep them in a separate compartment from apples.

The secret to even cooking is to cut the carrots into pieces of the same size.

3½ cups	thinly sliced carrots (sliced on the diagonal)	875 mL
¼ cup	finely chopped onion	60 mL
1 tbsp	butter or margarine	15 mL
½ tsp	dried thyme	2 mL
¼ tsp	salt	1 mL
	Freshly ground black pepper	

1. In a large nonstick skillet, combine carrots, onion, butter, thyme, salt, pepper to taste and ½ cup (125 mL) water. Bring to a boil over medium-high heat. Reduce heat and boil gently, stirring occasionally, for 7 to 9 minutes or until carrots are tender-crisp and water has evaporated.

Variation

Substitute 3 sprigs of fresh thyme for the dried thyme and finely chopped shallots for the onion. Discard thyme sprigs before serving. Garnish each serving with a fresh thyme sprig, if desired.

Health-Enhancing Tip

For a healthier, less inflammatory fat, use organic butter or ghee (see tip, page 312).

Nutrients per serving

Calories	76
Fat	3 g
Carbohydrate	12 g
Fiber	3 g
Protein	1 g
Vitamin A	18,804 IU
Iron	0.5 mg
Magnesium	15 mg
Zinc	0.3 mg
Selenium	0.2 mcg

Lemon Almond Sautéed Greens

Perk up your meal and boost your vitamin C and fiber with this quick, tasty, lemon-scented side dish. It's sure to become a favorite!

Makes 4 servings

TIPS

Wash greens well in a colander under cold running water. Drain, leaving the water clinging to the leaves. There's no need to spin or pat them dry.

One medium bunch of Swiss chard or an 8-oz (250 g) package of fresh spinach is just the right amount for this recipe. Avoid baby spinach, as it's too tender and cooks too quickly — save it for salads.

Toast almonds in a small dry skillet over medium heat, stirring constantly, for about 3 minutes or until golden and fragrant.

1 tbsp	vegetable oil	15 mL
1	clove garlic, minced	1
6 cups	lightly packed chopped Swiss chard (or 8 cups/2 L trimmed spinach)	1.5 L
1 cup	shredded cabbage	250 mL
1 tsp	grated lemon zest	5 mL
¼ tsp	salt	1 mL
¼ tsp	freshly ground black pepper	1 mL
1½ tsp	freshly squeezed lemon juice	7 mL
2 tbsp	sliced almonds, toasted (see tip, at left)	30 mL

1. In a large, deep skillet or wok, heat oil over medium-high heat. Sauté garlic for 30 seconds or until fragrant. Add Swiss chard, cabbage, lemon zest, salt and pepper; sauté for about 2 minutes or until chard is slightly wilted.

2. Stir in 1 tbsp (15 mL) water, cover and boil, stirring occasionally, for about 2 minutes or until vegetables are just tender.

3. Stir in lemon juice and sauté, uncovered, for 1 to 2 minutes or until vegetables are tender and most of the water has evaporated. Serve sprinkled with almonds.

Health-Enhancing Tip

For a healthier, less inflammatory fat, use melted virgin coconut oil or ghee (see tip, page 312) in place of the vegetable oil.

Nutrients per serving

Calories	64
Fat	5 g
Carbohydrate	4 g
Fiber	2 g
Protein	2 g
Vitamin A	3321 IU
Iron	1.2 mg
Magnesium	54 mg
Zinc	0.3 mg
Selenium	0.7 mcg

New Orleans Braised Onions

Here's a delicious way to obtain all the nutritional gifts onions have to offer: they reduce inflammation, help with allergies and feed healthy bacteria in the gut. With a small investment in preparation time, you'll get fantastic returns in improved health.

Makes 10 servings

TIPS

This is a great dish to serve with roasted poultry or meat. If your guests like spice, pass hot pepper sauce at the table.

When purchasing condensed beef broth, check the label to make sure it is gluten-free.

- **Medium to large (3½- to 5-quart) slow cooker**

2 to 3	large Spanish onions	2 to 3
6 to 9	whole cloves	6 to 9
½ tsp	salt	2 mL
½ tsp	cracked black peppercorns	2 mL
Pinch	ground thyme	Pinch
	Grated zest and juice of 1 orange	
½ cup	condensed beef broth, undiluted	125 mL
	Finely chopped fresh parsley (optional)	
	Hot pepper sauce (optional)	

1. Stud onions with cloves. Place in slow cooker stoneware and sprinkle with salt, peppercorns, thyme and orange zest. Pour orange juice and beef broth over onions, cover and cook on Low for 8 hours or on High for 4 hours, until onions are tender.

2. Keep onions warm. In a saucepan over medium heat, reduce cooking liquid by half.

3. When ready to serve, cut onions into quarters. Place on a deep platter and cover with sauce. Sprinkle with parsley, if desired, and pass the hot pepper sauce, if desired.

Nutrients per serving

Calories	13
Fat	0 g
Carbohydrate	3 g
Fiber	1 g
Protein	0 g
Vitamin A	26 IU
Iron	0.1 mg
Magnesium	3 mg
Zinc	0.1 mg
Selenium	0.2 mcg

Lentil-Stuffed Tomatoes

Prepare these tomatoes to serve as a side dish with oven-cooked meals. They can be stuffed up to 4 hours in advance, refrigerated, then heated (allow a longer heating time in this case).

Makes 4 servings

TIP

The amount of salt in canned legumes varies from brand to brand, so be sure to check the sodium value in the Nutrition Facts table. Draining and rinsing them before use removes about 50% of the sodium.

- **Preheat oven to 400°F (200°C)**
- **6- or 12-cup muffin pan**

4	firm tomatoes	4
¼ cup	finely chopped celery	60 mL
1 tbsp	finely chopped onion	15 mL
1 tbsp	finely chopped green bell pepper	15 mL
½ tsp	curry powder	2 mL
1 cup	rinsed drained canned brown lentils	250 mL
1 tbsp	freshly grated Parmesan cheese	15 mL

1. Core tomatoes and cut a thin slice from the top of each. Scoop pulp and juice into a skillet and mash pulp. Place tomato shells cut side down on a paper towel to drain.

2. Add celery, onion, green pepper and curry powder to tomato pulp and juice. Cook, stirring, over medium heat for about 5 minutes or until vegetables are tender. Add lentils and cook, stirring, until mixture is thickened.

3. Spoon lentil mixture into tomato shells. Sprinkle with Parmesan. Place stuffed tomatoes in 4 muffin cups. Set muffin pan on a baking sheet.

4. Bake in preheated oven for 10 minutes or until heated through.

Nutrients per serving

Calories	80
Fat	1 g
Carbohydrate	14 g
Fiber	6 g
Protein	6 g
Vitamin A	1054 IU
Iron	0.4 mg
Magnesium	15 mg
Zinc	0.3 mg
Selenium	0.3 mcg

Cherry Tomato and Zucchini Sauté

This colorful vegetable medley is a great summer side dish when markets are overflowing with squash and sweet tomatoes.

Makes 4 servings

TIP

To toast pine nuts, place nuts in a dry skillet over medium heat and cook, stirring, for 3 to 4 minutes or until fragrant and toasted. Watch carefully, as pine nuts burn easily.

2 tsp	extra virgin olive oil	10 mL
3	small zucchini, halved lengthwise and thinly sliced	3
2	green onions, sliced	2
2 cups	cherry tomatoes, halved	500 mL
½ tsp	ground cumin (optional)	2 mL
2 tsp	balsamic vinegar	10 mL
	Freshly ground black pepper	
2 tbsp	chopped fresh mint or basil	30 mL
2 tbsp	lightly toasted pine nuts (see tip, at left)	30 mL

1. In a large nonstick skillet, heat oil over medium-high heat. Add zucchini and cook, stirring, for 1 minute.

2. Add green onions, tomatoes, cumin (if using) and vinegar; cook, stirring, for 1 to 2 minutes or until zucchini is tender-crisp and tomatoes are heated through. Season to taste with pepper. Sprinkle with mint and pine nuts. Serve immediately.

Nutrients per serving

Calories	80
Fat	6 g
Carbohydrate	7 g
Fiber	2 g
Protein	2 g
Vitamin A	858 IU
Iron	0.9 mg
Magnesium	36 mg
Zinc	0.7 mg
Selenium	0.2 mcg

Mix 'n' Mash Vegetables

Say goodbye to boring mashed potatoes. This dish combines tasty winter vegetables to create a truly healing, delicious side dish.

Makes 4 servings

TIP

For a very smooth texture, purée the turnip mixture in a food processor or with an immersion blender. For a coarser texture, a regular potato masher will do.

1½ cups	chopped turnip or rutabaga	375 mL
1½ cups	chopped carrot	375 mL
1 cup	chopped peeled sweet potato	250 mL
2 tsp	margarine or butter	10 mL
¼ tsp	salt	1 mL
	Freshly ground black pepper	

1. In a pot of boiling water, cook turnip, carrot and sweet potato for about 20 minutes or until tender. Drain well and transfer to a bowl.

2. Mash or whip turnip mixture until smooth. Stir in margarine and salt. Season to taste with pepper.

Health-Enhancing Tip

For a healthier, less inflammatory fat, use organic butter or ghee (see tip, page 312) in place of the margarine.

Nutrients per serving

Calories	72
Fat	2 g
Carbohydrate	13 g
Fiber	3 g
Protein	1 g
Vitamin A	15,209 IU
Iron	0.6 mg
Magnesium	21 mg
Zinc	0.3 mg
Selenium	0.5 mcg

Steamed Vegetables with Toasted Almonds

Put your steamer basket to good use when preparing vegetables, and use this recipe as a guideline.

Makes 4 servings

TIP

To toast sliced almonds, place in a small nonstick skillet over medium heat and cook, stirring often, for 4 to 5 minutes or until golden and fragrant. Transfer to a bowl and let cool.

- **Steamer basket**

2 cups	cauliflower florets	500 mL
2 cups	broccoli florets	500 mL
½	red bell pepper, chopped	½
½	yellow or orange bell pepper, chopped	½
2 tsp	butter	10 mL
1	clove garlic, minced	1
2 tsp	freshly squeezed lemon juice	10 mL
3 tbsp	toasted sliced almonds	45 mL
1 tbsp	chopped fresh parsley	15 mL

1. Pour enough water into a large saucepan to come 1 inch (2.5 cm) up the side. Place steamer basket in pan, cover and bring to a boil over medium-high heat. Add cauliflower, broccoli, red pepper and yellow pepper; cover and steam for 5 to 7 minutes or until tender-crisp. Drain and transfer to a serving bowl.

2. Meanwhile, in a small saucepan, melt butter over medium heat, swirling pan occasionally, until butter turns a rich golden color (do not overcook or butter will burn.) Add garlic and cook, stirring, for 20 seconds or until fragrant. Stir in lemon juice.

3. Drizzle butter mixture over vegetables and sprinkle with almonds and parsley. Serve immediately.

Nutrients per serving

Calories	78
Fat	4 g
Carbohydrate	8 g
Fiber	3 g
Protein	4 g
Vitamin A	1717 IU
Iron	0.9 mg
Magnesium	34 mg
Zinc	0.5 mg
Selenium	1.7 mcg

TIP

The recipe can be easily doubled when you're serving a crowd, or save extras to throw into salads or other dishes.

Variation

Replace the cauliflower and broccoli with other vegetables you may have on hand, such as baby carrots, green beans, snap peas and zucchini. Estimate 1 cup (250 mL) raw vegetables per serving. Steam longer-cooking and denser vegetables, such as baby carrots, for 5 to 7 minutes or until almost fork-tender, then add the bell peppers and any shorter-cooking vegetables, such as snap peas, and steam for 3 to 5 minutes or until tender-crisp.

Health-Enhancing Tips

You can add more vegetables to this recipe if desired.

For a healthier fat, use organic butter or ghee (see tip, page 312).

Roasted Butternut Squash with Onion and Sage

Roasting brings out the best in winter squash. Roasted vegetables are also a great source of fiber and healing nutrients. Cook just until al dente to take advantage of resistant starches that feed the healthy bacteria in your gut.

Makes 4 servings

TIPS

Vegetable oil cooking sprays are sold in aerosol cans and pump sprays at supermarkets. You can also buy a spray pump mister and fill it with oil. Canola oil is a good all-purpose oil for both baking and roasting.

Most supermarkets now offer convenient packages of peeled, cubed ready-to-cook butternut squash in the produce department, making this dish a breeze to whip together.

- **Preheat oven to 375°F (190°C)**
- **11- by 7-inch (28 by 18 cm) glass baking dish, sprayed with vegetable oil cooking spray**

4 cups	cubed butternut squash (about 1 lb/500 g, cut into ¾-inch/2 cm cubes)	1 L
1	small onion, cut into thin wedges	1
1 tbsp	finely chopped fresh sage	15 mL
⅛ tsp	salt	0.5 mL
	Freshly ground black pepper	
2 tsp	extra virgin olive oil	10 mL

1. In baking dish, combine squash, onion, sage, salt, and pepper to taste. Drizzle with oil and toss to coat. Spread out in an even layer.

2. Roast in preheated oven for 30 to 35 minutes, stirring occasionally, until squash is just tender when pierced with a fork.

Variation

Roasted Butternut Squash with Sweet Spices: Replace the sage with ¼ tsp (1 mL) each ground cinnamon and ground cumin.

Nutrients per serving

Calories	91
Fat	2 g
Carbohydrate	18 g
Fiber	3 g
Protein	2 g
Vitamin A	14,893 IU
Iron	1.0 mg
Magnesium	50 mg
Zinc	0.3 mg
Selenium	0.8 mcg

Baked Sweet Potato Fries

Baked fries are a terrific alternative to the deep-fried variety, and when the[y]
sweet potatoes, you get added vitamins and fiber — and they taste great,

TIP

Sweet potatoes are sometimes incorrectly labeled "yams." True yams are larger than sweet potatoes and have fewer nutrients. Be sure to pick up sweet potatoes with orange-colored flesh. Store at room temperature for up to 1 week.

- Preheat oven to 400°F (200°C)
- Large baking sheet, lined with parchment paper

1	large sweet potato (about 1 lb/500 g)	1
1 tbsp	olive oil	15 mL
¼ tsp	salt	1 mL
	Freshly ground black pepper	

1. Peel sweet potato and rinse. Cut in half crosswise, then cut lengthwise into sticks about ½ inch (1 cm) square. Place on prepared baking sheet. Drizzle with oil and sprinkle with salt and pepper. Spread out in a single layer, leaving space between each fry.

2. Bake for about 30 minutes, flipping sweet potatoes halfway through, until browned and tender.

Variations

For a different flavor, try using melted virgin coconut oil in place of the olive oil.

You can also make this recipe with yams, parsnips, rutabagas or regular potatoes.

Nutrients per serving

Calories	127
Fat	3 g
Carbohydrate	23 g
Fiber	3 g
Protein	2 g
Vitamin A	16,088 IU
Iron	0.7 mg
Magnesium	28 mg
Zinc	0.3 mg
Selenium	0.7 mcg

Creamy Mashed Potatoes with Cauliflower

If you're craving a mound of creamy mashed potatoes, you won't feel deprived when you indulge in this delicious side dish that delivers all of the same great taste and appeal, but with the added bonus of cauliflower, a powerful cancer-fighting vegetable. This version is also lower in carbohydrate, to help you maintain your blood sugar levels.

Makes 4 servings

TIP

Do not use a food processor to mash the potatoes and cauliflower together, or you'll end up with a gooey mixture.

- **Steamer basket**
- **Food processor**

5 cups	cauliflower florets (about 1 lb/500 g)	1.25 L
4	small russet potatoes, peeled and quartered (about 1 lb/500 g)	4
1 tbsp	butter or soft margarine	15 mL
¼ cup	warm milk (approx.)	60 mL
¼ tsp	salt	1 mL
¼ tsp	freshly grated nutmeg	1 mL

1. Pour enough water into a large saucepan to come 1 inch (2.5 cm) up the side. Place steamer basket in pan, cover and bring to a boil over medium-high heat. Add cauliflower; cover and steam for 10 to 12 minutes or until very tender. Drain well.

2. Transfer cauliflower to food processor and purée. Set aside.

3. Add another 1 inch (2.5 cm) of water to the saucepan. Place steamer basket in pan, cover and bring to a boil over medium-high heat. Add potatoes; cover and steam for 20 to 25 minutes or until fork-tender. Drain well and return to saucepan. Place over low heat and dry for 1 minute.

4. Using a potato masher or an electric hand mixer on low speed, mash potatoes until very smooth. Mash in cauliflower purée, butter and enough of the milk to make a smooth mixture. Season with salt and nutmeg.

5. Return pan to medium-low heat and reheat mash, stirring often, until piping hot.

Nutrients per serving

Calories	156
Fat	4 g
Carbohydrate	28 g
Fiber	3 g
Protein	6 g
Vitamin A	121 IU
Iron	1.5 mg
Magnesium	47 mg
Zinc	0.7 mg
Selenium	1.3 mcg

Health-Enhancing Tip

For a healthier fat, use ghee (see tip, page 312) in place of the butter or margarine.

Savory Vegetarian Quinoa Pilaf

This delicious vegetarian dish is dotted with multicolored chunks of nutritious vegetables.

Makes 6 servings

TIPS

Quinoa is cooked when grains turn from white to transparent and the tiny spiral-like germ is separated.

For a richer, robust pilaf, substitute GF beef or chicken broth for the vegetable broth.

2 tsp	extra virgin olive oil	10 mL
1	stalk celery, diced	1
1	carrot, coarsely chopped	1
½	small onion, coarsely chopped	½
1½ cups	ready-to-use GF vegetable broth	375 mL
½ cup	quinoa	125 mL
1 tsp	dried basil	5 mL
	Salt and freshly ground black pepper	
1	red bell pepper, cut into ½-inch (1 cm) cubes	1
1	orange bell pepper, cut into ½-inch (1 cm) cubes	1
2	green onions, green tops only, chopped	2

1. In a large saucepan, heat olive oil over medium-low heat. Add celery, carrot and onion and cook, stirring frequently, for 8 to 10 minutes or until tender. Add broth, quinoa and basil and bring to a boil.

2. Reduce heat to low. Cover and simmer for 18 to 20 minutes or until water is absorbed and quinoa is tender. Season to taste with salt and pepper. Stir in red pepper, orange pepper and green onion. Let stand, covered, for 2 to 3 minutes.

Variation

Add small broccoli florets with the bell peppers. They add a tender-crisp texture.

Nutrients per serving

Calories	93
Fat	3 g
Carbohydrate	15 g
Fiber	3 g
Protein	3 g
Vitamin A	2443 IU
Iron	1.2 mg
Magnesium	37 mg
Zinc	0.6 mg
Selenium	1.4 mcg

Red Beans and Greens

Few meals could be more healthful than this delicious combination of hot leafy greens and flavorful beans. The smoked paprika makes the dish more robust, but it isn't essential. If you're cooking for a smaller group, make the full quantity of beans, spoon off what is needed, and serve with the appropriate quantity of cooked greens. Refrigerate or freeze the leftover beans for another meal.

Makes 10 servings

TIP

If you have time to make Basic Vegetable Stock (page 194), use it in place of the ready-to-use broth.

• **Medium to large (3½- to 6-quart) slow cooker**

2 cups	dried red kidney beans	500 mL
1 tbsp	olive oil	15 mL
2	large onions, finely chopped	2
2	stalks celery, finely chopped	2
4	cloves garlic, minced	4
1 tsp	dried oregano	5 mL
1 tsp	salt	5 mL
½ tsp	cracked black peppercorns	2 mL
½ tsp	dried thyme	2 mL
¼ tsp	ground allspice (or 6 whole allspice berries tied in a piece of cheesecloth)	1 mL
2	bay leaves	2
4 cups	ready-to-use GF vegetable broth	1 L
1 tsp	paprika, preferably smoked (optional)	5 mL

GREENS

2 lbs	dark leafy greens, such as collard greens or kale, thoroughly washed, stems removed and leaves chopped	1 kg
1 tbsp	olive oil	15 mL
1 tbsp	balsamic vinegar	15 mL
	Freshly ground black pepper	

1. Soak beans according to either method in Basic Beans (see page 255). Drain, rinse and set aside.

2. In a skillet, heat oil over medium heat for 30 seconds. Add onions and celery and cook, stirring, until softened, about 5 minutes. Add garlic, oregano, salt, peppercorns, thyme, allspice and bay leaves and cook, stirring, for 1 minute. Transfer to slow cooker stoneware. Add beans and broth.

3. Cover and cook on Low for 8 to 10 hours or on High for 4 to 5 hours, until beans are tender. Stir in smoked paprika (if using). Discard bay leaves (and allspice if using whole berries).

Nutrients per serving

Calories	144
Fat	2 g
Carbohydrate	25 g
Fiber	7 g
Protein	8 g
Vitamin A	244 IU
Iron	2.8 mg
Magnesium	44 mg
Zinc	1.0 mg
Selenium	1.4 mcg

MAKE AHEAD

This dish can be partially prepared before it is cooked. Complete steps 1 and 2. Cover and refrigerate for up to 2 days. When you're ready to cook, continue with the recipe.

4. *Greens:* In a large pot or steamer, steam greens until tender, about 10 minutes for collards. Toss with oil and balsamic vinegar. Season to taste with pepper. Add to beans and stir to combine. Serve immediately.

Health-Enhancing Tips

To increase the protein content of your meal, serve this dish with cooked tofu, chicken or fish.

To make this recipe more alkaline, substitute dried brown or green lentils for the beans. You will not need to soak the lentils. Cook on Low for 4 to 5 hours or on High for 2 to $2\frac{1}{2}$ hours, until lentils are tender.

Creamy Polenta

Polenta, the Italian version of cornmeal mush, is a magnificent way to add whole grains to your diet. When properly cooked, it is a soothing comfort food that functions like a bowl of steaming mashed potatoes, the yummy basis upon which more elaborate dishes can strut their stuff.

Makes 6 servings

TIPS

If you have trouble digesting cornmeal, try soaking it for at least 8 hours or overnight in warm non-chlorinated water (about 2 parts water to 1 part grain) with a spoonful or so of cider vinegar (preferably with the mother). Drain and rinse before cooking. Your polenta will be particularly creamy.

Grits are very sticky. Greasing the saucepan or using one with a nonstick finish helps with cleanup.

2½ cups	milk or cream	625 mL
2 cups	water or ready-to-use GF vegetable or chicken broth	500 mL
¼ tsp	salt	1 mL
1 cup	coarse stone-ground cornmeal or coarse stone-ground grits	250 mL
2 tbsp	freshly grated Parmesan cheese (optional)	30 mL

1. In a saucepan over medium heat, bring milk, water and salt to a boil. Gradually stir in cornmeal in a steady stream. If desired, stir in cheese. Cook, stirring constantly, until smooth and blended and mixture bubbles like lava, about 5 minutes.

2. Reduce heat to low (see tip, page 175). Continue cooking, stirring frequently, while the mixture bubbles and thickens, until the grains are tender and creamy, about 30 minutes for cornmeal and about 1 hour for grits. Serve immediately.

Variation

Oven Method: Use an ovenproof saucepan for step 1 or transfer mixture to a lightly greased baking dish after step 1. Instead of step 2, bake in a preheated 350°F (180°C) oven, covered, until cornmeal is tender and creamy, about 40 minutes for cornmeal or 1 hour for grits.

Nutrients per serving

Calories	140
Fat	1 g
Carbohydrate	26 g
Fiber	1 g
Protein	5 g
Vitamin A	255 IU
Iron	1.2 mg
Magnesium	20 mg
Zinc	0.6 mg
Selenium	6.1 mcg

Snacks and Desserts

Crispy-Coated Veggie Snacks 348

Steamed Sugar Snap Peas with Ginger 349

Oven-Baked Kale Chips 350

Spicy Cashews 351

Salty Almonds with Thyme 352

Spicy Tamari Almonds 353

Crunchy Peanut Butter Muffins 354

Lemon Blueberry Almond Muffins 356

Pumpkin Millet Muffins 358

Almond Sponge Cake 359

Pumpkin Date Bars 360

Homemade Crunchy Granola Bars 361

Peanut Butter Cookies 362

Cinnamon Crisps 363

Crispy-Coated Veggie Snacks

These healthier crispy baked tidbits are an appealing alternative to deep-fried fare. You could also use other vegetables, such as cauliflower, broccoli or white turnip. Serve with Broccoli Cilantro Pesto (page 329) for dipping.

Makes 36 pieces

TIP

Use any leftover savory bread to make the bread crumbs. For best results, the bread should be at least 1 day old. Using a food processor or blender, pulse until crumbs are of the desired consistency. For dry bread crumbs, spread the crumbs in a single layer on a baking sheet and bake at 350°F (180°C) for 6 to 8 minutes, shaking the pan frequently, until lightly browned, crisp and dry.

- **Preheat oven to 375°F (190°C)**
- **Baking sheet, lightly greased**

1	small zucchini	1
1	small sweet potato	1
12	small mushrooms	12
3 cups	dry GF bread crumbs (see tip, at left)	750 mL
1 cup	freshly grated Parmesan cheese	250 mL
1 tbsp	dried rosemary or thyme	15 mL
Pinch	cayenne pepper	Pinch
2 cups	plain yogurt	500 mL

1. Peel zucchini, cut in half crosswise and cut each half lengthwise into quarters.

2. Peel sweet potato, cut in half lengthwise and cut into slices $\frac{1}{4}$ inch (0.5 cm) thick.

3. Remove stems from mushrooms.

4. In a shallow dish or pie plate, combine bread crumbs, Parmesan cheese, rosemary and cayenne.

5. Working with a few pieces at a time, dip zucchini, sweet potato and mushroom caps into yogurt to generously coat. Then dip into crumb mixture, pressing to coat well.

6. Arrange on prepared baking sheet in a single layer. Bake in preheated oven for 20 to 25 minutes or until vegetables are tender and coating is golden.

7. Transfer to a serving plate and serve immediately.

Nutrients per 3 pieces (1 zucchini, 1 sweet potato and 1 mushroom)

Calories	158
Fat	6 g
Carbohydrate	21 g
Fiber	1 g
Protein	6 g
Vitamin A	1643 IU
Iron	0.5 mg
Magnesium	15 mg
Zinc	0.7 mg
Selenium	3.5 mcg

Steamed Sugar Snap Peas with Ginger

Here's a quick stir-fry with ginger and shallots that nicely complements the sweetness of emerald green sugar snap peas.

Makes 2 servings

TIPS

Keep fresh ginger on hand in your refrigerator and mince or grate it to use in a variety of dishes. Thanks to its vibrant taste, you'll find you can do away with salt in many dishes.

Snow peas can be prepared the same way. As they cook so quickly, reduce the steaming time to 1 minute or until bright green and crisp.

2 tsp	peanut or canola oil	10 mL
¼ cup	minced shallots	60 mL
2 tsp	minced gingerroot	10 mL
1 lb	sugar snap peas, strings removed	500 g
2 tbsp	water	30 mL

1. In a wok or large nonstick skillet, heat oil over medium-high heat. Stir-fry shallots and ginger for 1 minute.

2. Add peas and water; cover and steam for 3 minutes or until peas are just tender-crisp. Serve immediately.

Health-Enhancing Tips

For a healthier, less inflammatory fat, use sesame oil, ghee (see tip, page 312) or melted virgin coconut oil in place of the peanut or canola oil.

Use medium heat instead of medium-high, adjusting the cooking time as necessary.

Nutrients per serving

Calories	151
Fat	5 g
Carbohydrate	21 g
Fiber	6 g
Protein	7 g
Vitamin A	2703 IU
Iron	4.9 mg
Magnesium	60 mg
Zinc	0.7 mg
Selenium	1.8 mcg

Oven-Baked Kale Chips

In the past few years, kale chips have become very popular, with good reason. They are tasty and nutritious, perfect as a gluten-free dipper or on their own as a satisfying snack. And, if you make your own, you can be sure they don't contain any nasty additives. Increase the quantity to suit your needs.

Makes about 5 chips per stem

TIPS

When trimming the kale, remove the tough stem right to the end of the leaf (it has an unpleasantly chewy texture) and discard. Then cut the pieces crosswise into "chips."

The long, relatively solid leaves of lacinato kale (also known as black or dinosaur kale) allow for the creation of a "chip" that has enough heft to support a spread or to be used as a dipper. However, other types of kale also make delicious chips.

- **Preheat oven to 350°F (180°C)**

PER STEM OF KALE

1	leaf lacinato kale, trimmed and chopped (see tip, at left)	1
1 tsp	extra virgin olive oil	5 mL
	Fine sea salt	
	Sweet or hot paprika, regular or smoked (optional)	

1. In a salad spinner, thoroughly dry kale. Place olive oil in a bowl and add kale, in batches, as necessary. Using your hand, toss kale until evenly coated with oil.

2. Place on a baking sheet in a single layer. Bake in preheated oven until leaves crisp up, about 10 minutes. Remove from oven and sprinkle lightly with sea salt and paprika (if using).

Nutrients per 20 chips

Calories	49
Fat	4 g
Carbohydrate	3 g
Fiber	1 g
Protein	1 g
Vitamin A	4920 IU
Iron	0.6 mg
Magnesium	11 mg
Zinc	0.1 mg
Selenium	0.3 mcg

Spicy Cashews

Only slightly nippy with just a hint of cinnamon, these cashews are a tasty and nutritious treat any time of the year.

Makes about 2 cups (500 mL)

TIPS

Check your chili powder to make sure it doesn't contain gluten.

Sea salt is available in most supermarkets. It is much sweeter than table salt and is essential for this recipe — and not only because it is much better for you. Table salt would impart an unpleasant acrid taste to the nuts.

For a holiday gift, make up a batch or two and package in pretty jars. If well sealed, the nuts will keep for 10 days.

- **Small (maximum 3$\frac{1}{2}$-quart) slow cooker**

2 cups	raw cashews	500 mL
1 tsp	chili powder (see tip, at left)	5 mL
$\frac{1}{2}$ tsp	cayenne pepper	2 mL
$\frac{1}{4}$ tsp	ground cinnamon	1 mL
2 tsp	fine sea salt (see tip, at left)	10 mL
1 tbsp	extra virgin olive oil	15 mL

1. In slow cooker stoneware, combine cashews, chili powder, cayenne and cinnamon. Stir to combine thoroughly. Cover and cook on High for 1$\frac{1}{2}$ hours, stirring every 30 minutes, until nuts are nicely toasted.

2. In a small bowl, combine sea salt and olive oil. Add to nuts in slow cooker and stir to thoroughly combine. Transfer mixture to a serving bowl and serve hot or let cool.

Nutrients per 12 cashews

Calories	100
Fat	8 g
Carbohydrate	5 g
Fiber	1 g
Protein	3 g
Vitamin A	69 IU
Iron	1.0 mg
Magnesium	42 mg
Zinc	0.9 mg
Selenium	1.9 mcg

Salty Almonds with Thyme

You will want to eat these tasty almonds all the thyme. Enjoy this nutritious treat as a snack, sprinkled on salads or mixed into your favorite dish.

**Makes about
2 cups (500 mL)**

TIP

Sea salt is available in most supermarkets. It is much sweeter than table salt and is essential for this recipe — and not only because it is much better for you. Table salt would impart an unpleasant acrid taste to the nuts.

- **Small (maximum 3½-quart) slow cooker**

2 cups	unblanched almonds	500 mL
½ tsp	freshly ground white pepper	2 mL
1 tbsp	fine sea salt (or to taste)	15 mL
2 tbsp	extra virgin olive oil	30 mL
2 tbsp	fresh thyme leaves	30 mL

1. In slow cooker stoneware, combine almonds and pepper. Cover and cook on High for 1½ hours, stirring every 30 minutes, until nuts are nicely toasted.

2. In a bowl, combine salt, olive oil and thyme. Add to hot almonds in stoneware and stir thoroughly to combine. Spoon mixture into a small serving bowl and serve hot or let cool.

**Nutrients per
12 almonds**

Calories	112
Fat	10 g
Carbohydrate	4 g
Fiber	2 g
Protein	4 g
Vitamin A	14 IU
Iron	0.7 mg
Magnesium	46 mg
Zinc	0.5 mg
Selenium	0.4 mcg

Spicy Tamari Almonds

These tasty tidbits make great snacks or a perfect salad topper. Tamari is a wheat-free soy sauce, so they are naturally gluten-free.

Makes about 2 cups (500 mL)

TIP

For a holiday gift, make up a batch or two and package in pretty jars. If well sealed, the nuts will keep for 10 days.

- **Small (2- to 3½-quart) slow cooker**

2 cups	whole almonds	500 mL
¼ tsp	cayenne pepper	1 mL
2 tbsp	reduced-sodium tamari or liquid coconut amino acids	30 mL
1 tbsp	extra virgin olive oil	15 mL
	Fine sea salt	

1. In slow cooker stoneware, combine almonds and cayenne. Place a clean tea towel folded in half (so you will have two layers) over top of stoneware to absorb moisture. Cover and cook on High for 45 minutes.

2. In a small bowl, combine tamari and olive oil. Add to hot almonds and stir thoroughly to combine. Replace tea towel. Cover and cook on High for 1½ hours, until nuts are hot and fragrant, stirring every 30 minutes and replacing towel each time. Season to taste with salt. Store in an airtight container.

Nutrients per 12 almonds

Calories	112
Fat	10 g
Carbohydrate	4 g
Fiber	2 g
Protein	4 g
Vitamin A	11 IU
Iron	0.7 mg
Magnesium	45 mg
Zinc	0.5 mg
Selenium	0.4 mcg

Crunchy Peanut Butter Muffins

These gluten-free muffins are great for a quick breakfast or an afternoon snack. Peanuts not only add potent antioxidants, but also increase the protein content.

Makes 12 muffins

TIPS

Don't substitute dry-roasted peanuts — they may contain gluten.

To toast the peanuts, spread them in a single layer on a baking sheet and bake at 350°F (180°C) for 6 to 8 minutes, shaking the pan frequently, until fragrant and lightly browned.

- **12-cup muffin pan, lightly greased**

¾ cup	low-fat soy flour	175 mL
⅓ cup	whole bean flour	75 mL
¼ cup	tapioca starch	60 mL
1½ tsp	xanthan gum	7 mL
1 tbsp	GF baking powder	15 mL
½ tsp	salt	2 mL
1	large egg	1
½ cup	crunchy peanut butter, at room temperature	125 mL
⅓ cup	packed brown sugar	75 mL
1 tbsp	vegetable oil	15 mL
1¼ cups	water	300 mL
1 tsp	cider vinegar	5 mL
¾ cup	toasted coarsely chopped peanuts (see tips, at left)	175 mL

1. In a large bowl or plastic bag, combine soy flour, whole bean flour, tapioca starch, xanthan gum, baking powder and salt. Mix well and set aside.

2. In a separate bowl, using an electric mixer, beat egg, peanut butter, brown sugar and oil until combined. Add water and vinegar; mix until just combined. Add dry ingredients and peanuts; mix until just combined.

3. Spoon batter evenly into prepared muffin cups. Let stand for 30 minutes. Meanwhile, preheat oven to 350°F (180°C).

4. Bake for 18 to 20 minutes or until firm to the touch. Remove from pan immediately and let cool completely on a rack.

Nutrients per muffin

Calories	195
Fat	11 g
Carbohydrate	18 g
Fiber	4 g
Protein	9 g
Vitamin A	25 IU
Iron	1.4 mg
Magnesium	53 mg
Zinc	1.1 mg
Selenium	3.0 mcg

VARIATION

Substitute pea flour for the whole bean flour.

Health-Enhancing Tips

For a healthier, less inflammatory fat, substitute melted virgin coconut oil for the vegetable oil.

Use a peanut butter that lists peanuts as its only ingredient. Avoid peanut butters with added sugars and trans fats (listed as "partially hydrogenated oil" or "hydrogenated oil"). You may need to add a bit more melted virgin coconut oil in step 2 to reach the desired consistency.

Lemon Blueberry Almond Muffins

As the name promises, these muffins deliver an extra-refreshing burst of lemon in every bite. In addition, they provide the added nutritional benefits of blueberries.

Makes 12 muffins

TIPS

Keep a lemon in the freezer. Zest while frozen, then juice after warming in the microwave.

To toast slivered almonds, place in a small nonstick skillet over medium heat and cook, stirring often, for 4 to 5 minutes or until golden and fragrant. Transfer to a bowl and let cool.

- **12-cup muffin pan, lightly greased**

¾ cup	amaranth flour	175 mL
¾ cup	sorghum flour	175 mL
½ cup	almond flour	125 mL
⅓ cup	tapioca starch	75 mL
1½ tsp	xanthan gum	7 mL
1 tbsp	GF baking powder	15 mL
½ tsp	baking soda	2 mL
½ tsp	salt	2 mL
¾ cup	toasted slivered almonds (see tip, at left)	175 mL
2	large eggs	2
½ cup	milk	125 mL
⅓ cup	liquid honey	75 mL
2 tbsp	grated lemon zest	30 mL
⅓ cup	freshly squeezed lemon juice	75 mL
2 tbsp	vegetable oil	30 mL
½ tsp	GF almond extract	2 mL
1 cup	fresh or partially thawed frozen blueberries	250 mL

1. In a large bowl or plastic bag, combine amaranth flour, sorghum flour, almond flour, tapioca starch, xanthan gum, baking powder, baking soda, salt and almonds. Mix well and set aside.

2. In a separate bowl, using an electric mixer, beat eggs, milk, honey, lemon zest, lemon juice, oil and almond extract until combined. Add dry ingredients and mix until just combined. Carefully fold in blueberries.

3. Spoon batter evenly into prepared muffin cups. Let stand for 30 minutes. Meanwhile, preheat oven to 350°F (180°C).

4. Bake for 18 to 20 minutes or until firm to the touch. Remove from pan immediately and let cool completely on a rack.

Nutrients per muffin

Calories	195
Fat	9 g
Carbohydrate	26 g
Fiber	3 g
Protein	5 g
Vitamin A	73 IU
Iron	1.2 mg
Magnesium	36 mg
Zinc	0.4 mg
Selenium	4.9 mcg

Gently fold in the blueberries, rather than vigorously stirring them in; otherwise, you'll end up with blue muffins.

Variation

Substitute cranberries for the blueberries and chopped walnuts or pecans for the almonds.

Health-Enhancing Tips

For a healthier fat, substitute melted virgin coconut oil for the vegetable oil.

For more fiber, healthy omega-3 fats and protein, add 2 tbsp (30 mL) ground flax seeds (flaxseed meal) to the flour mixture in step 1.

For more protein, fold in 1 cup (250 mL) chopped nuts with the blueberries. Alternatively, add 2 scoops of protein powder (organic rice, organic pea, hemp or whey from grass-fed cows not given antibiotics or hormones) to the flour mixture in step 1; add 2 tbsp (30 mL) more milk in step 2.

To make the muffins dairy-free, replace the milk with unsweetened plain rice, almond or hemp milk.

Pumpkin Millet Muffins

These colorful, crunchy muffins carry well for lunch or a snack in any season.

Makes 12 muffins

TIPS

If you substitute pumpkin pie spice for the cinnamon, cloves and nutmeg, watch for hidden gluten.

If you purchase unroasted pumpkin seeds, toast them in a single layer in a large skillet over medium heat, shaking the pan frequently, for 5 to 8 minutes or until aromatic and lightly browned. Alternatively, you can buy roasted pumpkin seeds, in which case there's no need to toast. Either way, make sure the seeds are unsalted.

• **12-cup muffin pan, lightly greased**

¾ cup	sorghum flour	175 mL
¾ cup	whole bean flour	175 mL
¼ cup	tapioca starch	60 mL
1½ tsp	xanthan gum	7 mL
2 tsp	GF baking powder	10 mL
1 tsp	baking soda	5 mL
½ tsp	salt	2 mL
½ tsp	ground cinnamon	2 mL
¼ tsp	ground cloves	1 mL
¼ tsp	ground nutmeg	1 mL
½ cup	millet seeds	125 mL
¾ cup	green pumpkin seeds (pepitas), toasted (see tip, at left)	175 mL
2	large eggs	2
1 cup	pumpkin purée (not pie filling)	250 mL
½ cup	milk	125 mL
½ cup	GF sour cream	125 mL
⅓ cup	liquid honey	75 mL
¼ cup	vegetable oil	60 mL

1. In a large bowl or plastic bag, combine sorghum flour, whole bean flour, tapioca starch, xanthan gum, baking powder, baking soda, salt, cinnamon, cloves, nutmeg, millet seeds and pumpkin seeds. Mix well and set aside.

2. In a separate bowl, using an electric mixer, beat eggs, pumpkin purée, milk, sour cream, honey and oil until combined. Add dry ingredients and mix until just combined.

3. Spoon batter evenly into prepared muffin cups. Let stand for 30 minutes. Meanwhile, preheat oven to 350°F (180°C).

4. Bake for 18 to 20 minutes or until firm to the touch. Remove from pan immediately and let cool completely on a rack.

Nutrients per muffin

Calories	245
Fat	11 g
Carbohydrate	31 g
Fiber	4 g
Protein	8 g
Vitamin A	1119 IU
Iron	2.0 mg
Magnesium	56 mg
Zinc	0.9 mg
Selenium	4.3 mcg

Health-Enhancing Tip

To increase the protein without adding fat, add 2 scoops of protein powder to the flour mixture. Add 2 tbsp (30 mL) more milk or water to the egg mixture.

Almond Sponge Cake

The perfect lower-carbohydrate cake — light, airy, and not too sweet! Enjoy it on its own, or serve it topped with fresh fruit.

Makes 16 servings

TIPS

This is the ideal time to use liquid egg whites purchased in cartons. Substitute 1¼ cups (300 mL) liquid egg whites for the 10 egg whites.

Make sure the mixer bowl, wire whisk attachment, rubber spatula and tube pan are completely free of grease.

To slice without squishing cake, use dental floss or a knife with a serrated edge, such as an electric knife.

Nutrients per serving

Calories	85
Fat	3 g
Carbohydrate	11 g
Fiber	1 g
Protein	4 g
Vitamin A	61 IU
Iron	0.3 mg
Magnesium	13 mg
Zinc	0.1 mg
Selenium	6.6 mcg

- **Preheat oven to 350°F (180°C)**
- **10-inch (25 cm) tube pan, ungreased, bottom lined with parchment paper**

½ cup	almond or amaranth flour	125 mL
⅓ cup	cornstarch	75 mL
1 tsp	xanthan gum	5 mL
10	large egg whites, at room temperature	10
1 tbsp	freshly squeezed lemon juice	15 mL
1½ tsp	cream of tartar	7 mL
1 tsp	GF almond extract	5 mL
¼ tsp	salt	1 mL
⅓ cup	granulated sugar	75 mL
4	large egg yolks, at room temperature	4
¼ cup	granulated sugar	60 mL

1. In a small bowl or plastic bag, combine almond flour, cornstarch and xanthan gum. Set aside.

2. In a large bowl, using an electric mixer with wire whisk attachment, beat egg whites until foamy. While beating, add lemon juice, cream of tartar, almond extract and salt. Continue to beat until egg whites form stiff peaks. Gradually add the ⅓ cup (75 mL) sugar. Continue to beat until mixture is very stiff and glossy but not dry.

3. In a small deep bowl, using an electric mixer, beat egg yolks and the ¼ cup (60 mL) sugar until thick and pale lemon in color, approximately 5 minutes. Fold egg yolks into beaten egg white mixture. Sift in dry ingredients, one-third at a time. Gently fold in each addition until well blended. Spoon into prepared pan.

4. Bake in preheated oven for 25 to 30 minutes or until cake is golden and springs back when lightly touched. Invert pan over a funnel or bottle until completely cooled. Using a spatula, loosen the outside and inside edges of the pan and remove cake.

Pumpkin Date Bars

These quick and easy, moist bars are dotted with dates, nuts and a refreshing touch of orange. No need to frost — they're deliciously sweet just as they are.

Makes 24 bars

TIP

Store in an airtight container at room temperature for up to 5 days or freeze for up to 2 months.

- **9-inch (23 cm) square baking pan, lined with foil, lightly greased**

¾ cup	soy flour	175 mL
½ cup	packed brown sugar	125 mL
1½ tsp	xanthan gum	7 mL
2 tsp	GF baking powder	10 mL
½ tsp	salt	2 mL
2 tbsp	grated orange zest	30 mL
½ tsp	ground cinnamon	2 mL
½ tsp	ground nutmeg	2 mL
2	large eggs	2
½ cup	canned pumpkin purée (not pie filling)	125 mL
2 tbsp	vegetable oil	30 mL
¾ cup	chopped pitted dates	175 mL
½ cup	chopped walnuts	125 mL

1. In a large bowl or plastic bag, mix together soy flour, brown sugar, xanthan gum, baking powder, salt, orange zest, cinnamon and nutmeg. Set aside.

2. In another large bowl, using an electric mixer, beat eggs, pumpkin purée and oil until combined. Slowly beat in the dry ingredients and mix just until combined. Stir in dates and walnuts. Spoon into prepared pan. Using a moistened rubber spatula, spread to edges and smooth top. Let stand for 30 minutes. Meanwhile, preheat oven to 325°F (160°C).

3. Bake in preheated oven for 25 to 30 minutes or until a cake tester inserted in the center comes out clean. Let cool completely in the pan on a rack. Cut into small bars.

Variations

Substitute an equal amount of dried cranberries for the walnuts. This will increase the carbohydrate to 12 g and decrease the protein to 2 g.

For a stronger orange flavor, add ½ tsp (2 mL) orange extract.

Nutrients per bar

Calories	80
Fat	3 g
Carbohydrate	11 g
Fiber	2 g
Protein	3 g
Vitamin A	818 IU
Iron	0.6 mg
Magnesium	8 mg
Zinc	0.2 mg
Selenium	1.7 mcg

Homemade Crunchy Granola Bars

Store-bought granola bars are often high in sugar and other unhealthful ingredients. These homemade, wholesome bars will not only satisfy your sweet tooth, but will also nourish your body's craving for healthy nutrients.

Makes 12 bars

TIPS

To toast nuts, spread pecan or walnut halves or whole almonds on a baking sheet and bake in 350°F (180°C) oven for about 8 minutes, stirring once, until toasted and fragrant. Immediately transfer to a bowl and let cool. Chop, then measure the nuts.

Store granola bars in a cookie tin at room temperature for up to 1 week.

- Preheat oven to 350°F (180°C)
- 8-inch (20 cm) square metal baking pan, lined with foil or parchment paper, leaving a 2-inch (5 cm) overhang

1½ cups	certified GF quick-cooking rolled oats	375 mL
¼ cup	chopped toasted pecans, walnuts or almonds (see tip, at left)	60 mL
¼ cup	ground flax seeds (flaxseed meal)	60 mL
½ tsp	ground cinnamon	2 mL
⅓ cup	liquid honey	75 mL
¼ cup	vegetable oil	60 mL
½ tsp	GF vanilla extract	2 mL

1. In a large bowl, combine oats, pecans, flax seeds and cinnamon.

2. In a small bowl, whisk together honey, oil and vanilla. Pour over dry ingredients and stir until evenly coated. Using slightly moistened hands or a spatula, firmly press oat mixture into prepared pan.

3. Bake in preheated oven for 15 to 20 minutes or until golden brown and firm. Let cool in pan on a wire rack for 5 minutes. Using foil overhang as handles, transfer granola to a cutting board. Cut into bars and let cool on board until set and firm.

Nutrients per bar

Calories	144
Fat	8 g
Carbohydrate	16 g
Fiber	2 g
Protein	2 g
Vitamin A	2 IU
Iron	0.7 mg
Magnesium	12 mg
Zinc	0.2 mg
Selenium	0.8 mcg

Health-Enhancing Tip

For a healthier, less inflammatory fat, substitute melted virgin coconut oil for the vegetable oil.

Peanut Butter Cookies

A gluten-free version of everybody's absolute favorite cookie!

**Makes
3 dozen cookies**

TIP

For a chewy peanut butter cookie, add an extra egg.

MAKE AHEAD

Roll dough into logs 1½ inches (4 cm) in diameter. Wrap airtight and refrigerate for 1 week or freeze for up to 1 month to bake later. Thaw slightly and bake for 10 to 12 minutes. You decide the length of the log, depending on the number of cookies you want to bake. Cut partially thawed logs into ½-inch (1 cm) slices to bake.

- **Preheat oven to 350°F (180°C)**
- **Baking sheets, ungreased**

1 cup	soy flour	250 mL
½ cup	packed brown sugar	125 mL
½ cup	granulated sugar	125 mL
⅓ cup	cornstarch	75 mL
½ tsp	baking soda	2 mL
½ tsp	xanthan gum	2 mL
¼ tsp	salt	1 mL
½ cup	butter, softened	125 mL
½ cup	smooth peanut butter	125 mL
1	large egg	1
½ tsp	GF vanilla extract	2 mL
	Sweet rice flour (optional)	

1. In a bowl or plastic bag, combine soy flour, brown sugar, granulated sugar, cornstarch, baking soda, xanthan gum and salt. Mix well and set aside.

2. In a separate bowl, using an electric mixer, cream butter and peanut butter. Add egg and vanilla. Beat until light and fluffy. Slowly stir in the dry ingredients until combined. With a rubber spatula, scrape the bottom and sides of bowl.

3. Gather the dough into a large ball, kneading in any remaining dry ingredients. Roll into 1-inch (2.5 cm) balls. Place 1½ inches (4 cm) apart on the baking sheets. Flatten slightly with a fork dipped into sweet rice flour, if necessary, to prevent sticking. Bake in preheated oven for 10 to 15 minutes or until set. Transfer to a cooling rack immediately.

Variation

Substitute chunky peanut butter for smooth and add ½ cup (125 mL) chopped peanuts.

Health-Enhancing Tip

Use a peanut butter that lists peanuts as its only ingredient. Avoid peanut butters with added sugars and trans fats. You may need to add a bit more butter in step 2 to reach the desired consistency.

Nutrients per cookie

Calories	84
Fat	5 g
Carbohydrate	9 g
Fiber	1 g
Protein	2 g
Vitamin A	118 IU
Iron	0.3 mg
Magnesium	7 mg
Zinc	0.1 mg
Selenium	1.9 mcg

Cinnamon Crisps

Give cinnamon lovers these sweet, crunchy snacks anytime!

Makes 36 bars

TIPS

The dough is very stiff but still rolls out easily.

Cut bars while warm as they become too crisp to cut when they are cool.

- **Preheat oven to 300°F (150°C)**
- **15- by 10-inch (40 by 25 cm) jelly roll pan, greased**

1⅔ cups	soy flour	400 mL
⅓ cup	tapioca starch	75 mL
½ tsp	baking soda	2 mL
1 tsp	xanthan gum	5 mL
¼ tsp	salt	1 mL
1 tbsp	ground cinnamon	15 mL
1 cup	butter, softened	250 mL
½ cup	packed brown sugar	125 mL
½ cup	granulated sugar	125 mL
1	large egg, separated	1
1½ cups	chopped pecans	375 mL

1. In a bowl or plastic bag, combine soy flour, tapioca starch, baking soda, xanthan gum, salt and cinnamon. Mix well and set aside.

2. In a separate bowl, using an electric mixer, cream butter, brown sugar, granulated sugar and egg yolk until light and fluffy. Slowly beat in the dry ingredients until combined.

3. Form the dough into a large disk and place in the prepared pan. Cover with waxed paper. With a rolling pin, roll out the dough to fit the pan. Carefully remove the waxed paper.

4. In a small bowl, beat egg white with a fork just until foamy. Brush on top of dough. Sprinkle with pecans and press them in lightly. Let stand for 30 minutes. Bake in preheated oven for 35 to 45 minutes or until set. Immediately cut into bars. Let cool in the pan.

Variation

Make three kinds of cookies at the same time. Divide dough into thirds. Sprinkle one portion with chopped pecans. Then choose chocolate, butterscotch, peanut butter, raspberry or cinnamon chips for the other two portions.

Nutrients per bar

Calories	124
Fat	9 g
Carbohydrate	9 g
Fiber	1 g
Protein	3 g
Vitamin A	232 IU
Iron	0.6 mg
Magnesium	6 mg
Zinc	0.2 mg
Selenium	0.6 mcg

References

Journal Articles

Aakvaag A, Sand T, Opstad PK, Fonnum F. Hormonal changes in serum in young men during prolonged physical strain. *Eur J Appl Physiol Occup Physiol*, 1978 Oct 20; 39 (4): 283–91.

Abdou AM, Higashiguchi S, Horie K, et al. Relaxation and immunity enhancement effects of gamma-aminobutyric acid (GABA) administration in humans. *BioFactors*, 2006; 26 (3): 201–8.

Abraham GE. The bioavailability of iodine applied to the skin. *The Original Internist*, 2008; 15 (2): 77–79.

Aceves C, Anguiano B, Delgado G. Is iodine a gatekeeper of the integrity of the mammary gland? *J Mammary Gland Biol Neoplasia*, 2005; 10 (2): 189–96.

Akçay MN, Akçay G. The presence of the antigliadin antibodies in autoimmune thyroid diseases. *Hepatogastroenterology*, 2003 Dec; 50 Suppl 2:cclxxix-cclxxx.

Alsanea O, Clark OH. Treatment of Graves' disease: The advantages of surgery. *Endocrinol Metab Clin North Am*, 2000 Jun; 29 (2): 321–37.

American College of Obstetricians and Gynecologists. ACOG Practice Bulletin. Clinical management guidelines for obstetrician-gynecologists. Number 37, August 2002. (Replaces Practice Bulletin Number 32, November 2001). Thyroid disease in pregnancy. *Obstet Gynecol*, 2002 Aug; 100 (2): 387–96.

Antonelli A, Ferri C, Fallahi P, et al. CXCL10 and CCL2 chemokine serum levels in patients with hepatitis C associated with autoimmune thyroiditis. *J Interferon Cytokine Res*, 2009 Jun; 29 (6): 345–51.

Auf'mkolk M, Ingbar JC, Kubota K, et al. Extracts and auto-oxidized constituents of certain plants inhibit the receptor-binding and biological activity of Graves' immunoglobulins. *Endocrinology*, 1985 May; 116 (5): 1687–93.

Bártová J, Procházková J, Krátká Z, et al. Dental amalgam as one of the risk factors in autoimmune diseases. *Neuro Endocrinol Lett*, 2003 Feb–Apr; 24 (1–2): 65–67.

Bastemir M, Emral R, Erdogan G, Gullu S. High prevalence of thyroid dysfunction and autoimmune thyroiditis in adolescents after elimination of iodine deficiency in the Eastern Black Sea Region of Turkey. *Thyroid*, 2006 Dec; 16 (12): 1265–71.

Bastomsky CH. Enhanced thyroxine metabolism and high uptake goiters in rats after a single dose of 2,3,7,8-tetrachlorodibenzo-p-dioxin. *Endocrinology*, 1977 Jul; 101 (1): 292–96.

Beard JL, Borel MJ, Derr J. Impaired thermoregulation and thyroid function in iron-deficiency anemia. *Am J Clin Nutr*, 1990 Nov; 52 (5): 813–19.

Bégin ME, Langlois M F, Lorrain D, Cunnane SC. Thyroid function and cognition during aging. *Curr Gerontol Geriatr Res*, 2008; (12): 1–11.

Benvenga S, Amato A, Calvani M, Trimarchi F. Effects of carnitine on thyroid hormone action. *Ann N Y Acad Sci*, 2004 Nov; 1033: 158–167.

Benvenga S, Guarneri F, Vaccaro M, et al. Homologies between proteins of *Borrelia burgdorferi* and thyroid autoantigens. *Thyroid*, 2004 Nov; 14 (11): 964–66.

Benvenga S, Lakshmanan M, Trimarchi F. Carnitine is a naturally occurring inhibitor of thyroid hormone nuclear uptake. *Thyroid*, 2000 Dec; 10(12), 1043–1050.

Benvenga S, Ruggeri RM, Russo A, et al. Usefulness of L-carnitine, a naturally occurring peripheral antagonist of thyroid hormone action, in iatrogenic hyperthyroidism: A randomized, double-blind, placebo-controlled clinical trial. *J Clin Endocrinol Metab*, 2001 Aug; 86 (8), 3579–94.

Berry MJ, Larsen PR. The role of selenium in thyroid hormone action. *Endocr Rev*, 1992 May; 13 (2): 207–19.

Bianco AC, Salvatore D, Gereben B, et al. Biochemistry, cellular and molecular biology, and physiological roles of the iodothyronine selenodeiodinases. *Endocr Rev*, 2002 Feb; 23 (1): 38–89.

Blount BC, Pirkle JL, Osterloh JD, et al. Urinary perchlorate and thyroid hormone levels in adolescent and adult men and women living in the United States. *Environ Health Perspect*, 2006 Dec; 114 (12): 1865–71.

Boelen A, Kwakkel J, Fliers E. Beyond low plasma T3: Local thyroid hormone metabolism during inflammation and infection. *Endocr Rev*, 2011 Oct; 32 (5) : 670–93.

Brinker F. Inhibition of endocrine function by botanical agents I. *Boraginaceae* and *Labiatae*. *J Naturopath Med*, 1990; 1: 10–18.

Brown MM, Rhyne BC, Goyer RA. The intracellular effects of chronic arsenic exposure on renal proximal tubule cells. *J Toxicol Environ Health*, 1976 Jan; 1 (3): 505–14.

Brucker-Davis F. Effects of environmental synthetic chemicals on thyroid function. *Thyroid*, 1998 Sep; 8 (9): 827–56.

Brüngger M, Hulter HN, Krapf R. Effect of chronic metabolic acidosis on thyroid hormone homeostasis in humans. *Am J Physiol*, 1997 May; 272 (5 Pt 2): F648–53.

Brzezińska-Slebodzińska E. Fever induced oxidative stress: The effect on thyroid status and the 5'-monodeiodinase activity, protective role of selenium and vitamin E. *J Physiol Pharmacol*, 2001 Jun; 52 (2): 275–84.

Bunevicius R, Kazanavicius G, Zalinkevicius R, Prange AJ Jr. Effects of thyroxine as compared with thyroxine plus triiodothyronine in patients with hypothyroidism. *N Engl J Med*, 1999 Feb 11; 340 (6): 424–29.

Bürgi H, Siebenhüner L, Miloni E. Fluorine and thyroid gland function: A review of the literature. *Klin Wochenschr*, 1984 Jun 15; 62 (12): 564–69.

Cann SA, van Netten JP, van Netten C. Hypothesis: Iodine, selenium and the development of breast cancer. *Cancer Causes Control*, 2000 Feb; 11 (2): 121–27.

Caride A, Fernández-Pérez B, Cabaleiro T, et al. Cadmium chronotoxicity at pituitary level: Effects on plasma ACTH, GH, and TSH daily pattern. *J Physiol Biochem*, 2010 Sep; 66 (3): 213–20.

Cerqueira C, Knudsen N, Ovesen L, et al. Association of iodine fortification with incident use of antithyroid medication — A Danish nationwide study. *J Clin Endocrinol Metab*, 2009 Jul; 94 (7): 2400–2405.

Chatzipanagiotou S, Legakis JN, Boufidou F, et al. Prevalence of *Yersinia* plasmid-encoded outer protein (Yop) class-specific antibodies in patients with Hashimoto's thyroiditis. *Clin Microbiol Infect*, 2001 Mar; 7 (3): 138–43.

Chevrier J, Eskenazi B, Holland N, et al. Effects of exposure to polychlorinated biphenyls and organochlorine pesticides on thyroid function during pregnancy. *Am J Epidemiol*, 2008 Aug 1; 168 (3): 298–310.

Chisholm JJ Jr, Thomas DJ. Use of 2,3-dimercaptopropane-1-sulfonate in treatment of lead poisoning in children. *J Pharmacol Exp Ther*, 1985 Dec; 235 (3): 665–69.

Chopra IJ. Clinical review 86: Euthyroid sick syndrome: Is it a misnomer? *J Clin Endocrinol Metab*, 1997 Feb; 82 (2): 329–34.

Chopra IJ, Chopra U, Smith SR, et al. Reciprocal changes in serum concentrations of 3,3'5-triiodothyronine (T3) in systemic illnesses. *J Clin Endocrinol Metab*, 1975 Dec; 41 (6): 1043–49.

Chopra IJ, Huang TS, Beredo A, et al. Evidence for an inhibitor of extrathyroidal conversion of thyroxine to 3,5,3'-triiodothyronine in sera of patients with nonthyroidal illnesses. *J Clin Endocrinol Metab*, 1985 Apr; 60 (4): 666–72.

Clur A. Di-iodothyronine as part of the oestradiol and catechol oestrogen receptor — The role of iodine, thyroid hormones and melatonin in the aetiology of breast cancer. *Med Hypotheses*, 1988 Dec; 27 (4): 303–11.

Coceani M, Iervasi G, Pingitore A, et al. Thyroid hormone and coronary artery disease: From clinical correlations to prognostic implications. *Clin Cardiol*, 2009 Jul; 32 (7): 380–85.

Coiro V, Passeri M, Capretti L, et al. Serotonergic control of TSH and PRL secretion in obese men. *Psychoneuroendocrinology*, 1990; 15 (4): 261–68.

Corapçioğlu D, Tonyukuk V, Kiyan M, et al. Relationship between thyroid autoimmunity and *Yersinia enterocolitica* antibodies. *Thyroid*, 2002 Jul; 12 (7): 613–17.

Corssmit EP, Heyligenberg R, Endert E, et al. Acute effects of interferon-alpha administration on thyroid hormone metabolism in healthy men. *J Clin Endocrinol Metab*, 1995 Nov; 80 (11):3140–44.

Costa AJ. Interpreting thyroid tests. *Am Fam Physician*, 1995 Dec; 52 (8): 2325–30.

Cuoco L, Certo M, Jorizzo RA, et al. Prevalence and early diagnosis of coeliac disease in autoimmune thyroid disorders. *Ital J Gastroenterol Hepatol*, 1999 May; 31 (4): 283–87.

Darnerud PO, Aune M, Larsson L, Hallgren S. Plasma PBDE and thyroxine levels in rats exposed to Bromkal or BDE-47. *Chemosphere*, 2007 Apr; 67 (9): S386–92.

Davey JC, Nomikos AP, Wungjiranirun M, et al. Arsenic as an endocrine disruptor: Arsenic disrupts retinoic acid receptor- and thyroid hormone receptor-mediated gene regulation and thyroid hormone mediated amphibian tail metamorphosis. *Environ Health Perspect*, 2008 Feb; 116 (2): 165–72.

De La Viega A, Dohan O, Levy O, Carrasco N. Molecular analysis of the sodium/iodide symporter: Impact on thyroid and extrathyroid pathophysiology. *Physiol Rev*, 2000 Jul; 80 (3): 1083–1105.

Decherf S, Seugnet I, Fini JB, et al. Disruption of thyroid hormone-dependent hypothalamic set-points by environmental contaminants. *Mol Cell Endocrinol*, 2010 Jul 29; 323 (2): 172–82.

Desailloud R, Hober D. Viruses and thyroiditis: an update. *Virol J*, 2009 Jan 12; 6: 5.

Diamanti-Kandarakis E, Palioura E, Kandarakis SA, Koutsilieris M. The impact of endocrine disruptors on endocrine targets. *Horm Metab Res*, 2010 Jul; 42 (8): 543–52.

Divi RL, Chang HC, Doerge DR. Anti-thyroid isoflavones from soybean: Isolation, characterization, and mechanisms of action. *Biochem Pharmacol*, 1997 Nov 15; 54 (10): 1087–96.

Docter R, Krenning EP, de Jong M, Hennemann G. The sick euthyroid syndrome: Changes in thyroid hormone serum parameters and hormone metabolism. *Clin Endocrinol* (Oxf), 1993 Nov; 39 (5): 499–518.

Doerge DR, Chang HC. Inactivation of thyroid peroxidase by soy isoflavones, in vitro and in vivo. *J Chromatogr B Analyt Technol Biomed Life Sci*, 2002 Sep 25; 777 (1–2): 269–79.

Donders SH, Pieters GF, Heevel JG, et al. Disparity of thyrotropin (TSH) and prolactin responses to TSH-releasing hormone in obesity. *J Clin Endocrinol Metab*, 1985 Jul; 61 (1): 56–59.

Dong BJ. How medications affect thyroid function. *West J Med*, 2000 Feb; 172 (2): 102–6.

Duntas LH. The role of selenium in thyroid autoimmunity and cancer. *Thyroid*, 2006 May; 16 (5): 455–60.

Espino Montoro A, Medina Pérez M, González Martín MC, et al. [Subacute thyroiditis associated with positive antibodies to the Epstein-Barr virus.] [Article in Spanish.] *An Med Interna*, 2000 Oct; 17 (10): 546–48.

Fliers E, Alkemade A, Wiersinga W. The hypothalamic-pituitary-thyroid axis in critical illness. *Best Pract Res Clin Endocrinol Metab*, 2001 Dec; 15 (4): 453–64.

Gaby AR. Editorial: Iodine: A lot to swallow. *Townsend Letter for Doctors & Patients*, 2005 August/September.

Galletti PM, Joyet G. Effect of fluorine on thyroidal iodine metabolism in hyperthyroidism. *J Clin Endocrinol Metab*, 1958 Oct; 18 (10): 1102–10.

Gardner DF, Centor RM, Utiger RD. Effects of low dose iodide supplementation on thyroid function in normal men. *Clin Endocrinol* (Oxf), 1988 Mar; 28(3): 283–88.

Ghent WR, Eskin BA, Low DA, Hill LP. Iodine replacement in fibrocystic disease of the breast. *Can J Surg*, 1993 Oct; 36 (5): 453–60.

Goldey ES, Kehn LS, Lau C, et al. Developmental exposure to polychlorinated biphenyls (Aroclor 1254) reduces circulating thyroid hormone concentrations and causes hearing deficits in rats. *Toxicol Appl Pharmacol*, 1995 Nov; 135 (1): 77–88.

Greer MA, Goodman G, Pleus RC, Greer SE. Health effects assessment for environmental perchlorate contamination: The dose response for inhibition of thyroidal radioiodine uptake in humans. *Environ Health Perspect*, 2002 Sep; 110 (9): 927–37.

Gulland J. Iodine & breast health: Think beyond the thyroid. *Holistic Primary Care*, 2009 Spring; 10 (1): 14–15.

Hallgren S, Sinjari T, Håkansson H, Darnerud PO. Effects of polybrominated diphenyl ethers (PBDEs) and polychlorinated biphenyls (PCBs) on thyroid hormone and vitamin A levels in rats and mice. *Arch Toxicol*, 2001 Jun; 75 (4): 200–208.

Hammouda F, Messaoudi I, El Hani J, et al. Reversal of cadmium-induced thyroid dysfunction by selenium, zinc, or their combination in rat. *Biol Trace Elem Res*, 2008 Winter; 126 (1–3): 194–203.

Hashimoto H, Igarashi N, Yachie A, et al. The relationship between serum levels of interleukin-6 and thyroid hormone in children with acute respiratory infection. *J Clin Endocrinol Metab*, 1994 Feb; 78 (2): 288–91.

Heimeier RA, Das B, Buchholz DR, Shi YB. The xenoestrogen bisphenol A inhibits postembryonic vertebrate development by antagonizing gene regulation by thyroid hormone. *Endocrinology*, 2009 Jun; 150 (6): 2964–73.

Helfand M, Crapo L. Screening for thyroid disease. *Ann Intern Med*, 1990 Jun; 112 (11): 840–49.

Hellhammer J, Fries E, Buss C, et al. Effects of soy lecithin phosphatidic acid and phosphatidylserine complex (PAS) on the endocrine and psychological responses to mental stress. *Stress*, 2004 Jun; 7 (2): 119–26.

Hennemann G, Docter R, Friesema EC, et al. Plasma membrane transport of thyroid hormones and its role in thyroid hormone metabolism and bioavailability. *Endocr Rev*, 2001 Aug; 22 (4): 451–76.

Herbstman JB, Sjödin A, Apelberg BJ, et al. Birth delivery mode modifies the associations between prenatal polychlorinated biphenyl (PCB) and polybrominated diphenyl ether (PBDE) and neonatal thyroid hormone levels. *Environ Health Perspect*, 2008 Oct; 116 (10): 1376–82.

Hess SY. The impact of common micronutrient deficiencies on iodine and thyroid metabolism: The evidence from human studies. *Best Pract Res Clin Endocrinol Metab*, 2010 Feb; 24 (1): 117–32.

Hollowell JG, Staehling NW, Hannon WH, et al. Iodine nutrition in the United States. Trends and public health implications: Iodine excretion data from National Health and Nutrition Examination Surveys I and III (1971–1974 and 1988–1994). *J Clin Endocrinol Metab*, 1998 Oct; 83 (10): 3401–8.

Hou X, Chai C, Qian Q, et al. Determination of chemical species of iodine in some seaweeds. *Science of the Total Environment*, 1997 Oct; 204 (3): 215–21.

Hurrell RF. Bioavailability of iodine. *Eur J Clin Nutr*, 1997 Jan; 51 Suppl 1: S9–12.

Hybenova M, Hrda P, Procházková J, et al. The role of environmental factors in autoimmune thyroiditis. *Neuro Endocrinol Lett*, 2010; 31 (3): 283–89.

Iervasi G, Pingitore A, Landi P, et al. Low-T3 syndrome: A strong prognostic predictor of death in patients with heart disease. *Circulation*, 2003 Feb 11; 107 (5): 708–13.

Janssen OE, Mehlmauer N, Hahn S, et al. High prevalence of autoimmune thyroiditis in patients with polycystic ovary syndrome. *Eur J Endocrinol*, 2004 Mar; 150 (3): 363–69.

Jung KK, Kim SY, Kim TG, et al. Differential regulation of thyroid hormone receptor-mediated function by endocrine disruptors. *Arch Pharm Res*, 2007 May; 30 (5): 616–23.

Kannangai R, Sachithanandham J, Kandathil AJ, et al. Immune responses to Epstein-Barr virus in individuals with systemic and organ specific autoimmune disorders. *Indian J Med Microbiol*, 2010 Apr–Jun; 28 (2): 120–23.

Kapil U, Pathak P, Singh P. Benefits and safety of dietary iodine intake in India. *Pakistan J Nutr*, 2003; 2 (1): 43–45.

Karbownik M, Stasiak M, Zasada K, et al. Comparison of potential protective effects of melatonin, indole-3-proprionic acid, and propylthiouracil against lipid peroxidation caused by potassium bromate in the thyroid gland. *J Cell Biochem*, 2005 May 1; 95 (1): 131–38.

Kawada J, Nishida M, Yoshimura Y, Mitani K. Effects of organic and inorganic mercurials on thyroidal functions. *J Pharmacobiodyn*, 1980 Mar; 3 (3): 149–59.

Kelly GS. Peripheral metabolism of thyroid hormones: A review. *Altern Med Rev*, 2000 Aug; 5 (4): 306–33.

Kessler JH. The effect of supraphysiologic levels of iodine on patients with cyclic mastalgia. *Breast J*, 2004 Jul–Aug; 10 (4): 328–36.

Köhrle J. The deiodinase family: Selenoenzymes regulating thyroid hormone availability and action. *Cell Mol Life Sci*, 2000 Dec; 57 (13–14): 1853–63.

Konno N, Makita H, Yuri K, et al. Association between dietary iodine intake and prevalence of subclinical hypothyroidism in the coastal regions of Japan. *J Clin Endocrinol Metab*, 1994 Feb; 78 (2): 393–97.

Konno N, Yuri K, Taguchi H, et al. Screening for thyroid diseases in an iodine sufficient area with sensitive thyrotrophin assays, and serum thyroid autoantibody and urinary iodide determinations. *Clin Endocrinol* (Oxf), 1993 Mar; 38 (3): 273–81.

Koutras DA, Alexander WD, Harden RM, Wayne E. Effect of small iodine supplements on thyroid function in normal individuals. *J Clin Endocrinol Metab*, 1964 Sep; 24: 857–62.

Kuriyama K, Sze PY. Blood–brain barrier to H3-gamma-aminobutyric acid in normal and amino oxyacetic acid-treated animals. *Neuropharmacology*, 1971 Jan; 10 (1): 103–8.

Kurokawa Y, Maekawa A, Takahashi M, Hayashi Y. Toxicity and carcinogenicity of potassium bromate — A new renal carcinogen. *Environ Health Perspect*, 1990 Jul; 87: 309–35.

Lawrence J, Lamm S, Braverman LE. Low dose perchlorate (3 mg daily) and thyroid function. *Thyroid*, 2001 Mar; 11 (3): 295.

Lawrence JE, Lamm SH, Pino S, et al. The effect of short-term low-dose perchlorate on various aspects of thyroid function. *Thyroid*, 2000 Aug; 10 (8): 659–63.

Lazarus JH. The effects of lithium therapy on thyroid and thyrotropin-releasing hormone. *Thyroid*, 1998 Oct; 8(10): 909–13.

Li C, Cheng Y, Tang Q, et al. The association between prenatal exposure to organochlorine pesticides and thyroid hormone levels in newborns in Yancheng, China. *Environ Res*, 2014 Feb; 129: 47–51.

Lord RS, Bongiovanni B, Bralley JA. Estrogen metabolism and the diet-cancer connection: Rationale for assessing the ratio of urinary hydroxylated estrogen metabolites. *Alt Med Rev*, 2002 Apr; 7 (2): 112–29.

Mainardi E, Montanelli A, Dotti M. Thyroid-related autoantibodies and celiac disease: A role for a gluten-free diet? *J Clin Gastroenterol*, 2002 Sep; 35 (3): 245–48.

McHenry CR, Slusarczyk SJ. Hypothyroidism following hemithyroidectomy: Incidence, risk factors, and management. *Surgery*, 2000 Dec; 128 (6): 994–98.

Meier C, Trittibach P, Guglielmetti M, et al. Serum thyroid stimulating hormone in assessment of severity of tissue hypothyroidism in patients with overt primary thyroid failure: Cross sectional survey. *BMJ*, 2003 Feb 8; 326 (7384): 311–12.

Meletis CD, Zabriskie N. Iodine, a critically overlooked nutrient. *Alternative and Complementary Therapies*, 2007 June; 13 (3): 132–36.

Meltzer HM, Maage A, Ydersbond TA, et al. Fish arsenic may influence human blood arsenic, selenium, and T4:T3 ratio. *Biol Trace Elem Res*, 2002 Winter; 90 (1–3): 83–98.

Miller DW. Extrathyroid benefits of iodine. *J Amer Physicians and Surgeons*, 2006 Winter; 11 (4): 106–10.

Mitchell HA, Weinshenker D. Good night and good luck: Norepinephrine in sleep pharmacology. *Biochem Pharmacol*, 2010 Mar 15; 79 (6). 801–9.

Mittendorf EA, McHenry CR. Thyroidectomy for selected patients with thyrotoxicosis. *Arch Otolaryngol Head Neck Surg*, 2001 Jan; 127 (1): 61–65.

Moriyama K, Tagami T, Akamizu T, et al. Thyroid hormone action is disrupted by bisphenol A as an antagonist. *J Clin Endocrinol Metab*, 2002 Nov; 87 (11): 5185–90.

Moss J. A perspective on high dose iodine supplementation, Part V — The Japanese experiment with dietary iodine. *Moss Nutrition Report #218*, 2007 Dec.

Murai K, Okamura K, Tsuji H, et al. Thyroid function in "yusho" patients exposed to polychlorinated biphenyls (PCB). *Environ Res*, 1987 Dec; 44 (2): 179–87.

Nagataki S. The average of dietary iodine intake due to the ingestion of seaweeds is 1.2 mg/day in Japan. *Thyroid*, 2008 Jun; 18 (6): 667–68.

Nagataki S, Shizume K, Nakao K. Thyroid function in chronic excess iodide ingestion: Comparison of thyroidal absolute iodine uptake and degradation of thyroxine in euthyroid Japanese subjects. *J Clin Endocrinol Metab*, 1967 May; 27 (5): 638–47.

Nam KH, Yoon JH, Chang HS, Park CS. Optimal timing of surgery in well-differentiated thyroid carcinoma detected during pregnancy. *J Surg Oncol*, 2005 Sep 1; 91 (3): 199–203.

Niepomniszcze H, Pitoia F, Katz SB, et al. Primary thyroid disorders in endogenous Cushing's syndrome. *Eur J Endocrinol*, 2002 Sep; 147 (3): 305–11.

Nishida M, Matsumoto H, Asano A, et al. Direct evidence for the presence of methylmercury bound in the thyroid and other organs obtained from mice given methylmercury; differentiation of free and bound methylmercuries in biological materials determined by volatility of methylmercury. *Chem Pharm Bull* (Tokyo), 1990 May; 38 (5): 1412–13.

Nishiyama S, Futagoishi-Suginohara Y, Matsukura M, et al. Zinc supplementation alters thyroid hormone metabolism in disabled patients with zinc deficiency. *J Am Coll Nutr*, 1994 Feb; 13 (1): 62–67.

O'Reilly DS. Thyroid hormone replacement: An iatrogenic problem. *Int J Clin Pract*, 2010 Jun; 64 (7): 991–94.

Obál F Jr, Krueger JM. The somatotropic axis and sleep. *Rev Neurol* (Paris), 2001 Nov; 157 (11 Pt 2): S12–15.

Obut TA, Saryg SK, Erdynieva TA, Dement'eva Tiu. [Changes in the thyroid activity and influence of dehydroepiandrosterone-sulfate under the cold and not cold influence.] [Article in Russian.] *Ross Fiziol Zh Im I M Sechenova*, 2009 Nov; 95 (11): 1234–41.

Orrego A, Kumar RS, Dowling JT. Inhibition by cortisol of deiodination of thyroxine by rat liver in vitro. *Nature*, 1967 Nov 25; 216 (5117): 820–21.

Palit TK, Miller CC 3rd, Miltenburg DM. The efficacy of thyroidectomy for Graves' disease: A meta-analysis. *J Surg Res*, 2000 May 15; 90 (2): 161–65.

Pallav K, Leffler DA, Tariq S, et al. Noncoeliac enteropathy: The differential diagnosis of villous atrophy in contemporary clinical practice. *Aliment Pharmacol Ther*, 2012 Feb; 35 (3): 380–90.

Panossian A, Wikman G. Evidence-based efficacy of adaptogens in fatigue, and molecular mechanisms related to their stress-protective activity. *Curr Clin Pharmacol*, 2009 Sep; 4 (3): 198–219.

Pansini F, Bassi P, Cavallini AR, et al. Effect of the hormonal contraception on serum reverse triiodothyronine levels. *Gynecol Obstet Invest*, 1987; 23 (2): 133–34.

Papanastasiou L, Vatalas IA, Koutras DA, Mastorakos G. Thyroid autoimmunity in the current iodine environment. *Thyroid*, 2007 Aug; 17 (8): 729–39.

Paul T, Meyers B, Witorsch RJ, et al. The effect of small increases in dietary iodine on thyroid function in euthyroid subjects. *Metabolism*, 1988 Feb; 37 (2): 121–24.

Pavelka S. Metabolism of bromide and its interference with the metabolism of iodine. *Physiol Res*, 2004; 53 (Suppl 1): S81–90.

Pearce CJ, Himsworth RL. Total and free thyroid hormone concentrations in patients receiving maintenance replacement treatment with thyroxine. *Br Med J (Clin Res Ed)*, 1984 Mar 3; 288 (6418), 693–95.

Pearce EN, Gerber AR, Gootnick DB, et al. Effects of chronic iodine excess in a cohort of long-term American workers in West Africa. *J Clin Endocrinol Metab*, 2002 Dec; 87 (12):5499–502.

Pedersen IB, Laurberg P, Knudsen N, et al. An increased incidence of overt hypothyroidism after iodine fortification of salt in Denmark: A prospective population study. *J Clin Endocrinol Metab*, 2007 Aug; 92 (8): 3122–27.

Peeters RP, van der Geyten S, Wouters PJ, et al. Tissue thyroid hormone levels in critical illness. *J Clin Endocrinol Metab*, 2005 Dec; 90 (12): 6498–507.

Peeters RP, Wouters PJ, Kaptein E, et al. Reduced activation and increased inactivation of thyroid hormone in tissues of critically ill patients. *J Clin Endocrinol Metab*, 2003 Jul; 88 (7): 3202–11.

Peeters RP, Wouters PJ, van Toor H, et al. Serum 3,3',5'-triiodothyronine (rT3) and 3,5,3'-triiodothyronine/rT3 are prognostic markers in critically ill patients and are associated with postmortem tissue deiodinase activities. *J Clin Endocrinol Metab*, 2005 Aug; 90 (8): 4559–65.

Peuhkuri K, Sihvola N, Korpela R. Dietary factors and fluctuating levels of melatonin. *Food Nutr Res*, 2012; 56.

Pittman CS, Suda AK, Chambers JB Jr, et al. Abnormalities of thyroid hormone turnover in patients with diabetes mellitus before and after insulin therapy. *J Clin Endocrinol Metab*, 1979 May; 48 (5): 854–60.

Prochazkova J, Sterzl I, Kucerova H, et al. The beneficial effect of amalgam replacement on health in patients with autoimmunity. *Neuro Endocrinol Lett*, 2004 Jun; 25 (3): 211–18.

Pucci E, Chiovato L, Pinchera A. Thyroid and lipid metabolism. *Int J Obes Relat Metab Disord*, 2000 Jun; 24 Suppl 2: S109–12.

Rallison ML, Dobyns BM, Meikle AW, et al. Natural history of thyroid abnormalities: Prevalence, incidence, and regression of thyroid disease in adolescents and young adults. *Am J Med*, 1991 Oct; 91 (4): 363–70.

Rezzonico J, Rezzonico M, Pusiol E, et al. Introducing the thyroid gland as another victim of the insulin resistance syndrome. *Thyroid*, 2008 Apr; 18 (4): 461–64.

Richardson VM, Staskal DF, Ross DG, et al. Possible mechanisms of thyroid hormone disruption in mice by BDE 47, a major polybrominated diphenyl ether congener. *Toxicol Appl Pharmacol*, 2008 Feb 1; 226 (3): 244–50.

Riedel W, Layka H, Neeck G. Secretory pattern of GH, TSH, thyroid hormones, ACTH, cortisol, FSH, and LH in patients with fibromyalgia syndrome following systemic injection of the relevant hypothalamic-releasing hormones. *Z Rheumatol*, 1998; 57 Suppl 2: 81–87.

Ristic-Medic D, Piskackova Z, Hooper L, et al. Methods of assessment of iodine status in humans: A systematic review. *Am J Clin Nutr*, 2009 Jun; 89 (6): 2052S–69S.

Rogan EG, Badawi AF, Devanesan PD, et al. Relative imbalances in estrogen metabolism and conjugation in breast tissue of women with carcinoma: Potential biomarkers of susceptibility to cancer. *Carcinogenesis*, 2003 Apr; 24 (4): 697–702.

Sahu S, Ray K, Yogendra Kumar MS, et al. *Valeriana wallichii* root extract improves sleep quality and modulates brain monoamine level in rats. *Phytomedicine*, 2012 Jul 15; 19 (10): 924–29.

Saito T, Endo T, Kawaguchi A, et al. Increased expression of the Na+/I- symporter in cultured human thyroid cells exposed to thyrotrophin and in Graves' thyroid tissue. *J Clin Endocrinol Metab*, 1997 Oct; 82 (10): 3331–36.

Salay E, Garabrant D. Polychlorinated biphenyls and thyroid hormones in adults: A systematic review appraisal of epidemiological studies. *Chemosphere*, 2009 Mar; 74 (11): 1413–19.

Sangster B, Blom JL, Sekhuis VM, et al. The influence of sodium bromide in man: A study in human volunteers with special emphasis on the endocrine and the central nervous system. *Food Chem Toxicol*, 1983 Aug; 21 (4): 409–19.

Sangster B, Krajnc EI, Loeber JG, et al. Study of sodium bromide in human volunteers, with special emphasis on the endocrine system. *Hum Toxicol*, 1982 Oct; 1 (4): 393–402.

Santini G, Patrignani P, Sciulli MG, et al. The human pharmacology of monocyte cyclooxygenase 2 inhibition by cortisol and synthetic glucocorticoids. *Clin Pharmacol Ther*, 2001 Nov; 70 (5): 475–83.

Saunders J, Hall SE, Sönksen PH. Thyroid hormones in insulin requiring diabetes before and after treatment. *Diabetologia*, 1978 Jun; 15 (1): 29–32.

Schaff L, Pohl T, Schmidt R, et al. Screening for thyroid disorders in a working population. *Clin Investig*, 1993 Feb; 71 (2): 126–31.

Schantz SL, Widholm JJ, Rice DC. Effects of PCB exposure on neuropsychological function in children. *Environ Health Perspect*, 2003 Mar; 111 (3): 357–576.

Schröder-van der Elst JP, Smit JW, Romijn HA, van der Heide D. Dietary flavonoids and iodine metabolism. *Biofactors*, 2003; 19 (3–4): 171–76.

Schuetz P, Müller B. The hypothalamic-pituitary-adrenal axis in critical illness. *Endocrinol Metab Clin North Am*, 2006 Dec; 35 (4): 823–38.

Shaw K, Turner J, Del Mar C. Tryptophan and 5-hydroxytryptophan for depression. *Cochrane Database Syst Rev*, 2002; (1): CD003198.

Shen DH, Kloos RT, Mazzaferri EL, Jhian SM. Sodium iodide symporter in health and disease. *Thyroid*, 2001 May; 11 (5): 415–25.

Skare S, Frey HM. Iodine induced thyrotoxicosis in apparently normal thyroid glands. *Acta Endocrinologica* (Copenh), 1980 Jul; 94 (3): 332–36.

Slebodzinski AB. Ovarian iodide uptake and triiodothyronine generation in follicular fluid: The enigma of the thyroid ovary interaction. *Domest Anim Endocrinol*, 2005 Jul; 29 (1): 97–103.

Smyth PP. Role of iodine in antioxidant defence in thyroid and breast disease. *Biofactors*, 2003; 1 (3–4): 121–30.

Smyth PP. The thyroid, iodine and breast cancer. *Breast Cancer Res*, 2003; 5 (5): 235–38.

Smyth PP, Dwyer RM. The sodium iodide symporter and thyroid disease. *Clin Endocrinol* (Oxf), 2002 Apr; 56 (4): 427–29.

Stadel BV. Dietary iodine and risk of breast, endometrial, and ovarian cancer. *Lancet*, 1976 Apr 24; 1 (7965): 890–91.

Stasiak M, Lewiński A, Karbownik-Lewińska M. [Relationship between toxic effects of potassium bromate and endocrine glands.] [Article in Polish.] *Endokrynol Pol*, 2009 Jan–Feb; 60 (1): 40–50.

Stechova K, Pomahacova R, Hrabak J, et al. Reactivity to *Helicobacter pylori* antigens in patients suffering from thyroid gland autoimmunity. *Exp Clin Endocrinol Diabetes*, 2009 Sep; 117 (8): 423–31.

Stefanić M, Papić S, Suver M, et al. Association of vitamin D receptor gene 3'-variants with Hashimoto's thyroiditis in the Croatian population. *Int J Immunogenet*, 2008 Apr; 35 (2): 125–31.

Steinmaus C, Miller MD, Howd R. Impact of smoking and thiocyanate on perchlorate and thyroid hormone associations in the 2001–2002 National Health and Nutrition Examination Survey. *Environ Health Perspect*, 2007 Sep; 115 (9): 1333–38.

Sterzl I, Hrdá P, Procházková J, et al. [Reactions to metals in patients with chronic fatigue and autoimmune endocrinopathy.] [Article in Czech.] *Vnitr Lek*, 1999 Sep; 45 (9): 527–31.

Sterzl I, Procházková J, Hrdá P, et al. Mercury and nickel allergy: Risk factors in fatigue and autoimmunity. *Neuro Endocrinol Lett*, 1999; 20 (3–4): 221–28.

Sterzl I, Prochazkova J, Hrda P, et al. Removal of dental amalgam decreases anti-TPO and anti-Tg autoantibodies in patients with autoimmune thyroiditis. *Neuro Endocrinol Lett*, 2006 Dec; 27 Suppl 1: 25–30. Erratum in: *Neuro Endocrinol Lett*, 2007 Oct; 28 (5): iii.

Stewart PM, Wallace AM, Valentino R, et al. Mineralocorticoid activity of liquorice: 11-beta-hydroxysteroid dehydrogenase deficiency comes of age. *Lancet*, 1987 Oct 10; 2 (8563): 821–24.

Stewart PW, Lonky E, Reihman J, et al. The relationship between prenatal PCB exposure and intelligence (IQ) in 9-year-old children. *Environ Health Perspect*, 2008 Oct; 116 (10): 1416–22.

Stewart PW, Reihman J, Lonky EI, et al. Cognitive development in preschool children prenatally exposed to PCBs and MeHg. *Neurotoxicol Teratol*, 2003 Jan–Feb; 25 (1): 11–22.

Stoddard FR 2nd, Brooks AD, Eskin BA, Johannes GJ. Iodine alters gene expression in the MCF7 breast cancer cell line: Evidence for an anti-estrogen effect of iodine. *Int J Med Sci*, 2008 Jul; 5 (4): 189–96.

Stouthard JM, van der Poll T, Endert E, et al. Effects of acute and chronic interleukin-6 administration on thyroid hormone metabolism in humans. *J Clin Endocrinol Metab*, 1994 Nov; 79 (5), 1342–46.

Sun H, Shen OX, Wang XR, et al. Anti-thyroid hormone activity of bisphenol A, tetrabromobisphenol A and tetrachlorobisphenol A in an improved reporter gene assay. *Toxicol In Vitro*, 2009 Aug; 23 (5): 950–54.

Surks MI, Ortiz E, Daniels GH, et al. Subclinical thyroid disease: Scientific review and guidelines for diagnosis and management. *JAMA*, 2004 Jan 14; 291 (2): 228–38.

Szot P, Wilkinson CW, White SS, et al. Chronic cortisol suppresses pituitary and hypothalamic peptide message expression in pigtailed macaques. *Neuroscience*, 2004; 126 (1): 241–46.

Tajiri J, Higashi K, Morita M, et al. Studies of hypothyroidism in patients with high iodine intake. *J Clin Endocrinol Metab*, 1986 Aug; 63 (2): 412–17.

Tan SW, Meiller JC, Mahaffey KR. The endocrine effects of mercury in humans and wildlife. *Crit Rev Toxicol*, 2009; 39 (3): 228–69.

Teng X, Shi X, Shan Z, et al. Safe range of iodine intake levels: A comparative study of thyroid diseases in three women population cohorts with slightly different iodine intake levels. *Biol Trace Elem Res*, 2008 Jan; 121 (1): 23–30.

Thomas D, Karachaliou F, Kallergi K, et al. Herpes virus antibodies seroprevalence in children with autoimmune thyroid disease. *Endocrine*, 2008 Apr; 33 (2): 171–75.

Todd CH, Dunn JT. Intermittent oral administration of potassium iodide solution for the correction of iodine deficiency. *Am J Clin Nutr*, 1998 Jun; 67 (6): 1279–83.

Tomer Y, Davies TF. Infection, thyroid disease, and autoimmunity. *Endocr Rev*, 1993 Feb; 14 (1): 107–20.

Tseng LH, Li MH, Tsai SS, et al. Developmental exposure to decabromodiphenyl ether (PBDE 209): Effects on thyroid hormone and hepatic enzyme activity in male mouse offspring. *Chemosphere*, 2008 Jan; 70 (4): 640–47.

Valentino R, Savastano S, Maglio M, et al. Markers of potential coeliac disease in patients with Hashimoto's thyroiditis. *Eur J Endocrinol*, 2002 Apr; 146 (4): 479–83.

Valentino R, Savastano S, Tommaselli AP, et al. Prevalence of coeliac disease in patients with thyroid autoimmunity. *Horm Res*, 1999; 51 (3): 124–27.

van der Poll T, Romijn JA, Wiersinga WM, Sauerwein HP. Tumor necrosis factor: A putative mediator of the sick euthyroid syndrome in man. *J Clin Endocrinol Metab*, 1990 Dec; 71 (6): 1567–72.

van Leeuwen FX, den Tonkelaar EM, van Logten MJ. Toxicity of sodium bromide in rats: Effects on endocrine system and reproduction. *Food Chem Toxicol*, 1983 Aug; 21 (4): 383–89.

Vas J, Monestier M. Immunology of mercury. *Ann N Y Acad Sci*, 2008 Nov; 1143: 240–67.

Velický J, Titlbach M, Dusková J, et al. Potassium bromide and the thyroid gland of the rat: Morphology and immunochemistry, RIA and INAA analysis. *Ann Anat*, 1997 Oct; 179 (5): 421–31.

Venturi S. Is there a role for iodine in breast diseases? *Breast*, 2001 Oct; 10 (5): 379–82.

Vgontzas AN, Bixler EO, Lin HM, et al. Chronic insomnia is associated with nyctohemeral activation of the hypothalamic-pituitary-adrenal axis: Clinical implications. *J Clin Endocrinol Metab*, 2001 Aug; 86 (8): 3787–94.

Viljoen M, Panzer A, Willemse N. Gastro intestinal hyperpermeability: A review. *East Afr Med J*, 2003 Jun; 80 (6): 324–30.

Vini L, Hyer S, Pratt B, Harmer C. Management of differentiated thyroid cancer diagnosed during pregnancy. *Eur J Endocrinol*, 1999 May; 140(5): 404–6.

Visser TJ. Role of sulfation in thyroid hormone metabolism. *Chem Biol Interact*, 1994 Jun; 92 (1–3): 293–303.

Vobecký M, Babický A. Effect of enhanced bromide intake on the concentration ratio I/Br in the rat thyroid gland. *Biol Trace Elem Res*, 1994 Fall; 43–45: 509–16.

Vobecký M, Babický A, Lener J, Svandová E. Interaction of bromine with iodine in the rat thyroid gland at enhanced bromide intake. *Biol Trace Elem Res*, 1996 Sep; 54 (3): 207–12.

Wagner H, Hörhammer L, Frank U. [Lithospermic acid, the antihormonally active principle of *Lycopus europaeus L.* and *Symphytum officinale*. 3. Ingredients of medicinal plants with hormonal and antihormonal-like effect.] [Article in German.] *Arzneimittelforschung*, 1970 May; 20 (5): 705–13.

Wagner H, Nörr H, Winterhoff H. Plant adaptogens. *Phytomedicine*, 1994 Jun; 1 (1): 63–76.

Wang J, Zhang W, Liu H, et al. Parvovirus B19 infection associated with Hashimoto's thyroiditis in adults. *J Infect*, 2010 May; 60 (5): 360–70.

Wartofsky L, Burman KD. Alterations in thyroid function in patients with systemic illness: The "euthyroid sick syndrome." *Endocr Rev*, 1982 Spring; 3 (2): 164–217.

Werga-Kjellman P, Zedenius J, Tallstedt L, et al. Surgical treatment of hyperthyroidism: A ten-year experience. *Thyroid*, 2001 Feb; 11 (2): 187–92.

Wiederkehr M, Krapf R. Metabolic and endocrine effects of metabolic acidosis in humans. *Swiss Med Wkly*, 2001 Mar 10; 131 (9–10): 127–32.

Williamson M. Thyroid dysfunction and its somatic reflection: A preliminary report. *J Am Osteopath Assoc*, 1973 Mar; 72 (7): 731–37.

Winterhoff H, Gumbinger HG, Vahlensieck U, et al. Endocrine effects of *Lycopus europaeus L.* following oral application. *Arzneimittlforschung*, 1994 Jan; 44 (1): 41–45.

Wise A, O'Brien K, Woodruff T. Are oral contraceptives a significant contributor to the estrogenicity of drinking water? *Environ Sci Technol*, 2011 Jan 1; 45 (1): 51–60.

Witte J, Goretzki PE, Dotzenrath C, et al. Surgery for Graves' disease: Total versus subtotal thyroidectomy — Results of a prospective randomized trial. *World J Surg*, 2000 Nov; 24 (11): 1303–11.

Wurtman RJ, Wurtman JJ, Regan MM, et al. Effects of normal meals rich in carbohydrates or proteins on plasma tryptophan and tyrosine ratios. *Am J Clin Nutr*, 2003 Jan; 77 (1): 128–32.

Yen PM. Molecular basis of resistance to thyroid hormone. *Trends Endocrinol Metab*, 2003 Sep; 14 (7): 327–33.

Zimmermann MB, Köhrle J. The impact of iron and selenium deficiencies on iodine and thyroid metabolism: Biochemistry and relevance to public health. *Thyroid*, 2002 Oct; 12 (10): 867–78.

Zoeller RT. Environmental chemicals impacting the thyroid: Targets and consequences. *Thyroid*, 2007 Sep; 17 (9): 811–17.

Zoeller RT. Thyroid toxicology and brain development: Should we think differently? *Environ Health Perspect*, 2003 Sep; 111 (12): A628.

Zoeller RT, Dowling AL, Vas AA. Developmental exposure to polychlorinated biphenyls exerts thyroid hormone-like effects on the expression of RC3/ neurogranin and myelin basic protein messenger ribonucleic acids in the developing rat brain. *Endocrinology*, 2000 Jan; 141 (1). 181–89.

Zoeller TR. Environmental chemicals targeting thyroid. *Hormones* (Athens), 2010 Jan–Mar; 9 (1): 28–40.

Zois C, Stavrou I, Kalogera C, et al. High prevalence of autoimmune thyroiditis in schoolchildren after elimination of iodine deficiency in northwestern Greece. *Thyroid*, 2003 May; 13 (5): 485–89.

Zois C, Stavrou I, Svarna E, et al. Natural course of autoimmune thyroiditis after elimination of iodine deficiency in northwestern Greece. *Thyroid*, 2006 Mar; 16 (3): 289–93.

Zulewski H, Müller B, Exer P, et al. Estimation of tissue hypothyroidism by a new clinical score: evaluation of patients with various grades of hypothyroidism and controls. *J Clin Endocrinol Metab*, 1997 Mar; 82 (3): 771–76.

Books

Baker SM, Bennett P, Bland JS, et al. *The Textbook of Functional Medicine*. Gig Harbor, WA: Institute for Functional Medicine, 2005.

Barnes BO. *Hypothyroidism: The Unsuspected Illness* New York: Harper & Row, 1976.

Berkow R, Fletcher AJ (eds.). *The Merck Manual of Diagnosis and Therapy*, 16th ed. Rahway, NJ: Merck Research Laboratories, 1992.

Blumenthal M, Busse WR, Goldberg A, et al. (eds.). *The Complete Commission E Monographs: Therapeutic Guide to Herbal Medicines*. Boston: Integrative Medicine Communications, 1998.

Braverman LE, Utiger RD. *Werner and Ingbar's The Thyroid: A Fundamental and Clinical Text*. Philadelphia: Lippincott Williams & Wilkins, 2000.

Fischbach F. *A Manual of Laboratory & Diagnostic Tests*, 5th ed. Philadelphia: J.B. Lippincott, 1996.

Guyton AC, Hall JE. *Textbook of Medical Physiology*, 9th ed. Philadelphia: W.B. Saunders, 1996.

Werbach MR. *Nutritional Influences on Illness*, 2nd ed. Tarzana, CA: Third Line Press, 1996.

Zoeller RT. Polychlorinated biphenyls as disruptors of thyroid hormone action. In Robertson LW, Hansen LG (eds.). *PCBs: Recent Advances in Environmental Toxicology and Health Effects*. Lexington, KY: University Press of Kentucky, 2001: 265–72.

Websites

American Association of Restorative Medicine. Table of Adaptogenic Herbs to Treat Adrenal Gland Dysfunction. Available at: http://restorativemedicine. org/books/fundamentals-of-naturopathic- endocrinology/professionals/adrenal-metabolism- disorders/table-of-adaptogenic-herbs-used-to-treat- adrenal-gland-dysfunction.

Linus Pauling Institute Micronutrient Information Center, Oregon State University. Vitamin B_{12}. Available at: http://lpi.oregonstate.edu/infocenter/ vitamins/vitaminB12.

Resources

Recommended Websites

Renew Your Health Naturally
Dr. Nikolas Hedberg's website
www.drhedberg.com

About Health: Thyroid Disease
Mary Shomon's website through About.com
thyroid.about.com

American Association of Clinical Endocrinologists
www.aace.com

AACE Thyroid Awareness
www.thyroidawareness.com

American Thyroid Association
www.thyroid.org

Environmental Working Group
An environmental toxin resource
www.ewg.org

EWG's Skin Deep Cosmetics Database
The Environmental Working Group's database
for thyroid-disrupting chemicals in cosmetics
www.ewg.org/skindeep

HypothyroidMom
A great blog with lots of resources
www.hypothyroidmom.com

International Academy of Oral Medicine and Toxicology
Where to find a mercury-free dentist
www.iaomt.org

National Academy of Hypothyroidism
A group of thyroidologists led by Dr. Kent Holtorf
www.nahypothyroidism.org

Stop the Thyroid Madness
Another great website for information
www.stopthethyroidmadness.com

Thyroid Change
Sign the petition so your voice is heard
www.thyroidchange.org

Thyroid Nation
A great site for thyroid information
www.thyroidnation.com

Thyroid UK
www.thyroiduk.org.uk

Recommended Books

Barnes, Broda O., and Lawrence Galton. *Hypothyroidism: The Unsuspected Illness.* New York: Harper, 1976.

Cohen, Suzy. *Thyroid Healthy: Lose Weight Look Beautiful and Live the Life You Imagine.* Boulder, CO: Dear Pharmacist Inc., 2014.

Shomon, Mary J. *Living Well with Hypothyroidism,* revised edition. New York: HarperCollins, 2005.

Wentz, Isabella, with Marta Nowosadzka. *Hashimoto's Thyroiditis: Lifestyle Interventions for Finding and Treating the Root Cause.* La Vergne, TN: Lightning Source, 2013.

Contributing Authors

Julia Aitken
Julia Aitkin's Easy Entertaining Cookbook
A recipe from this book is found on page 331.

Alexandra Anca, MHSc, RD, with Theresa Santandrea-Cull
Complete Gluten-Free Diet and Nutrition Guide
Recipes from this book are found on pages 180, 188, 202, 210, 231, 252, 253, 282, 285 and 324.

Byron Ayanoglu
The New Vegetarian Gourmet
A recipe from this book is found on page 212.

The Best Low-Carb Cookbook
A recipe from this book is found on page 224.

Johanna Burkhard and Barbara Allan, RD, CDE
The Diabetes Prevention & Management Cookbook
Recipes from this book are found on pages 176, 183, 197, 206–9, 222, 223, 234, 241, 244, 245, 247, 248 (bottom), 249, 283, 284, 286, 288, 304, 318, 325, 330, 349, 336, 338–40 and 342.

Dietitians of Canada
Cook Great Food
A recipe from this book is found on page 220.

Judith Finlayson
150 Best Slow Cooker Recipes
Recipes from this book are found on pages 312 and 327.

Judith Finlayson
The Complete Gluten-Free Whole Grains Cookbook
Recipes from this book are found on pages 173, 175, 178, 203, 214, 228, 254, 267, 281, 290, 298 and 346.

Judith Finlayson
Delicious & Dependable Slow Cooker Recipes
A recipe from this book is found on page 334.

Judith Finlayson
The Healthy Slow Cooker
A recipe from this book is found on page 322.

Judith Finlayson
The Healthy Slow Cooker, Second Edition
Recipes from this book are found on pages 174, 177, 181, 194–96, 198–201, 204, 242, 255–59, 280, 287, 294, 297, 305–8, 314, 320 and 350–53.

Judith Finlayson with Barbara Selley, BA, RD, Nutrition Editor
The Best Diabetes Slow Cooker Recipes
Recipes from this book are found on pages 250, 344, 260–63 and 310.

Margaret Howard
The 250 Best 4-Ingredient Recipes
A recipe from this book is found on page 271.

Sobia Khan, MSc, RD
150 Best Indian, Asian, Caribbean & More Diabetes Recipes
Recipes from this book are found on pages 190, 221, 230, 268, 278, 279, 292, 301, 313 and 319.

Linda Stephen
The Best Convection Oven Cookbook
A recipe from this book is found on page 226.

Suneeta Vaswani
Easy Indian Cooking, Second Edition
A recipe from this book is found on page 182.

Donna Washburn and Heather Butt
125 Best Gluten-Free Recipes
Recipes from this book are found on pages 186, 237, 238, 248 (top), 264, 296, 316, 362 and 363.

Donna Washburn and Heather Butt
250 Gluten-Free Favorites
Recipes from this book are found on pages 211, 216, 232, 236, 240, 272, 354–56 and 358.

Donna Washburn and Heather Butt
The Best Gluten-Free Family Cookbook
Recipes from this book are found on pages 184, 300, 329, 343, 348, 359 and 360.

Katherine E. Younker, Editor
America's Complete Diabetes Cookbook
Recipes from this book are found on pages 274, 277, 302, 309 and 326.

Sharon Zeiler, BSc, MBA, RD, editor
Canada's 250 Essential Diabetes Recipes
Recipes from this book are found on pages 218, 225, 270, 276, 317, 328, 332, 333, 335, 337, 341 and 361.

Library and Archives Canada Cataloguing in Publication

Hedberg, Nikolas R., 1977–, author
    The complete thyroid health & diet guide : understanding and managing thyroid disease / Dr. Nikolas R. Hedberg, DC, DABCI, DACBN, BCNP; Danielle Cook, MS, RD, CDE.

Includes index.
ISBN 978-0-7788-0504-5 (pbk.)

    1. Thyroid gland—Diseases. 2. Thyroid gland—Diseases—Diet therapy.
I. Cook, Danielle, 1975-, author II. Title. III. Title: Complete thyroid health and diet guide.

RC655.H43 2015   616.4'4   C2015-901360-7

Index

A

acetylation, 61
Achilles tendon reflex test, 30
achlorhydria, 105
acid/alkali balance, 135–41
    improving, 136–37
ACTH (adrenocorticotropic hormone), 80
adaptogens, 82–83
Addison's disease, 80
adrenal fatigue, 73, 76–77, 79, 81–85
adrenal glands, 14–15, 17, 29, 74–76
    dysfunctional, 76–77
    and other organs, 80, 81
adrenaline, 14, 74, 75
albumin, 16
alcohol, 49
aldosterone, 75
almonds and almond flour, 160
    Almond Sponge Cake, 359
    Black Sticky Rice Congee with Coconut, 177
    Crunchy Almond Chicken, 296
    Grain-Free Granola, 172
    Lemon Almond Sautéed Greens, 333
    Lemon Blueberry Almond Muffins, 356
    Salty Almonds with Thyme, 352
    Spicy Tamari Almonds, 353
    Spinach with Almonds, 252
    Steamed Vegetables with Toasted Almonds, 338
    Vanilla Almond Milk, 189
alpha lipoic acid (ALA), 84
aluminum, 67
amaranth, 160–61
    Almond Sponge Cake, 359
    Hot Millet Amaranth Cereal, 173
    Lemon Blueberry Almond Muffins, 356
amino acids, 20, 37, 132, 136–37
    as supplements, 62, 116, 133
amiodarone, 32
amphetamines, 30
anaphylaxis, 56, 57
androgens, 15
anemia (pernicious), 47
antacids, 44
antibacterial products, 68, 72

antibiotics, 40, 44
antibodies, 27, 32, 48, 49
anti-gliadin antibody test, 143
Anti-inflammatory Hummus, 243
antithyroglobulin, 48
apples
    Curried Squash and Apple Soup, 206
    Kale and Pear Salad with Warmed Shallot Dressing, 222
Armour Thyroid, 102
arsenic, 67
artichokes
    Artichoke and White Bean Spread, 242
    French Basil Chicken, 297
    Stuffed Artichokes, 324
ashwagandha, 82, 117
asparagus, 161
    Asparagus with Lemon and Garlic, 326
    Roasted Asparagus, 325
autoimmune thyroiditis. See thyroiditis
avocado
    Salmon and Wild Rice Cakes with Avocado-Chili Topping, 281
    Spanish Orange and Avocado Salad, 221
    Tomato Avocado Salsa, 249

B

bacon and pancetta
    Minestrone (variation), 211
    Zesty Braised Beef with New Potatoes, 314
bacteria, 39–41, 55
barrier hyperpermeability, 41–46
Basic Beans, 255
Basic Pesto, 246
Basic Tomato Sauce, 250
Basic Vegetable Stock, 194
basil, 161
    Basic Pesto, 246
    Broccoli Cilantro Pesto with Pasta, 329
    Cherry Tomato and Zucchini Sauté, 336
    Creamy Basil Pesto, 247
    French Basil Chicken, 297
    Herb-Glazed Brussels Sprouts, 331

    Pan-Roasted Trout with Fresh Tomato Basil Sauce, 286
    Parsley Pesto Sauce, 248
baths (alkalizing), 136
beans, 97, 161. See also beans, green; bean sprouts
    Artichoke and White Bean Spread, 242
    Basic Beans, 255
    Breakfast Burritos, 188
    Butternut Chili, 260
    Chili Black Bean Dip, 241
    Fassolada (Greek Bean Soup), 212
    Lentil Squash Salad (variation), 232
    Minestrone, 211
    Red Beans and Greens, 344
    Roasted Garlic Dip, 240
    Turkey Ratatouille Chili, 309
beans, green
    Catalan Beef Stew, 313
    Indian Peas and Beans, 258
    Minestrone (variation), 211
bean sprouts
    Shrimp and Vegetable Spring Rolls, 288
    Tofu Chop Suey, 270
beef
    Beef and Quinoa Soup, 216
    Butternut Chili, 260
    Catalan Beef Stew, 313
    Country Supper Cabbage Rolls, 317
    Hearty Beef Stock, 196
    Meatballs for Everyday, 316
    Minestrone (variation), 211
    Segovia-Style Lamb, 319
    Zesty Braised Beef with New Potatoes, 314
beets
    Beet Soup with Lemongrass and Lime, 198
    Cumin Beets, 327
    Kasha and Beet Salad with Celery and Feta, 228
Bengali Fish Curry, 279
berberine, 83
beta-glucuronidase, 54, 62
betaine hydrochloride, 55
beverages, 141, 142, 189–92
bexarotene, 30
bile, 59, 60, 63
bile acid sequestrants, 105
biotin, 84

bisphenol A (BPA), 64–65, 66, 159
bisphosphonates, 105
black cohosh, 119
Black Sticky Rice Congee with Coconut, 177
bladderwrack, 97–98
Bland, Jeffrey, 55
blood–brain barrier, 45
blood sugar, 78, 85, 114
  balancing, 83–84, 126–28
blood sugar–adrenal–thyroid axis, 78–80
blueberries, 162
  Buckwheat Walnut Bread (variation), 186
  Cranberry Quinoa Porridge (variation), 175
  Lemon Blueberry Almond Muffins, 356
  Power Smoothie 1, 191
blue flag, 106
body burden, 68, 72
body type, 123–25
Borrelia burgdorferi, 39
Brazil nuts, 48, 162
breads, 130, 138–39
Breakfast Burritos, 188
breakfasts, 171–92
breastfeeding, 95, 110
breast health, 94
breathing (deep), 113, 136
broccoli, 162
  Asparagus with Lemon and Garlic (tip), 326
  Broccoli Cilantro Pesto with Pasta, 329
  Garden-Fresh Frittata, 184
  Marinated Vegetable Medley, 225
  Potato, Leek and Broccoli Soup, 202
  Sautéed Broccoli and Red Peppers, 328
  Savory Vegetarian Quinoa Pilaf (variation), 343
  Steamed Vegetables with Toasted Almonds, 338
bromine, 92, 98, 111
Brussels sprouts
  Braised Brussels Sprouts, 330
  Herb-Glazed Brussels Sprouts, 331
buckwheat, 162
  Buckwheat Walnut Bread, 186
  Buttermilk Buckwheat Pancakes, 178
  Kasha and Beet Salad with Celery and Feta, 228
  Butternut Chili, 260
B vitamins, 18, 47

C

cabbage
  Country Supper Cabbage Rolls, 317
  Lemon Almond Sautéed Greens, 333
  Minestrone (variation), 211
  Miso Mushroom Chicken with Chinese Cabbage, 305
  Shrimp and Vegetable Spring Rolls, 288
Cactus Salad, 230
cadmium, 67, 70
caffeine, 50, 77, 85
calcium, 46
calcium d-glucarate, 86, 91
calorie intake, 125–26
Candida albicans, 40–41
carbimazole, 104
carbohydrates, 20, 122, 127–28, 142
L-carnitine, 38, 84
carrots. See also vegetables
  Basic Tomato Sauce, 250
  Beef and Quinoa Soup, 216
  Gingery Chicken and Wild Rice Soup, 214
  Lamb with Lentils and Chard, 322
  Mix 'n' Mash Vegetables, 337
  Moroccan-Spiced Carrot Soup, 197
  Shrimp and Vegetable Spring Rolls, 288
  Spinach Salad with Carrots and Mushrooms, 223
case histories
  adrenal fatigue, 73
  autoimmune thyroiditis, 36–37
  dietary changes, 12, 58, 122
  excess estrogen, 86–87
  food sensitivities, 51
  Hashimoto's thyroiditis, 51
  hypothyroidism, 111
  infections, 51
  iodine deficiency, 92
  lifestyle changes, 111
  medication, 102
  supplements, 12, 58, 86
  tests, 23
cashews
  Grain-Free Granola, 172
  Spicy Cashews, 351
Catalan Beef Stew, 313
cation-exchange resins (Kayexalate/Kalexate), 105
cauliflower
  Cauliflower Pizza Crust, 266
  Creamy Mashed Potatoes with Cauliflower, 342

Marinated Vegetable Medley, 225
Steamed Vegetables with Toasted Almonds, 338
celery, 162–63. See also vegetables
  Baked Salmon Patties, 282
  Curried Squash and Apple Soup, 206
  Gingery Chicken and Wild Rice Soup, 214
  Kasha and Beet Salad with Celery and Feta, 228
  Tofu Chop Suey, 270
celery root
  Celery Root and Mushroom Lasagna, 262
  Vichyssoise with Celery Root and Watercress, 200
celiac disease, 43, 105, 143
cereals, 130, 172–77
chamomile (German), 118
cheese. See also cheese, Parmesan
  Baked Salmon Patties, 282
  Breakfast Burritos, 188
  Cactus Salad, 230
  Celery Root and Mushroom Lasagna, 262
  Creamy Basil Pesto, 247
  Crustless Dill Spinach Quiche with Mushrooms and Cheese, 274
  Fast and Easy Greek Salad, 220
  Garden-Fresh Frittata, 184
  Kasha and Beet Salad with Celery and Feta, 228
  Quinoa-Stuffed Tomatoes, 267
  Vegetable Quiche with Oat Groat Crust, 272
  Wild Rice Cakes, 254
  Zucchini Patties, 253
cheese, Parmesan
  Artichoke and White Bean Spread, 242
  Basic Pesto, 246
  Broccoli Cilantro Pesto with Pasta, 329
  Crispy-Coated Veggie Snacks, 348
  Parsley Pesto Sauce, 248
  Western Omelet, 183
chelation, 70
chemicals (thyroid-disrupting), 63–66, 68, 69, 72
Cherry Tomato and Zucchini Sauté, 336
chicken. See also turkey
  Crunchy Almond Chicken, 296
  French Basil Chicken, 297
  Gingery Chicken and Wild Rice Soup, 214
  Homemade Chicken Stock, 195

Indian-Style Chicken with Puréed Spinach, 306
Indian-Style Grilled Chicken Breasts, 302
Italian-Style Chicken in White Wine with Olives and Polenta, 298
Jerk Chicken, 301
Lemon Garlic Chicken, 300
Minestrone (variation), 211
Miso Mushroom Chicken with Chinese Cabbage, 305
Spicy Peanut Chicken, 308
Tandoori Chicken with Cucumber Mint Raita, 304
chickpeas. *See also* beans
Anti-inflammatory Hummus, 243
Sautéed Broccoli and Red Peppers (variation), 328
Spicy Lamb with Chickpeas, 320
Chili Black Bean Dip, 241
chlordanes, 66
cholesterol, 28, 32, 134
chromium, 83
cilantro, 163
Broccoli Cilantro Pesto with Pasta, 329
Cactus Salad, 230
Chili Black Bean Dip (variation), 241
Cucumber Mint Raita, 248
Mexican-Style Seafood Stew with Hominy, 290
Pan-Roasted Trout with Fresh Tomato Basil Sauce (variation), 286
Pork Quinoa Salad with Indian Dressing, 236
Shrimp and Vegetable Spring Rolls, 288
Spicy Peanut Chicken, 308
Sweet Potato Coconut Curry with Shrimp, 287
Turkey Mole, 310
cinnamon, 163
Cinnamon Crisps, 363
Grain-Free Granola, 172
ciprofloxacin, 105
circadian rhythm, 75, 114
cirrhosis (biliary), 105
cleanses, 71
coconut, 163
Grain-Free Granola, 172
coconut milk
Black Sticky Rice Congee with Coconut, 177
Coconut Pancakes, 179
Gingery Red Lentils with Spinach and Coconut, 256

Poached Eggs on Spicy Lentils, 181
Spicy Peanut Chicken, 308
Sweet Potato Coconut Curry with Shrimp, 287
Thai-Style Pumpkin Soup, 204
coffee, 105. *See also* caffeine
Coindet, Jean-François, 94
condiments, 140–41
constipation, 40, 43, 50, 55
copper, 70
corn and hominy
Fish Fillets with Corn and Red Pepper Salsa, 277
Mexican-Style Seafood Stew with Hominy, 290
cortisol, 15, 17, 75, 79–80
effects, 18, 28, 53, 75, 77
cosmetic products, 68, 72
Country Supper Cabbage Rolls, 317
Courtois, Bernard, 94
cranberries, 97
Cranberry Quinoa Porridge, 175
Hot Oat Bran and Flax Porridge, 176
Lemon Blueberry Almond Muffins (variation), 356
Lentil Squash Salad, 232
Pumpkin Date Bars (variation), 360
Spinach Salad with Carrots and Mushrooms, 223
cream. *See* milk and cream
Creamy Basil Pesto, 247
Creamy Mashed Potatoes with Cauliflower, 342
Creamy Polenta, 346
Crêpes, 180
cretinism, 48
CRH (corticotropin-releasing hormone), 80
Crispy-Coated Veggie Snacks, 348
Crunchy Almond Chicken, 296
Crunchy Peanut Butter Muffins, 354
Crustless Dill Spinach Quiche with Mushrooms and Cheese, 274
cucumber
Cucumber Mint Raita, 248
Fast and Easy Greek Salad, 220
Grilled Salmon and Romaine Salad, 234
Marinated Vegetable Medley, 225
Pork Quinoa Salad with Indian Dressing, 236
Cumin Beets, 327
Curried Squash and Apple Soup, 206

D

dairy products, 130, 132–33, 140
DDT, 65, 66
dental amalgams, 45, 66
Depo-Provera, 89
desserts, 359–63
detoxification, 59, 60–61, 62, 70–71. *See also* liver
DHEA (dehydroepiandrosterone), 75–76, 84, 88
diabetes, 31, 79
Dicke, Willem-Karel, 143
diet. *See also* eating habits; foods; nutrients
body type and, 123–25
elimination, 43, 49
gluten challenge, 144
and hormone levels, 83, 85, 90
low-carbohydrate, 122, 127
paleo, 56
proteins in, 58, 132–33, 137, 159
vegan, 97, 132
vegetarian, 58, 132
digestive system. *See* gastrointestinal (GI) tract
diindolylmethane (DIM), 86, 90, 91
dioxins, 65, 66
dips and spreads, 238, 240–45
dopamine, 30
dysbiosis, 40, 52

E

eating habits, 141–44. *See also* diet; foods
ectomorphs, 123–24
eggs, 97
Almond Sponge Cake, 359
Breakfast Burritos, 188
Coconut Pancakes, 179
Garden-Fresh Frittata, 184
Indian Scrambled Eggs, 182
Poached Eggs on Spicy Lentils, 181
Tofu Vegetable Quiche, 271
Vegetable Quiche with Oat Groat Crust, 272
Western Omelet, 183
Zucchini Patties, 253
eleuthero, 83
endocrine system, 13–15. *See also specific hormones*
endomorphs, 123, 124
energy equilibrium (homeostasis), 125–26
enzymes, 20
epinephrine. *See* adrenaline
Epsom salts, 136
Epstein-Barr virus, 36, 37, 39, 54

essential fatty acids (EFAs), 82, 133–35

estrogen, 15, 89–90, 94. *See also* DHEA
  in environment, 90, 91
  excess, 17, 39, 49, 86–87, 90, 91

euthyroid sick syndrome, 31

exercise, 121, 126
  deep breathing, 113, 136
  effects, 83, 88, 120–21

F

Fassolada (Greek Bean Soup), 212

Fast and Easy Greek Salad, 220

fasting, 127

fat
  body, 91
  dietary, 20, 133–35, 140, 159

fatty liver disease, 62

fennel, 164
  Roasted Portobello Mushroom and Fennel Salad, 226

ferritin levels, 58

fiber (dietary), 86, 105, 159

fibrocystic breast disease, 92, 94

fibroids (uterine), 92

fish, 97. *See also* salmon; seafood
  Bengali Fish Curry, 279
  Crunchy Almond Chicken (variation), 296
  Fish Chowder, 218
  Fish Fillets with Corn and Red Pepper Salsa, 277
  Fish for the Sole, 285
  Mediterranean-Style Mahi-Mahi, 280
  Mexican-Style Seafood Stew with Hominy, 290
  Pan-Roasted Trout with Fresh Tomato Basil Sauce, 286
  Peruvian Ceviche, 278
  Poached Fish, 276
  Sardine Spread, 245

flame retardants, 64, 72

flavorings, 140–41

flax seeds
  Homemade Crunchy Granola Bars, 361
  Hot Oat Bran and Flax Porridge, 176
  Power Smoothie 1, 191

flours, 138–39. *See also* gluten-free flours

flu, 39

fluorine, 98–99

foods, 72, 158–59
  allergies/sensitivities to, 42–43, 49, 51, 55, 56–57

  healing, 160–69

low-glycemic-index, 128–31
  organic, 91, 128, 158

4R protocol, 55

French Basil Chicken, 297

French lilac, 83

fruit, 127, 129, 137. *See also* fruit, dried; *specific fruits*
  Black Sticky Rice Congee with Coconut, 177
  Kale and Pear Salad with Warmed Shallot Dressing, 222
  Mango Yogurt Smoothie, 190

fruit, dried, 97. *See also specific fruits*
  Cranberry Quinoa Porridge, 175
  Pork Quinoa Salad with Indian Dressing, 236
  Pumpkin Date Bars, 360
  Spinach Salad with Carrots and Mushrooms, 223

fungicides, 65

G

GABA (gamma-aminobutyric acid), 117

gallbladder. *See* bile; hepatic system

GALT (gut-associated lymphoid tissue), 53, 81

Garden-Fresh Frittata, 184

garlic, 164
  Anti-inflammatory Hummus, 243
  Basic Pesto, 246
  Creamy Basil Pesto, 247
  Hearty Beef Stock, 196
  Lentil and Spinach Soup, 210
  Lentil Tapenade, 244
  Parsley Pesto Sauce, 248
  Pork Vindaloo, 312
  Roasted Garlic and Sun-Dried Tomato Dressing, 238
  Sweet Potato Coconut Curry with Shrimp, 287
  Zucchini Patties, 253

gastrointestinal (GI) tract, 51–57, 81. *See also* leaky gut syndrome
  treating dysfunction in, 55, 57, 105

GI–estrogen–thyroid axis, 54

ginger, 164
  Baked Salmon with Ginger and Lemon, 283
  Beet Soup with Lemongrass and Lime, 198
  Bengali Fish Curry, 279
  Curried Squash and Apple Soup, 206

Gingery Chicken and Wild Rice Soup, 214

Gingery Red Lentils with Spinach and Coconut, 256

Indian-Style Grilled Chicken Breasts, 302

Onion-Braised Shrimp, 294

Peruvian Ceviche, 278

Poached Eggs on Spicy Lentils, 181

Spicy Lamb with Chickpeas, 320

Spinach and Tofu Curry, 268

Steamed Sugar Snap Peas with Ginger, 349

Sweet Potato Coconut Curry with Shrimp, 287

Tandoori Chicken with Cucumber Mint Raita, 304

Thai-Inspired Peanut and Wild Rice Soup, 203

Thai-Style Pumpkin Soup, 204

ginseng (Korean), 82

glands, 13. *See also specific glands*

glucocorticoids, 30

glucuronidation, 18, 61

glutathione, 18, 61, 72

gluten-free flours
  Buckwheat Walnut Bread, 186
  Cinnamon Crisps, 363
  Crêpes, 180
  Crunchy Peanut Butter Muffins, 354
  Lemon Blueberry Almond Muffins, 356
  Peanut Butter Cookies, 362
  Pumpkin Date Bars, 360
  Pumpkin Millet Muffins, 358
  Thin Pizza Crust, 264

gluten intolerance, 43, 47, 49, 143–44

glycemic index, 128

glycine, 18

glycine conjugation, 61

goiter, 14, 93

gonads, 15

Grain-Free Granola, 172

grains, 131, 136, 138–39, 144. *See also* flours; *specific grains*

grapefruit juice, 105

Graves' disease, 38, 48

Green Goddess Salad Dressing, 237

greens, leafy, 136. *See also* kale; spinach
  Lamb with Lentils and Chard, 322
  Lemon Almond Sautéed Greens, 333
  Red Beans and Greens, 344
  Vichyssoise with Celery Root and Watercress, 200

greens, salad
  Grilled Salmon and Romaine Salad, 234
  Roasted Portobello Mushroom and Fennel Salad, 226
  Shrimp and Vegetable Spring Rolls, 288
  Spanish Orange and Avocado Salad, 221
guggul, 98
gut barrier, 42–44, 50, 55

H

H2 receptor antagonists, 105
hair analysis, 69
halides, 98–99
Hashimoto's thyroiditis, 37–38, 51, 96, 102
HCB (hexachlorobenzene), 65, 66
heart disease, 19
Hearty Beef Stock, 196
Helicobacter pylori, 40, 51, 53, 81
hemithyroidectomy (thyroid lobectomy), 108
hepatic system, 59–62, 72. *See also* liver
hepatitis C, 39
herbal remedies, 36, 38, 117
  for blood sugar balance, 83
  for sleep, 116–20
  for thyroid dysfunction, 106, 107
herbs, 160. *See also specific herbs*
  Crustless Dill Spinach Quiche with Mushrooms and Cheese, 274
  Garden-Fresh Frittata, 184
  Green Goddess Salad Dressing, 237
  Grilled Salmon with Lemon Oregano Pesto, 284
  Herb-Glazed Brussels Sprouts, 331
  Meatballs for Everyday, 316
  Roasted Garlic and Sun-Dried Tomato Dressing, 238
Homemade Chicken Stock, 195
Homemade Crunchy Granola Bars, 361
honey
  Grain-Free Granola, 172
  Homemade Crunchy Granola Bars, 361
  Lemon Blueberry Almond Muffins, 356
hops, 118
hormone replacement therapy (HRT), 89
hormones, 13–16. *See also* endocrine system; hormones, thyroid; *specific hormones*
  adrenal, 14, 74–76
  balancing, 91
  chemicals and, 63
  circadian rhythm and, 75
  imbalance in, 17, 86–91
  liver and, 60
  as supplements, 84, 89
  tests for, 87, 91
hormones, thyroid, 16, 87. *See also specific hormones*
  conversion of, 17–18, 28, 29, 52, 53, 54
  and diabetes, 79
  elimination of, 18–19
  and energy equilibrium, 126
  and hepatic system, 59–60
  iodine and, 92–93
  medications and, 18–19, 30
  natural vs. synthetic, 102, 103
  during pregnancy, 30–31
  replacing, 103–4, 105
  resistance to, 28
  as supplements, 84, 103–4, 105, 107
  tests for, 27–31
Hot Millet Amaranth Cereal, 173
Hot Oat Bran and Flax Porridge, 176
hydrochloric acid, 52–53, 55, 106
5-hydroxytryptophan (5-HTP), 116
hyperpermeability, 41–46
hyperthyroidism, 24, 95
  treatments for, 104, 108, 109–10
hypocalcemia, 108
hypoglycemia, 79
hypothalamic–pituitary–adrenal (HPA) axis, 80
hypothalamic–pituitary–thyroid axis, 13–14, 103
hypothalamus, 13–14, 87
hypothyroidism, 24, 31, 111. *See also* iodine deficiency
  after treatments, 108, 109
  low-carbohydrate diets and, 122, 127, 128
  medications for, 103–4
  screening for, 32–33

I

immune system, 21, 36–50, 81
immunoglobulin A (IgA), 57
immunoglobulin E (IgE) antibody response, 56
immunoglobulin G (IgG) food sensitivities, 49, 57
Indian Peas and Beans, 258
Indian Scrambled Eggs, 182
Indian-Style Chicken with Puréed Spinach, 306
Indian-Style Grilled Chicken Breasts, 302
infections, 36–37, 39, 49, 52
inflammation, 62
influenza, 39
insomnia. *See* sleep
insulin, 15, 17, 18
insulin resistance, 62, 78–79, 91
interleukin, 30
intrinsic factor, 47
iodine, 16, 92–99
  deficiency of, 92, 93–96
  excess, 93, 94
  hormones and, 80, 94
  radioactive, 109–10
  sources, 93, 95, 96–98
  as supplement, 47, 49, 86, 93, 96, 99
  tests for, 99
  and thyroid hormones, 92–93
iron supplements, 58
islets of Langerhans, 15
isolation (social), 112
Italian-Style Chicken in White Wine with Olives and Polenta, 298

J

Jerk Chicken, 301

K

kale, 164
  Kale and Pear Salad with Warmed Shallot Dressing, 222
  Oven-Baked Kale Chips, 350
  Power Smoothie 1, 191
  Power Smoothie 2, 192
Kasha and Beet Salad with Celery and Feta, 228
kava, 118
Kayexalate/Kalexate, 105
kelp, 97–98
Kocher, Emil Theodor, 94

L

lamb
  Grilled Lamb Chops with Rosemary Mustard Baste, 318
  Lamb with Lentils and Chard, 322
  Segovia-Style Lamb, 319
  Spicy Lamb with Chickpeas, 320
lavender, 119
lead, 67, 70
leaky gut syndrome, 41–44, 56, 62, 70, 81

leeks. *See also* vegetables
Catalan Beef Stew, 313
Garden-Fresh Frittata, 184
Gingery Chicken and Wild Rice Soup, 214
Potato, Leek and Broccoli Soup, 202
Vichyssoise with Celery Root and Watercress, 200
legumes, 130. *See also* beans; lentils; peas
lemon
Baked Salmon with Ginger and Lemon, 283
Grilled Salmon with Lemon Oregano Pesto, 284
Lemon Almond Sautéed Greens, 333
Lemon Blueberry Almond Muffins, 356
Lemon Garlic Chicken, 300
Sardine Spread, 245
lemon balm, 119
lemongrass
Beet Soup with Lemongrass and Lime, 198
Thai-Inspired Peanut and Wild Rice Soup, 203
Thai-Style Pumpkin Soup, 204
lentils, 161
Basic Beans (variation), 255
Gingery Red Lentils with Spinach and Coconut, 256
Lamb with Lentils and Chard, 322
Lentil and Spinach Soup, 210
Lentil Squash Salad, 232
Lentil-Stuffed Tomatoes, 335
Lentil Tapenade, 244
Mushroom Lentil Soup, 209
Poached Eggs on Spicy Lentils, 181
leptin, 87–88
Levothroid, 104
levothyroxine (Sythnroid), 8, 102, 103
Levoxyl, 104
licorice, 106
lifestyle changes, 50, 111–21. *See also* exercise; sleep; thyroid diet
lime
Beet Soup with Lemongrass and Lime, 198
Cactus Salad, 230
Pan-Roasted Trout with Fresh Tomato Basil Sauce (variation), 286
Peruvian Ceviche, 278
Shrimp and Vegetable Spring Rolls, 288

Thai-Inspired Peanut and Wild Rice Soup, 203
Thai-Style Pumpkin Soup, 204
lithium, 32, 64
liver, 15, 59, 60–61, 62, 80. *See also* detoxification; hepatic system
lung barrier, 45
Lyme disease, 39

M

macronutrients, 20, 125
magnesium, 18, 50, 83, 114
magnesium glycinate, 137
magnolia, 82
Mango Yogurt Smoothie, 190
Marinated Vegetable Medley, 225
Marine, David, 94
Meatballs for Everyday, 316
medications, 44, 93, 102–7. *See also* herbal remedies; *specific drugs*
and thyroid hormones, 18–19, 30
meditation, 112
Mediterranean-Style Mahi-Mahi, 280
melatonin, 14, 114–16
menopause, 76, 89, 119
menstrual problems, 90
mercury, 45, 67–68
selenium and, 48, 70
mesomorphs, 124
metabolism, 18, 19–21
metals (toxic), 18, 41, 45, 66–68
eliminating, 70–71
tests for, 69
metformin, 30, 83
methimazole (Tapazole), 104
methionine, 18
methylation, 61
methylparaben, 65
Mexican-Style Seafood Stew with Hominy, 290
micronutrients, 20–21, 83
milk and cream (dairy or non-dairy), 97
Creamy Polenta, 346
Crêpes, 180
Fish Chowder, 218
Hot Oat Bran and Flax Porridge, 176
Mango Yogurt Smoothie, 190
Power Smoothie 1, 191
Power Smoothie 2, 192
Steel-Cut Oats (tip), 174
Vichyssoise with Celery Root and Watercress, 200
millet, 165
Hot Millet Amaranth Cereal, 173

Pumpkin Millet Muffins, 358
Quinoa-Stuffed Tomatoes (variation), 267
minerals (dietary), 21, 83. *See also specific minerals*
Minestrone, 211
mint
Cherry Tomato and Zucchini Sauté, 336
Cucumber Mint Raita, 248
Herb-Glazed Brussels Sprouts, 331
Spanish Orange and Avocado Salad, 221
Miso Mushroom Chicken with Chinese Cabbage, 305
mitochondria, 19
Mix 'n' Mash Vegetables, 337
molybdenum, 18
Moroccan-Spiced Carrot Soup, 197
muffins, 354–58
mushrooms, 165
Celery Root and Mushroom Lasagna, 262
Crispy-Coated Veggie Snacks, 348
Crustless Dill Spinach Quiche with Mushrooms and Cheese, 274
Garden-Fresh Frittata, 184
Miso Mushroom Chicken with Chinese Cabbage, 305
Mushroom Lentil Soup, 209
Roasted Portobello Mushroom and Fennel Salad, 226
Segovia-Style Lamb, 319
Spinach Salad with Carrots and Mushrooms, 223
Turkey Ratatouille Chili, 309
Warm Spinach and Mushroom Salad, 224
Western Omelet, 183

N

N-acetylcysteine, 18
Nature-Throid, 104
New Orleans Braised Onions, 334
nickel carbonyl, 70
noradrenaline (norepinephrine), 74
NSAIDs (nonsteroidal anti-inflammatory drugs), 44, 50
nutrients
for blood sugar balance, 83–84
deficiencies of, 17, 44, 47–48
essential, 19, 82, 133–35
for liver detoxification, 59, 61
need for, 19–21

nuts and nut butters, 140, 165.
    See also specific nuts
    Homemade Crunchy Granola
        Bars, 361
    Kale and Pear Salad with
        Warmed Shallot Dressing,
        222
    Power Smoothie 1, 191
    Power Smoothie 2, 192

O

oats and oat bran, 165
    Homemade Crunchy Granola
        Bars, 361
    Hot Oat Bran and Flax
        Porridge, 176
    Oat Groat Crust, 273
    Steel-Cut Oats, 174
obesity, 31
oils (cooking), 134, 140
Old-Fashioned Split Pea Soup, 208
olives, 165–66
    Italian-Style Chicken in
        White Wine with Olives and
        Polenta, 298
    Lentil Tapenade, 244
omega-3 fatty acids, 82, 133–35
onions, 166. *See also* vegetables
    Basic Tomato Sauce, 250
    Bengali Fish Curry, 279
    New Orleans Braised Onions,
        334
    Onion-Braised Shrimp, 294
    Roasted Butternut Squash with
        Onion and Sage, 340
    Shrimp and Vegetable Spring
        Rolls, 288
    Sweet Potato Coconut Curry
        with Shrimp, 287
    Warm Spinach and Mushroom
        Salad, 224
opiates, 30
orange
    Grilled Salmon and Romaine
        Salad, 234
    New Orleans Braised Onions,
        334
    Pumpkin Date Bars, 360
    Spanish Orange and Avocado
        Salad, 221
oregano, 166
    Catalan Beef Stew, 313
    Grilled Salmon with Lemon
        Oregano Pesto, 284
orlistat, 105
Oven-Baked Kale Chips, 350

P

pancetta. *See* bacon and pancetta
pantethine, 82

parabens, 65
parasites, 41
parathyroid glands, 108
parsley
    Green Goddess Salad Dressing,
        237
    Grilled Salmon and Romaine
        Salad, 234
    Mediterranean-Style Mahi-
        Mahi, 280
    Parsley Pesto Sauce, 248
parsnips
    Baked Sweet Potato Fries
        (variation), 341
    Spicy Lamb with Chickpeas,
        320
parvovirus B19 (fifth disease),
    39
passionflower, 119
pasta, 130
    Broccoli Cilantro Pesto with
        Pasta, 329
    Celery Root and Mushroom
        Lasagna, 262
    Minestrone, 211
PBDEs (polybrominated diphenyl
    ethers), 64
PCBs (polychlorinated biphenyls),
    63–64, 66
PCOS (polycystic ovarian
    syndrome), 78, 88
peanuts and peanut butter, 166
    Crunchy Peanut Butter
        Muffins, 354
    Peanut Butter Cookies, 362
    Pork Quinoa Salad with Indian
        Dressing (variation), 236
    Shrimp and Vegetable Spring
        Rolls, 288
    Spicy Peanut Chicken, 308
    Thai-Inspired Peanut and Wild
        Rice Soup, 203
peas, dried. *See also* beans;
        chickpeas
    Basic Beans (variation), 255
    Indian Peas and Beans, 258
    Lentil Squash Salad, 232
    Split Pea Soup, Old-Fashioned,
        208
peas, green
    Quinoa Salad, 231
    Spicy Peanut Chicken, 308
    Steamed Sugar Snap Peas with
        Ginger, 349
    Valencia Seafood Paella, 292
pecans
    Cinnamon Crisps, 363
    Lemon Blueberry Almond
        Muffins (variation), 356
peppers, bell. *See also* vegetables
    Beet Soup with Lemongrass
        and Lime, 198

Fish Fillets with Corn and Red
    Pepper Salsa, 277
French Basil Chicken, 297
Quinoa Salad, 231
Red Pepper Coulis, 254
Sardine Spread, 245
Sautéed Broccoli and Red
    Peppers, 328
Shrimp and Vegetable Spring
    Rolls, 288
Spanish Orange and Avocado
    Salad, 221
Tofu Chop Suey, 270
Valencia Seafood Paella, 292
Western Omelet, 183
peppers, chile
    Beet Soup with Lemongrass
        and Lime, 198
    Bengali Fish Curry, 279
    Breakfast Burritos, 188
    Butternut Chili, 260
    Cactus Salad, 230
    Chili Black Bean Dip
        (variation), 241
    Indian Scrambled Eggs, 182
    Indian-Style Chicken with
        Puréed Spinach, 306
    Jerk Chicken, 301
    Mexican-Style Seafood Stew
        with Hominy, 290
    Onion-Braised Shrimp, 294
    Pan-Roasted Trout with
        Fresh Tomato Basil Sauce
        (variation), 286
    Quinoa-Stuffed Tomatoes, 267
    Spinach and Tofu Curry, 268
    Thai-Inspired Peanut and Wild
        Rice Soup, 203
    Tomato Avocado Salsa, 249
    Turkey Mole, 310
perchlorates, 65, 66
perilla oil, 82
Peruvian Ceviche, 278
pesticides, 65
pH, 135–41
phellodendron, 82
phenols, 64–65, 66
phosphatidylserine, 82, 117
phthalates, 64, 66
pineal gland, 14
pine nuts
    Basic Pesto, 246
    Cherry Tomato and Zucchini
        Sauté, 336
    Roasted Portobello Mushroom
        and Fennel Salad, 226
pituitary gland, 13–14, 28, 29–30,
    80
    and other glands, 13–14, 80,
        103
Pizza Crust, Thin, 264
plastics, 64–65, 66, 72

polycystic ovarian syndrome (PCOS), 78, 88
pork
  Country Supper Cabbage Rolls, 317
  Meatballs for Everyday, 316
  Pork Quinoa Salad with Indian Dressing, 236
  Pork Vindaloo, 312
  Turkey Ratatouille Chili (variation), 309
porphyrin testing, 69
post-workout recipes
  main dishes, 292, 309, 320–22
  salads, 230–33
  side dishes, 340–46
  soups, 208–15
  vegetarian, 254–65
potassium bicarbonate, 137
potatoes, 97, 166
  Baked Sweet Potato Fries (variation), 341
  Creamy Mashed Potatoes with Cauliflower, 342
  Fish Chowder, 218
  Gingery Red Lentils with Spinach and Coconut, 256
  Potato, Leek and Broccoli Soup, 202
  Turkey Ratatouille Chili, 309
  Zesty Braised Beef with New Potatoes, 314
Power Smoothie 1, 191
Power Smoothie 2, 192
prebiotics, 40, 44
prednisone, 105
pregnancy, 30–31, 95, 108, 110
pregnenolone, 76, 84, 91
probiotics, 41, 44, 50, 55
progesterone, 89, 90. See also DHEA
propylthiouracil, 104
prostate health, 94
proteins, 16, 20, 139
  in diet, 58, 132–33, 137, 159
proton pump inhibitors, 105
Provera, 89
pumpkin, 207. See also squash
  Curried Squash and Apple Soup, 206
  Pumpkin Date Bars, 360
  Pumpkin Millet Muffins, 358
  Thai-Style Pumpkin Soup, 204

Q

quiches, 271–74
quinoa, 166–67
  Beef and Quinoa Soup, 216
  Cranberry Quinoa Porridge, 175
  Quinoa Salad, 231
  Quinoa-Stuffed Tomatoes, 267
  Savory Vegetarian Quinoa Pilaf, 343

R

raloxifene, 105
Red Beans and Greens, 344
rheumatoid factor, 29
rhodiola, 82
rice and wild rice
  Black Sticky Rice Congee with Coconut, 177
  Country Supper Cabbage Rolls, 317
  Gingery Chicken and Wild Rice Soup, 214
  Kasha and Beet Salad with Celery and Feta (variation), 228
  Salmon and Wild Rice Cakes with Avocado-Chili Topping, 281
  Thai-Inspired Peanut and Wild Rice Soup, 203
  Valencia Seafood Paella, 292
  Wild Rice Cakes, 254
Rickettsia, 39
ritonavir, 30
rosemary, 137, 160
  Grilled Lamb Chops with Rosemary Mustard Baste, 318
  Vegetable Quiche with Oat Groat Crust, 272
rT3 (reverse T3), 17, 18, 54
  cortisol and, 53, 79
  tests for, 23, 27
rubella, 39
rutabaga
  Baked Sweet Potato Fries (variation), 341
  Mix 'n' Mash Vegetables, 337

S

Saccharomyces boulardii, 55
sage
  Italian-Style Chicken in White Wine with Olives and Polenta, 298
  Roasted Butternut Squash with Onion and Sage, 340
  Roasted Garlic Dip, 240
St. John's wort, 30
salad dressings, 236–38
salads, 220–34
salmon, 167
  Baked Salmon Patties, 282
  Baked Salmon with Ginger and Lemon, 283
  Grilled Salmon and Romaine Salad, 234
  Grilled Salmon with Lemon Oregano Pesto, 284
  Salmon and Wild Rice Cakes with Avocado-Chili Topping, 281
salt, 85, 93, 95, 97, 136, 160
  Salty Almonds with Thyme, 352
sardines, 167
  Sardine Spread, 245
sauces, 246–50
Savory Vegetarian Quinoa Pilaf, 343
seafood, 97. See also fish
  Mexican-Style Seafood Stew with Hominy, 290
  Onion-Braised Shrimp, 294
  Shrimp and Vegetable Spring Rolls, 288
  Sweet Potato Coconut Curry with Shrimp, 287
  Valencia Seafood Paella, 292
seaweed, 97–98
seeds, 140, 168
  Grain-Free Granola, 172
  Hot Oat Bran and Flax Porridge, 176
  Kale and Pear Salad with Warmed Shallot Dressing (variation), 222
  Lentil Squash Salad, 232
  Power Smoothie 2, 192
  Pumpkin Millet Muffins, 358
  Spinach Salad with Carrots and Mushrooms, 223
Segovia-Style Lamb, 319
selenium, 48, 70
selenomethionine, 48, 49, 70
shallots
  Kale and Pear Salad with Warmed Shallot Dressing, 222
  Steamed Sugar Snap Peas with Ginger, 349
SHBG (sex hormone–binding globulin), 32, 88
skin barrier, 45
skullcap, 119
sleep, 50, 85, 113–21
  exercise and, 120–21
  supplements to support, 114–16
snacks, 131, 348–53
sorghum, 167–68. See also gluten-free flours
soups, 193–218
sour cream
  Chili Black Bean Dip, 241
  Green Goddess Salad Dressing, 237
  Pumpkin Millet Muffins, 358
  Roasted Garlic and Sun-Dried Tomato Dressing, 238